Minimal Access Cardiac Surgery: State of the Art and Future Perspectives

Minimal Access Cardiac Surgery: State of the Art and Future Perspectives

Guest Editor

Jason Ali

MDPI

Basel • Beijing • Wuhan • Barcelona • Belgrade • Novi Sad • Cluj • Manchester

Guest Editor
Jason Ali
Department of Cardiothoracic
Surgery
Royal Papworth Hospital
NHS Foundation Trust
Cambridge
UK

Editorial Office
MDPI AG
Grosspeteranlage 5
4052 Basel, Switzerland

This is a reprint of the Special Issue, published open access by the journal *Journal of Cardiovascular Development and Disease* (ISSN 2308-3425), freely accessible at: https://www.mdpi.com/journal/jcdd/special_issues/GG8CZ69WRI.

For citation purposes, cite each article independently as indicated on the article page online and as indicated below:

Lastname, A.A.; Lastname, B.B. Article Title. *Journal Name* **Year**, *Volume Number*, Page Range.

ISBN 978-3-7258-6528-4 (Hbk)
ISBN 978-3-7258-6529-1 (PDF)
https://doi.org/10.3390/books978-3-7258-6529-1

Contents

About the Editor

Jason Ali

Jason Ali is a Consultant Cardiac Surgeon at Royal Papworth Hospital and an Affiliated Assistant Professor at the University of Cambridge. Jason obtained his medical qualification with distinction from the University of Cambridge in 2008 and went on to complete a PhD focusing on the immune response to transplanted organs, earning several prestigious research prizes along the way, including the Surgical Research Society's Patey Prize. He was appointed as a consultant cardiothoracic surgeon in 2022.

Jason holds a Master's in Medical Education and has several local and national roles in education. He is a Fellow and Director of Studies for Clinical Medicine at Churchill College, University of Cambridge. He was appointed as the Clinical Subdean for Royal Papworth Hospital, leading the medical student education programme.

Jason actively contributes to the advancement of medical knowledge through his extensive research endeavours. With over 130 peer-reviewed publications, he has made significant contributions. His influence extends to editorial roles, where he serves as a valued member of the Editorial Board for the *Journal of Thoracic Disease*. One of his notable projects is his leadership role as Co-Lead on the EuroSCORE III project. This initiative is focused on developing a cardiac surgical risk calculator, which already holds international significance.

Journal of
Cardiovascular Development and Disease

MDPI

Editorial

Shaping the Future of Cardiac Surgery: The Rise of Minimal-Access Techniques

Heen Shamaz [1,*] and Jason Ali [2]

[1] Edinburgh Medical School, College of Medicine and Veterinary Medicine, The University of Edinburgh, Edinburgh EH16 4SB, UK
[2] Department of Cardiothoracic Surgery, Royal Papworth Hospital NHS Foundation Trust, Cambridge Biomedical Campus, Cambridge CB2 0AY, UK; jason.ali@nhs.net
* Correspondence: h.shamaz@sms.ed.ac.uk; Tel.: +44-7884930868

Minimal access techniques are increasingly shaping the landscape of cardiac surgery. Once considered niche, these approaches have become more widespread, shifting how cardiac surgeons offer surgical options to their patients. While enthusiasm grows, so too does the responsibility to critically evaluate the evidence base, technical demands, and implications for patient outcomes.

The traditional median sternotomy remains the most commonly used approach in cardiac surgery, owing to its familiarity and safety record [1]. However, considerations re-guarding postoperative pain, recovery time, and cosmesis have driven interest in less invasive approaches [2,3], perhaps further driven by the evolution of interventional procedures such as transcatheter aortic valve implantation and mitral valve transcatheter edge-to-edge repairs. These have resulted in patients and their referrers desiring less invasive surgical alternatives to the median sternotomy.

In our special series, the breadth of cardiac surgery has been considered, and it is evident that minimal access procedures are emerging throughout the specialty. It has been understood that much of the invasiveness of cardiac surgery stems not from the incision, but from the systemic inflammatory effects of cardiopulmonary bypass (CPB) itself [4]. In this regard, when surgeons talk about minimal invasive cardiac surgery, what they often mean is minimal access. However, advances in CPB do offer the opportunity to reduce the invasiveness of cardiac surgery. Modern mini-CPB circuits aim to reduce haemodilution, inflammatory activation, and coagulation disruption. Encouraging clinical data shows reduced rates of atrial fibrillation, renal complications, and transfusion requirements. It is also noteworthy that many studies have cautioned that minimal access does not always equate to minimal invasiveness. Indeed, the technical complexity of working through reduced incisions may in fact prolong CPB or cross-clamp time, potentially offsetting the benefits of smaller incisions (Contribution 1).

Minimal access coronary revascularisation is an appealing method for treating coronary artery disease; however, the large variation in nomenclature complicates interpretation of the literature and makes comparisons with other techniques challenging. The ideal method would reap the benefits of surgical revascularisation with advantages typically seen in off-pump surgery and percutaneous coronary interventions, such as reduced pain, shorter hospital stays, faster mobilisation, and earlier return to work (Contribution 2). Minimal access techniques must not compromise the long-term patency of grafts that traditional surgical approaches reliably provide.

Valvular procedures are also seeing a shift towards minimal access techniques. Minimally invasive mitral valve surgery (MIMVS), thoracotomy or robotic techniques are becoming a popular choice in patients with low-risk degenerative valve disease (Contribution 3). Studies suggest that when appropriately selected, patients can benefit from MIMVS with durable long-term outcomes [5] (contribution 4). Similarly, minimal-access tricuspid valve surgery, whether performed via direct vision, endoscopy, or robotic methods, offers a promising solution for early intervention (Contribution 5]). In recent years we have seen the debate around open vs. transcatheter aortic valve replacement. Concerns remain regarding prosthesis durability, conduction disturbances, and stroke risk; however, as these risks are mitigated, the role of minimal-access surgical aortic valve replacement becomes increasingly attractive (Contribution 6).

The field of congenital cardiac surgery has also seen significant innovation. Techniques such as percutaneous device closure for atrial septal defects have demonstrated similar outcomes to open surgery in survival, with the added benefits of shorter hospital stays and better cosmetic outcomes (Contribution 7, Contribution 8). For younger patients, these factors are particularly relevant, and the long-term psychological impact of a less invasive approach should not be underestimated.

Robotic technologies are having a significant impact on the evolution of minimal access surgery across all surgical specialties offering precision and reduced tissue trauma. This trend towards robotic surgery is starting to gain traction in cardiac surgery. Studies have shown that while robotic techniques promise smaller incisions, faster recovery, and greater patient satisfaction, their adoption to widespread use remains limited by financial barriers, the need for specialised training, and longer operative times (Contribution 9). The evidence base is growing for these innovations; however, randomised evidence is scarce and as we know there is less room for error. Overall, the available evidence suggests that the learning curve in robotic cardiac surgery is complex and dependent on various factors, including the surgeon's prior experience, the surgical team's experience (consisting of cardiac anaesthesia, surgical assistants, surgical nurses, and technicians), the patient population, and the specific surgical techniques used (Contribution 10). Understanding these dynamics can inform the planning and management of surgical transitions, ensuring optimal patient care and continued improvement in surgical outcomes.

In today's world of cardiac surgery, patient outcomes are not only related to surgical expertise. They also relate to the presence of excellent competencies in areas such as an aesthesia, intensive care, perfusion, and physical rehabilitation. Cardiac surgery is a team effort. Postoperative recovery is often cited as a key advantage of minimal access surgery, with benefits such as reduced blood loss, shorter ICU and hospital stays, improved pain management, and earlier return to baseline functional status (Contribution 11, Contribution 12). However, success depends upon careful patient selection, and a multidisciplinary learning curve is to be expected as we start integrating more of these new techniques. Alongside these challenges, Enhanced Recovery After Surgery protocols are still naïve in cardiac surgery which can cause variability in postoperative outcomes from centre to centre. In summary, minimally invasive and minimal-access techniques appear to be the future of cardiac surgery, increasingly desired by patients who perceive superiority. The articles in this Special Issue demonstrate the expanding capabilities of these techniques while also exploring the challenges in developing a balanced approach to adopting innovations. As we move forward, the goal is not merely smaller incisions, but smarter surgery which is tailored to our patients' needs and enriched by evidence-based advancement.

Conflicts of Interest: The author declares no conflict of interest.

List of Contributions:

1. Carrel, T. Reduced invasiveness of cardiopulmonary bypass: The mini-circuit and the micro-cardioplegia. *J. Cardiovasc. Dev. Dis.* **2023**, *10*, 290.
2. Purmessur, R.; Wijesena, T.; Ali, J. Minimal-access coronary revascularization: Past, present, and future. *J. Cardiovasc. Dev. Dis.* **2023**, *10*, 326.
3. Oezpekar, U.C.; Barbieri, F.; Höfer, D.; Gollmann-Tepeköylü, C.; Holfeld, J.; Sommerauer, F.; Wagner, J.; Rajsic, S.; Ersahin, S.; Bonaros, N.; et al. An individualized, less-invasive surgical approach algorithm improves outcome in elderly patients undergoing mitral valve surgery. *J. Cardiovasc. Dev. Dis.* **2023**, *10*, 28.
4. Kawajiri, H.; Schaff, H.V.; Dearani, J.A.; Daly, R.C.; Greason, K.L.; Arghami, A.; Rowse, P.G.; Viehman, J.K.; Lahr, B.D.; Gallego-Navarro, C.; et al. Clinical outcomes of mitral valve repair for degenerative mitral regurgitation in elderly patients. *Eur. J. Cardiothorac. Surg.* **2022**, *62*, ezac299.
5. Sauvé, J.-A.; Wu, Y.-S.; Ghatanatti, R.; Zacharias, J. Minimal access tricuspid valve surgery. *J. Cardiovasc. Dev. Dis.* **2023**, *10*, 118.
6. Kirmani, B.H.; Akowuah, E. Minimal access aortic valve surgery. *J. Cardiovasc. Dev. Dis.* **2023**, *10*, 281.
7. Hardman, G.; Zacharias, J. Minimal-access atrial septal defect (ASD) closure. *J. Cardiovasc. Dev. Dis.* **2023**, *10*, 206.
8. Lo Rito, M.; Brindicci, Y.C.M.; Moscatiello, M.; Varrica, A.; Reali, M.; Saracino, A.; Chessa, M.; Aloisio, T.; Isgrò, G.; Giamberti, A. Minimally invasive surgery for simple congenital heart defects: Preserving aesthetics without jeopardizing patient safety. *J. Cardiovasc. Dev. Dis.* **2023**, *10*, 452.
9. Faerber, G.; Mukharyamov, M.; Doenst, T. Is there a future for minimal access and robots in cardiac surgery? *J. Cardiovasc. Dev. Dis.* **2023**, *10*, 380.
10. Khairallah, S.M.; Rahouma, M.; Mick, S.L. Transferring surgical expertise: Analyzing the learning curve of robotic cardiac surgery operative time reduction when surgeon moves from one experienced center to another. *J. Cardiovasc. Dev. Dis.* **2024**, *11*, 81.
11. Aston, D.; Zeloof, D.; Falter, F. Anaesthesia for minimally invasive cardiac surgery. *J. Cardiovasc. Dev. Dis.* **2024**, *10*, 462.
12. Krüger, A.; Flo Forner, A.; Ender, J.; Janai, A.; Roufail, Y.; Otto, W. Enhanced recovery after cardiac surgery. *J. Cardiovasc. Dev. Dis.* **2024**, *10*, 263.

References

1. Kun, H.; Yang, X. Median sternotomy closure: Review and update research. *J. Med. Coll. PLA* **2009**, *24*, 112–117. [CrossRef]
2. Mazezeffi, M.; Khelemsky, Y. Poststernotomy pain: A clinical review. *J. Cardiothorac. Vasc. Anesth.* **2011**, *25*, 1163–1178. [CrossRef] [PubMed]
3. King, M.; Stambulic, T.; Hassan, S.M.A.; Norman, P.A.; Derry, K.; Payne, D.M.; El Diasty, M. Median sternotomy pain after cardiac surgery: To block, or not? A systematic review and meta-analysis. *J. Card. Surg.* **2022**, *37*, 3729–3742. [PubMed]
4. Butler, J.; Rocker, G.M.; Westaby, S. Inflammatory response to cardiopulmonary bypass. *Ann. Thorac. Surg.* **1993**, *55*, 552–559. [CrossRef] [PubMed]
5. Götte, J.; Zittermann, A.; Hakim-Meibodi, K.; Hata, M.; Schramm, R.; Bleiziffer, S.; Parsa, M.A.; Gummert, J.; Renner, A. Long-term clinical outcome in elderly patients undergoing mitral valve repair. *Thorac. Cardiovasc. Surg.* **2022**, *70*, 93–99. [CrossRef] [PubMed]

Journal of
Cardiovascular Development and Disease

MDPI

Review

Is There a Future for Minimal Access and Robots in Cardiac Surgery?

Gloria Faerber, Murat Mukharyamov and Torsten Doenst *

Department of Cardiothoracic Surgery, Jena University Hospital, Friedrich Schiller University, Am Klinikum 1, 07747 Jena, Germany
* Correspondence: doenst@med.uni-jena.de; Tel.: +49-3641-9322965; Fax: +49-3641-9322902

Abstract: Minimally invasive techniques in cardiac surgery have found increasing use in recent years. Both patients and physicians often associate smaller incisions with improved outcomes (i.e., less risk, shorter hospital stay, and a faster recovery). Videoscopic and robotic assistance has been introduced, but their routine use requires specialized training and is associated with potentially longer operating times and higher costs. Randomized evidence is scarce and transcatheter treatment alternatives are increasing rapidly. As a result, the concept of minimally invasive cardiac surgery may be viewed with skepticism. In this review, we examine the current status and potential future perspectives of minimally invasive and robotic cardiac surgery.

Keywords: cardiac surgery; minimal access; robotic surgery

1. Introduction

It has been more than 70 years since cardiac surgery evolved from a "risky endeavor" with limited chance of success to a standardized procedure used to predictably treat patients with heart disease. The introduction of cardiopulmonary bypass and the implementation of myocardial protection techniques have led to remarkable progress in the field, practically providing a full spectrum of surgical treatment options for all main cardiac pathologies [1]. Over time, techniques have been refined. Surgeons and patients alike began to prioritize reducing surgical trauma and improving cosmetic results. This focus led to the development of less invasive procedures in the cardiac surgical field for valve repair [2,3] and coronary artery bypass graft surgery [4]. During this process, robotic technologies were developed, primarily as a telemanipulator and with improved instrument maneuverability [5]. In more recent years, transcatheter technologies emerged as even less invasive alternatives, which now enable the interventional treatment of coronary and/or valve pathologies as an isolated or combined procedure [6]. As a result, the current times are characterized by a plethora of methods and technologies that are available to treat cardiac diseases. This is a new situation, specifically for cardiac surgery, for which the initial developments had practically no reasonable alternative [1]. Thus, efforts to achieve the same surgical result with a smaller incision or the use of a telemanipulator may be questioned, if there is a fully interventional alternative. In this context, we here review the available evidence for minimally invasive and robotically assisted surgery. We will demonstrate that minimally invasive surgical treatment options are far from becoming obsolete, but are valuable tools for the multidisciplinary heart team and their task to optimize individual patient treatment.

2. Definition of Minimally Invasive Cardiac Surgery

There is no universal definition for the term minimally invasive cardiac surgery. In general, normal invasiveness is characterized by the use of sternotomy as an access route to the heart and the use of cardiopulmonary bypass. Thus, off-pump procedures have often been termed minimally invasive cardiac surgery, although sternotomy is still the main access route [7]. However, in the context of this article, minimally invasive cardiac surgery refers to operations with smaller incisions and access to the heart either through partial sternotomy or through mini-thoracotomies.

Figure 1 shows a graphic categorization of the different invasive approaches used to treat heart disease. The marked area encompasses the procedures that are generally summarized as minimally invasive cardiac surgery. These minimally invasive approaches can be sub-classified in partial sternotomy or sternotomy-free approaches. The use of videoscopic or robotic technology is more common in sternotomy-free approaches. Figure 2 schematically illustrates the minimally invasive access routes to the heart in relation to the respective cardiac surgical procedure. For the mitral valve, a mini-thoracotomy has become routine in many centers (60% of all isolated mitral cases were accessed through mini-thoracotomies in Germany in 2022). For the aortic valve, access through partial sternotomy is becoming increasingly popular, with up to 40% of cases in Germany performed through this route [7]. In addition, some centers use parasternal, mini-thoracotomy approaches as their primary access route to the aortic valve [8] Again, modified approaches allow us to address combined pathologies involving not only the mitral and tricuspid valves but also simultaneously correcting the aortic valve [9]. Moreover, in recent years, reports have emerged that describe the combination of two mini-thoracotomies for simultaneous interventions on valves and coronaries, such as bypass grafting of one or two branches of the left coronary artery and correction of mitral/tricuspid valve or aortic valve pathologies [10]. However, the number of patients receiving a minimally invasive heart operation is certainly influenced by a strong selection bias, since experience and surgical expertise affect patient selection.

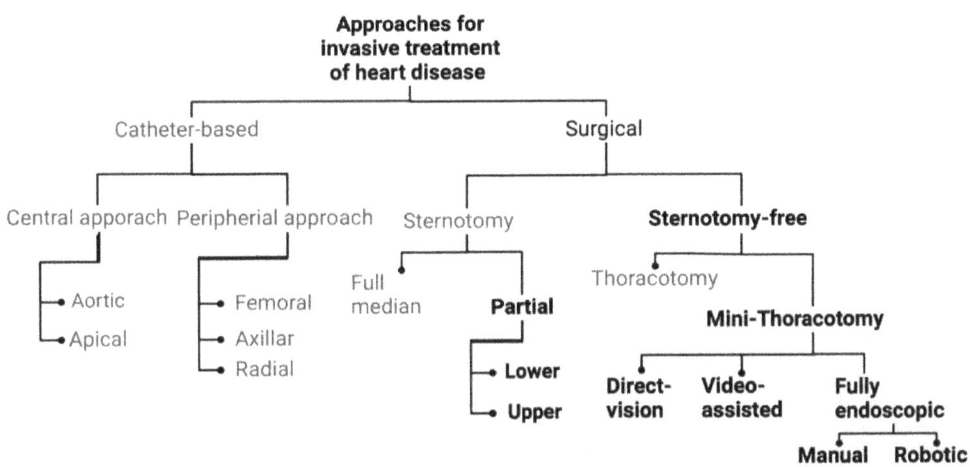

Figure 1. Graphic categorization of the different approaches used for the invasive treatment of heart disease.

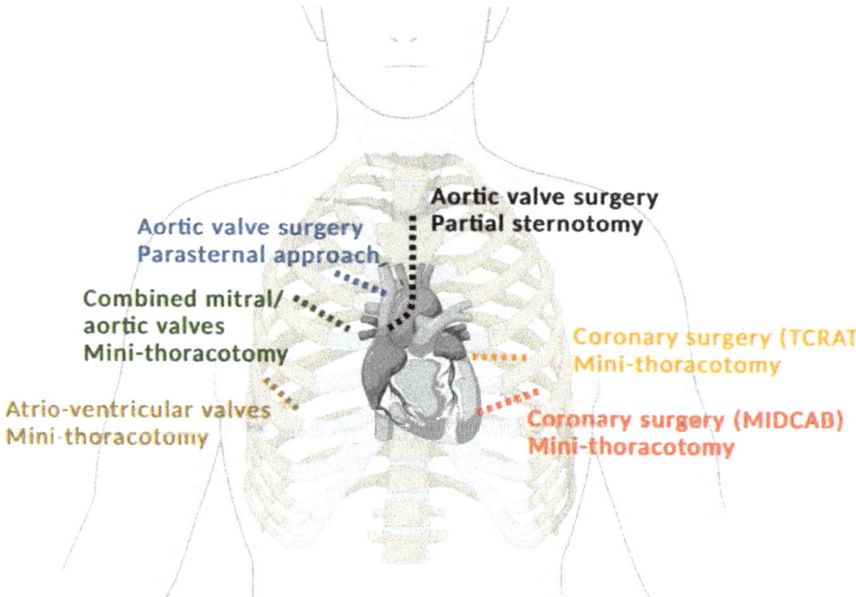

Figure 2. Schematic illustration of minimally invasive access routes to the heart in relation to the intended cardiac surgical procedure.

In the coronary field, a left anterolateral mini-thoracotomy in the fifth intercostal space is the standard access point when grafting the LIMA to the LAD [11]. This procedure is generally performed off-pump. Advancements in this technique led to the performance of multiple bypass grafting through the same approach [12], and some specialized centers even use both internal thoracic arteries when using this approach [13,14]. Telemanipulators offer great visibility and maneuverability for ITA harvesting and are favored by some surgeons [15]. Although MIDCAB approaches allow all coronary vessels to be targeted, the LAD is the best target and these techniques are often used in the context of additional coronary stenting (also known as hybrid procedures) [16]. Most recently, anterior throacotomies (TCRAT) have been proposed [17] to perform complete bypass operations including the use of cardiopulmonary bypass and classic aortic clamp techniques, allowing secure grafting of all coronary targets without the need to operate off-pump.

Minimally invasive approaches require cardiopulmonary bypass (except for off-pump CABG cases) which is often established through peripheral (mostly groin) cannulation. Despite the initial skepticism regarding a presumed increase in stroke rates [18] (for return of flow in the descending artery) this technique has proven its safety [19]. Percutaneous cannulation of the femoral vessels, among other benefits, accelerates the operation and reduces the number of peri-operative complications [20]. Surgical techniques and myocardial protection generally align with those used in conventional, sternotomy cardiac surgery, with some technical differences, such as the use of specialized long-shafted instruments and retractors. It is important to realize that it has always been the goal, with any of the minimal-access approaches to the heart, to deliver the same surgical procedure to the heart, just through a smaller incision. Advantages may come from causing less surgical trauma and disadvantages may come from the greater surgical challenge of performing the same procedure through a smaller incision and from potentially longer operating times. Thus, assessing the impact of using minimal-access approaches to the heart on outcomes is important.

3. Scientific Evidence

Minimally invasive cardiac surgery, when compared to traditional approaches, exhibits fundamentally different characteristics, with these differences being more or less noticeable at all perioperative stages, from the actual surgery itself to the early postoperative period and intermediate outcomes. In general, randomized evidence is scarce. The available randomized trials are summarized in Table 1. In minimally invasive surgery, operative, cardiopulmonary bypass, and aortic cross-clamp times have been described to be longer [21–23]. We and others demonstrated that longer aortic cross-clamp times increase the risk of perioperative mortality in conventional sternotomy cardiac surgery [24,25]. However, despite longer myocardial ischemia times for minimally invasive procedures, no difference in mortality was observed compared to the same procedures performed through sternotomy in several investigations [26]. To the contrary, despite longer operative times, early operative secondary endpoints such as ventilation times [22] or right ventricular function [27] were better in the minimally invasive cardiac surgery group. These differences further translated into a trend towards shorter patient stay in the intensive care unit and earlier discharge from the hospital [22]. We recently demonstrated that the relationship of cross-clamp time and mortality can also be found in minimally invasive mitral valve surgery [24], suggesting that this mini-approach must convey some protective effects to counteract the negative impact of elongated clamp times and explain the above-described advantages.

Table 1. Summary of current randomized data comparing conventional, less invasive, or interventional procedures for heart valve diseases.

Author	Journal/ Year	Valve	Comparison	Number of Randomized Observations	Result	Mortality
Rodríguez-Caulo et al. [28]	STCVS 2021	Aortic	Sternotomy vs. MICS	100	Better QOL at 1 year in MIC arm	No difference
Vukovic et al. [29]	JCS 2019	Aortic	Sternotomy vs. MICS	100	Lower hospital stay in MICS arm	No difference
Hancock et al. [30]	BMJ 2021	Aortic	Sternotomy vs. MICS	270	Equal transfusions rate	No difference
Dalen et al. [27]	ICVTS 2018	Aortic	Sternotomy vs. MICS	40	Higher postoperative TAPSE in MICS arm	No difference
Feldman et al. [31]	NEJM 2011	Mitral	Sternotomy vs. MitraClip	279	Less re-do surgeries and residual MR in surgical arm	No difference
Nasso et al. [22]	Cardiology 2014	Mitral	Sternotomy vs. MICS	160	Longer operative, bypass and cross-clamp times, but shorter ventilation, ICU and in-hospital stay in MICS arm	No difference
Akowuah et al. [23]	2023	Mitral	Sternotomy vs. MICS	330	No difference in QOL in 3 months	Lower in MICS

Randomized trials have yielded contradictory results regarding patients' quality of life and satisfaction at different time points after surgery. The most recent Mini-Mitral trial reported better quality of life and satisfaction at 1 month for patients undergoing minimally invasive mitral valve surgery versus sternotomy, although the primary endpoint at three months was no different [28]. Other reports support the absence of a difference at 3 months [23]. A possible explanation for this observation might be that the influence of the surgical approach becomes less important as time after surgery increases. In the initial postoperative course, sternotomy-free approaches may benefit from quicker physical recovery compared to sternotomy, where bone and wound healing usually takes longer. Postoperative healing is the primary focus in the initial phase, while freedom from symptoms and durability of the cardiac procedure counts in the long-run. Unfortunately, long-term comparisons or functional analyses of thoracic integrity between sternotomy and mini-thoracotomy approaches are not available. However, the above-described goal of delivering the same surgical results through minimized access makes these findings only plausible. A long-term survival benefit for patients undergoing minimally invasive cardiac surgery may not be expected if the surgical result is intended to be the same.

The interventional field is the area in which the "non-inferiority concept" has been the basis of their development. Classic surgical thinking has been guided by the logic that change is required if results are superior. With the development of interventional techniques, change was massive in all areas with an approach for which not being worse was the primary target. The current situation is therefore characterized by steadily growing numbers of interventional techniques and shrinking numbers in classic cardiac surgery in both coronary and valve procedures [7]. The question of whether these transcatheter interventions hold their promise of not being worse has sparked a great discussion in the community [32].

Interestingly, the ability of an interventional approach to allow a procedure to be performed without general anesthesia and cardiopulmonary bypass and via a purely percutaneous access route even raised the expectations of improved results, although the statistical designs have always tested for non-inferiority [33]. A prime example to support this statement is the US Corevalve trial that indeed demonstrated the superiority of transcatheter Corevalve placement over classic surgical aortic valve replacement (SAVR) over a three-year period [34]. However, none of the other TAVI vs. SAVR trials could statistically repeat such superiority [35,36]. Any differences that may have been initially observed in favor of TAVI disappeared (mainly in the first year), the latest after 5 years, and a significant survival advantage of SAVR emerged in both randomized and non-randomized evidence for SAVR in the long-run (Figure 3). Since most trials do not follow their patients long-term, the available information sparks the concern that techniques with potentially inferior long-term outcomes are favored over their superior alternatives for the perceived lesser invasiveness. A similar development can be seen in other areas where interventional techniques are increasingly being used [37]. Often times, new interventions are even being tested against medial therapy, although surgery is considered the current gold standard [38,39]. Since most patients are more afraid of classic sternotomy operations today than they may have been before the availability of interventional alternatives, sternotomy-free approaches move into the center of attention in classic cardiac surgery. The development of these approaches, specifically at a time at which valve interventions emerge, underscores this statement. Figure 4 illustrates the development of cardiac surgery over the past 70 years together with the advent of interventional and minimally invasive surgical procedures. Thus, for optimal patient care, heart team discussions are required to provide recommendations that balance short-term outcomes and long-term results.

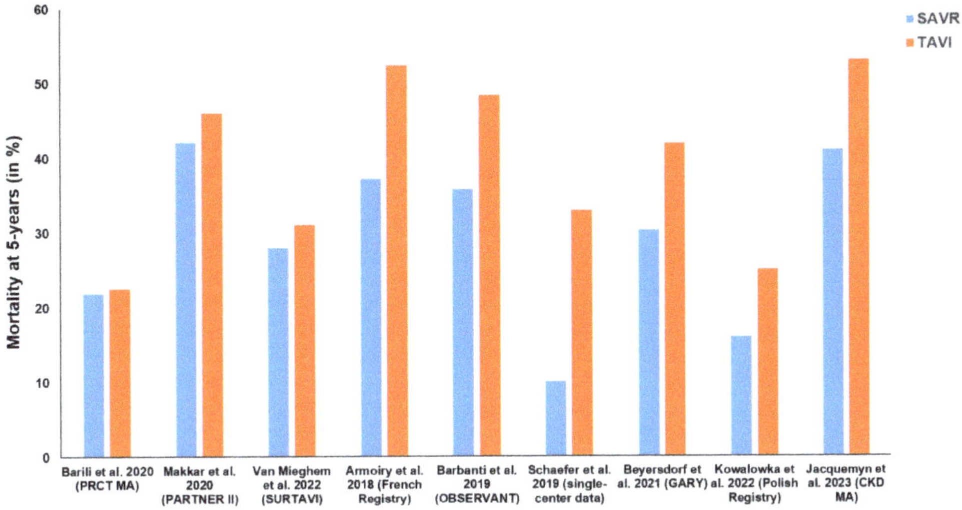

Figure 3. Composition of mortality rates of SAVR and TAVI comparisons from randomized studies and propensity matched registry analyses demonstrating 5-year outcomes. (SAVR—surgical aortic valve replacement, TAVI—transcatheter aortic valve implantation) [35,40–47].

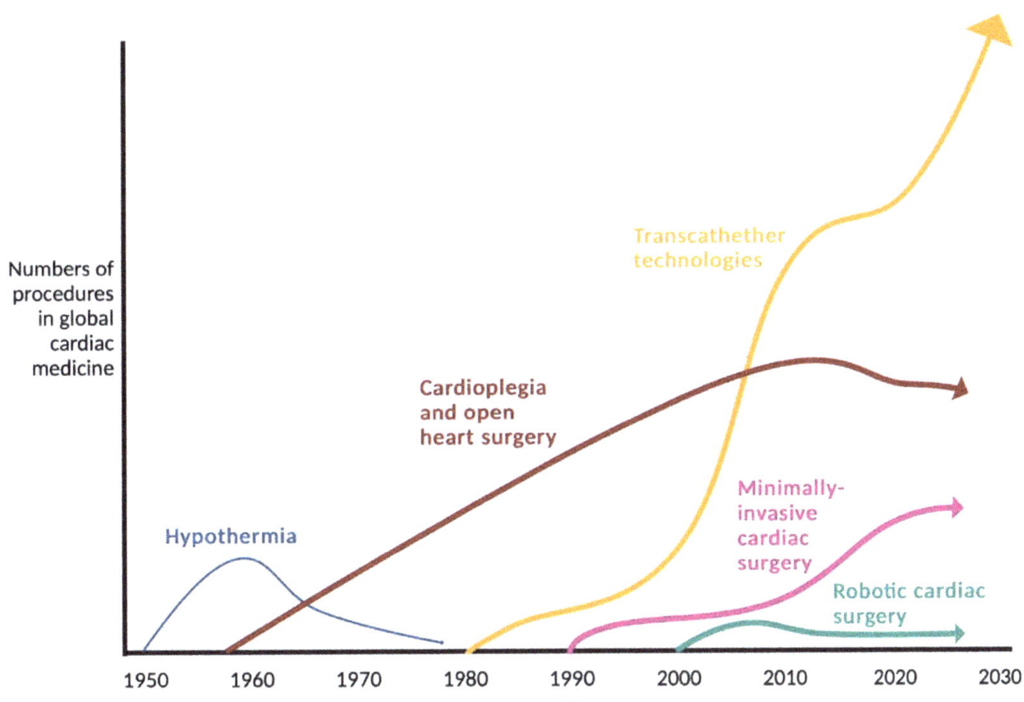

Figure 4. Simplified illustration of the development of the invasive treatment of heart disease with surgical and interventional means over the last 70 years.

4. Minimally Invasive Cardiac Surgery Requires Specific Training

The increasing demand for minimally invasive cardiac surgical procedures requires surgeons to adapt not only to the different approach, but also to the different tools needed to treat these cases (e.g., specific instruments, techniques, and imaging modalities), different learning curves and different ways to teach these techniques to the young.

Compared to conventional sternotomy, minimally invasive approaches are technically more demanding. There is less room for error, because minor complications may require a conversion to sternotomy or aggravate the course of the operation significantly. The limited visibility through the small incision also limits a teacher's ability to supervise and correct the performance of surgical trainees. Here, endoscopic and robotically assisted approaches provide a substantial advantage. Specifically, the master–slave concept with the da Vinci system requires mentioning; in this approach, a junior and a senior surgeon sit on two separate consoles and the senior can (similar to a driving instructor) supervise, guide, and even take over the surgical procedure performed by the junior surgeon. However, if the interest in teaching is high enough, with direct supervision, a team of junior and senior surgeons can perform and teach a case safely [48]

Since a minimally invasive procedure usually requires more time even in experienced hands, simulator training becomes more and more attractive and important in order to minimize learning curves and optimize the speed of performance. In addition, familiarizing novices with repair concepts in theory further adds to the safety of surgery by increasing the likelihood that initial repairs will immediately generate success (that is why we have created the motto "cardiac surgery is thinking with your hands" [1]).

The need to reorganize training and qualification for minimally invasive cardiac surgery finds evidence in the literature by studies demonstrating that outcomes of mitral valve surgery are related to the specific expertise of surgeons and centers [49], and that learning curves are long and may be surgeon specific [50]. It may therefore be necessary to rethink our current approach of training novice surgeons through sternotomy approaches first and then expose them to the minimal access later. Individual experiences support the notion that primary training with minimally invasive access is reasonable and safe. In any case, specialized centers (for instance for valve repair surgeries) have the potential to routinely provide outcomes that are excellent [51,52]. In addition, different approaches in general usually expand a field's horizon. In line with this statement, there is evidence that the minimally invasive approach to cardiac valves also broadened our surgical horizon and provides new perspectives.

5. Perspectives of Minimally Invasive Cardiac Surgery

In addition to maintaining thoracic cage integrity, faster recovery and better quality of life in the early recovery period, experience with minimally invasive approaches may allow us to perform procedures that have been considered too risky through (often times redo-) sternotomy. A prime example is the presence of mitral valve regurgitation or stenosis in patients who have previously undergone aortic valve surgery or coronary artery bypass grafting. If the aortic valve is competent, the procedure may be performed via thoracotomy on the beating and/or fibrillating heart, without the need to dissect fragile bypass grafts or divide severe adhesions from previous sternotomies [53,54] (given the required surgical experience is present [21]). Considering that such approaches may allow the establishment of a mechanical result that has the currently best potential for long-term durability, these options are valuable, since the currently available interventional alternatives appear to have not demonstrated their long-term potential and the initial results are questionable [55].

Table 2 summarizes the scenarios in which minimally invasive approaches have the potential to provide advantages for the conduct of classic cardiac surgery. With today's patients presenting with increased age and number of comorbidities, it must be the goal for surgical procedures to correct the required problem without causing additional harm. Since an operation on a patient without additional morbidities and normal peripheral organ function will likely be the same as addressing the same pathology in a patient with substantial comorbidities and peripheral organ dysfunction, the additional risk in the latter patient is likely to be caused by the trauma created by anesthesia and surgery alike. It appears less dependent on the specific surgical procedure. Thus, in today's cardiac surgery, the outcomes are not only related to surgical expertise but also to the presence of excellent competencies in areas such as anesthesia, ICU care, perfusion, and physical rehabilitation. In other words, cardiac surgery today is a team effort. Interventional techniques are beginning to replace surgical procedures to some degree, but they are also a valuable adjunct to the current practice of cardiac surgery. Heart team recommendations are becoming the standard for individualized decision making. In these discussions, minimally invasive access surgery has gained a growing role, in which recommendations not only consist of an interventional or surgical approach, but they may also consist of hybrid approaches, minimally invasive versus sternotomy approaches, or even staged procedures. Thus, the options to balance peri-procedural risk and long-term benefits have never been greater than they are today, but it is up to us to master the surgical and interventional skills and work together in order to deliver those skills to the individual patient.

Table 2. The potential of minimally invasive approaches to provide advantages for the conduct of classic cardiac surgery.

Surgical Scenarios in Which Minimally Invasive Approaches Have Provided Advantages for the Conduct of Classic Cardiac Surgery through Sternotomy (Modified from Doenst and Lamelas [21])
Tricuspid valve: surgery without sternotomy, as a redo without pericardial dissection, with or without cross-clamping
Mitral valve: surgery without sternotomy, as a redo (specifically with patent mammary) with or without pericardial dissection, with or without cross-clamping, beating heart/fibrillating heart.
Redo cases with previous sternal wound infection (specifically those with loss of sternal bone)
Cases with morbid obesity
Frail patients with or without significant osteoporosis
Patients with large breast implants

Funding: This research received no external funding.

Data Availability Statement: Represented data available in a publicly accessible biomedical databases.

Conflicts of Interest: The authors declare no conflict of interest.

Abbreviations

CABG	Coronary Artery Bypass Grafting.
CKD	Chronic Kidney Disease.
ICU	Intensive Care Unit.
LAD	Left Anterior Descending.
LIMA	Left Internal Mammary Artery.
MA	Meta-Analysis.
MICS	Minimally Invasive Cardiac Surgery.
MIDCAB	Minimally Invasive Direct Coronary Artery Bypass.
PRCT	Prospective Randomized Clinical Trial.
QOL	Quality of Life.
SAVR	Surgical Aortic Valve Replacement.
TAPSE	Tricuspid Annular Plane Systolic Excursion.
TAVI	Transcatheter Aortic Valve Implantation.
TCRAT	Total coronary revascularization via left anterior thoracotomy.

References

1. Doenst, T.; Schlensak, C.; Schibilsky, D.; Faerber, G. Do we need basic research in cardiac surgery? *Thorac. Cardiovasc. Surg.* **2018**, *7*, 002–006.
2. Carpentier, A.; Loulmet, D.; Le Bret, E.; Haugades, B.; Dassier, P.; Guibourt, P. Open heart operation under videosurgery and minithoracotomy. First case (mitral valvuloplasty) operated with success. *Comptes Rendus L'academie Sci. Ser. III Sci. Vie* **1996**, *319*, 219–223.
3. Mohr, F.; Onnasch, J.; Falk, V.; Walther, T.; Diegeler, A.; Krakor, R.; Schneider, F.; Autschbach, R. The evolution of minimally invasive mitral valve surgery—2 year experience. *Eur. J. Cardio-Thorac. Surg.* **1999**, *15*, 233–239. [CrossRef]
4. Calafiore, A.M.; Di Giammarco, G.; Teodori, G.; Bosco, G.; D'Annunzio, E.; Barsotti, A.; Maddestra, N.; Paloscia, L.; Vitolla, G.; Sciarra, A. Left anterior descending coronary artery grafting via left anterior small thoracotomy without cardiopulmonary bypass. *Ann. Thorac. Surg.* **1996**, *61*, 1658–1665. [CrossRef] [PubMed]
5. Falk, V.; Diegler, A.; Walther, T.; Autschbach, R.; Mohr, F.W. Developments in robotic cardiac surgery. *Curr. Opin. Cardiol.* **2000**, *15*, 378–387. [CrossRef] [PubMed]
6. Penkalla, A.; Pasic, M.; Drews, T.; Buz, S.; Dreysse, S.; Kukucka, M.; Mladenow, A.; Hetzer, R.; Unbehaun, A. Transcatheter aortic valve implantation combined with elective coronary artery stenting: A simultaneous approach. *Eur. J. Cardio-Thorac. Surg.* **2015**, *47*, 1083–1089. [CrossRef] [PubMed]
7. Beckmann, A.; Meyer, R.; Lewandowski, J.; Markewitz, A.; Blaßfeld, D.; Böning, A. German Heart Surgery Report 2022: The Annual Updated Registry of the German Society for Thoracic and Cardiovascular Surgery. *Thorac. Cardiovasc. Surg.* **2023**, *71*, 340–355. [CrossRef]
8. Tkebuchava, S.; Färber, G.; Sponholz, C.; Fuchs, F.; Heinisch, P.; Bauer, M.; Doenst, T. Minimally-invasive parasternal aortic valve replacement-A slow learning curve towards improved outcomes. *J. Card. Surg.* **2020**, *35*, 544–548. [CrossRef]
9. Faerber, G.; Gieck, K.; Diab, M.; Doenst, T. Minimally invasive aortic and mitral valve surgery with or without tricuspid valve surgery performed via right anterior thoracotomy approach. *Thorac. Cardiovasc. Surg.* **2016**, *64*, ePP80. [CrossRef]
10. Smit, P.; Shariff, M.A.; Nabagiez, J.P.; Khan, M.A.; Sadel, S.M.; McGinn, J.T., Jr. Experience with a minimally invasive approach to combined valve surgery and coronary artery bypass grafting through bilateral thoracotomies. *Heart Surg. Forum* **2013**, *16*, E125–E131. [CrossRef]
11. Detter, C.; Reichenspurner, H.; Boehm, D.H.; Thalhammer, M.; Raptis, P.; Schütz, A.; Reichart, B. Minimally invasive direct coronary artery bypass grafting (MIDCAB) and off-pump coronary artery bypass grafting (OPCAB): Two techniques for beating heart surgery. *Heart Surg. Forum* **2002**, *5*, 157–162. [PubMed]
12. Ruel, M.; Shariff, M.A.; Lapierre, H.; Goyal, N.; Dennie, C.; Sadel, S.M.; Sohmer, B.; McGinn, J.T., Jr. Results of the minimally invasive coronary artery bypass grafting angiographic patency study. *J. Thorac. Cardiovasc. Surg.* **2014**, *147*, 203–209. [CrossRef]
13. Diab, M.; Färber, G.; Sponholz, C.; Tasar, R.; Lehmann, T.; Tkebuchava, S.; Franz, M.; Doenst, T. Coronary artery bypass grafting using bilateral internal thoracic arteries through a left-sided minithoracotomy: A single-center starting experience. *Thorac. Cardiovasc. Surg.* **2019**, *67*, 437–443. [CrossRef] [PubMed]
14. Kikuchi, K.; Une, D.; Kurata, A.; Ruel, M. Off-pump minimally invasive coronary artery bypass grafting using the bilateral internal thoracic arteries and the right gastroepiproic artery. *Eur. J. Cardio-Thorac. Surg.* **2016**, *49*, 1285–1286. [CrossRef] [PubMed]
15. Balkhy, H.H.; Wann, L.S.; Krienbring, D.; Arnsdorf, S.E. Integrating coronary anastomotic connectors and robotics toward a totally endoscopic beating heart approach: Review of 120 cases. *Ann. Thorac. Surg.* **2011**, *92*, 821–827. [CrossRef] [PubMed]
16. Puskas, J.D.; Halkos, M.E.; DeRose, J.J.; Bagiella, E.; Miller, M.A.; Overbey, J.; Bonatti, J.; Srinivas, V.; Vesely, M.; Sutter, F. Hybrid coronary revascularization for the treatment of multivessel coronary artery disease: A multicenter observational study. *J. Am. Coll. Cardiol.* **2016**, *68*, 356–365. [CrossRef] [PubMed]
17. Babliak, O.; Demianenko, V.; Melnyk, Y.; Revenko, K.; Pidgayna, L.; Stohov, O. Complete coronary revascularization via left anterior thoracotomy. *Innovations* **2019**, *14*, 330–341. [CrossRef]
18. Bedeir, K.; Reardon, M.; Ramchandani, M.; Singh, K.; Ramlawi, B. Elevated stroke risk associated with femoral artery cannulation during mitral valve surgery. *Semin. Thorac. Cardiovasc. Surg.* **2015**, *27*, 97–103. [CrossRef]
19. Lamelas, J.; Williams, R.F.; Mawad, M.; LaPietra, A. Complications associated with femoral cannulation during minimally invasive cardiac surgery. *Ann. Thorac. Surg.* **2017**, *103*, 1927–1932. [CrossRef]
20. Moschovas, A.; Amorim, P.A.; Nold, M.; Faerber, G.; Diab, M.; Buenger, T.; Doenst, T. Percutaneous cannulation for cardiopulmonary bypass in minimally invasive surgery is associated with reduced groin complications. *Interact. Cardiovasc. Thorac. Surg.* **2017**, *25*, 377–383. [CrossRef]
21. Doenst, T.; Lamelas, J. Do we have enough evidence for minimally-invasive cardiac surgery? A critical review of scientific and non-scientific information. *J. Cardiovasc. Surg.* **2017**, *58*, 613–623. [CrossRef] [PubMed]
22. Nasso, G.; Bonifazi, R.; Romano, V.; Bartolomucci, F.; Rosano, G.; Massari, F.; Fattouch, K.; Del Prete, G.; Riccioni, G.; Del Giglio, M. Three-year results of repaired Barlow mitral valves via right minithoracotomy versus median sternotomy in a randomized trial. *Cardiology* **2014**, *128*, 97–105. [CrossRef] [PubMed]
23. Akowuah, E.F.; Maier, R.H.; Hancock, H.C.; Kharatikoopaei, E.; Vale, L.; Fernandez-Garcia, C.; Ogundimu, E.; Wagnild, J.; Mathias, A.; Walmsley, Z. Minithoracotomy vs. Conventional Sternotomy for Mitral Valve Repair: A Randomized Clinical Trial. *JAMA* **2023**, *329*, 1957–1966. [CrossRef] [PubMed]

24. Doenst, T.; Berretta, P.; Bonaros, N.; Savini, C.; Pitsis, A.; Wilbring, M.; Gerdisch, M.; Kempfert, J.; Rinaldi, M.; Folliguet, T. Aortic cross-clamp time correlates with mortality in the Mini-mitral International Registry. *Eur. J. Cardio-Thorac. Surg.* **2023**, *63*, ezad147. [CrossRef] [PubMed]
25. Al-Sarraf, N.; Thalib, L.; Hughes, A.; Houlihan, M.; Tolan, M.; Young, V.; McGovern, E. Cross-clamp time is an independent predictor of mortality and morbidity in low-and high-risk cardiac patients. *Int. J. Surg.* **2011**, *9*, 104–109. [CrossRef] [PubMed]
26. Hancock, H.C.; Maier, R.H.; Kasim, A.S.; Mason, J.M.; Murphy, G.J.; Goodwin, A.T.; Owens, W.A.; Kirmani, B.H.; Akowuah, E.F. Mini-sternotomy versus conventional sternotomy for aortic valve replacement. *J. Am. Coll. Cardiol.* **2019**, *73*, 2491–2492. [CrossRef] [PubMed]
27. Dalén, M.; Da Silva, C.O.; Sartipy, U.; Winter, R.; Franco-Cereceda, A.; Barimani, J.; Bäck, M.; Svenarud, P. Comparison of right ventricular function after ministernotomy and full sternotomy aortic valve replacement: A randomized study. *Interact. Cardiovasc. Thorac. Surg.* **2018**, *26*, 790–797. [CrossRef]
28. Rodríguez-Caulo, E.A.; Guijarro-Contreras, A.; Guzón, A.; Otero-Forero, J.; Mataró, M.J.; Sánchez-Espín, G.; Porras, C.; Villaescusa, J.M.; Melero-Tejedor, J.M.; Jiménez-Navarro, M. Quality of life after ministernotomy versus full sternotomy aortic valve replacement. *Semin. Thorac. Cardiovasc. Surg.* **2021**, *33*, 328–334. [CrossRef]
29. Vukovic, P.M.; Milojevic, P.; Stojanovic, I.; Micovic, S.; Zivkovic, I.; Peric, M.; Milicic, M.; Milacic, P.; Milojevic, M.; Bojic, M. The role of ministernotomy in aortic valve surgery—A prospective randomized study. *J. Card. Surg.* **2019**, *34*, 435–439. [CrossRef]
30. Hancock, H.C.; Maier, R.H.; Kasim, A.; Mason, J.; Murphy, G.; Goodwin, A.; Owens, W.A.; Akowuah, E. Mini-sternotomy versus conventional sternotomy for aortic valve replacement: A randomised controlled trial. *BMJ Open.* **2021**, *11*, e041398. [CrossRef]
31. Feldman, T.; Foster, E.; Glower, D.D.; Kar, S.; Rinaldi, M.J.; Fail, P.S.; Smalling, R.W.; Siegel, R.; Rose, G.A.; Engeron, E.; et al. EVEREST II Investigators. Percutaneous repair or surgery for mitral regurgitation. *N. Engl. J. Med.* **2011**, *14*, 1395–1406. [CrossRef] [PubMed]
32. Vahanian, A.; Beyersdorf, F.; Praz, F.; Milojevic, M.; Baldus, S.; Bauersachs, J.; Capodanno, D.; Conradi, L.; De Bonis, M.; De Paulis, R. 2021 ESC/EACTS Guidelines for the management of valvular heart disease: Developed by the Task Force for the management of valvular heart disease of the European Society of Cardiology (ESC) and the European Association for Cardio-Thoracic Surgery (EACTS). *Eur. Heart J.* **2022**, *43*, 561–632. [CrossRef] [PubMed]
33. Barili, F.; Brophy, J.M.; Ronco, D.; Myers, P.O.; Uva, M.S.; Almeida, R.M.; Marin-Cuartas, M.; Anselmi, A.; Tomasi, J.; Verhoye, J.-P. Risk of Bias in Randomized Clinical Trials Comparing Transcatheter and Surgical Aortic Valve Replacement: A Systematic Review and Meta-analysis. *JAMA Netw. Open* **2023**, *6*, e2249321. [CrossRef] [PubMed]
34. Reardon, M.J.; Van Mieghem, N.M.; Popma, J.J.; Kleiman, N.S.; Søndergaard, L.; Mumtaz, M.; Adams, D.H.; Deeb, G.M.; Maini, B.; Gada, H. Surgical or transcatheter aortic-valve replacement in intermediate-risk patients. *N. Engl. J. Med.* **2017**, *376*, 1321–1331. [CrossRef] [PubMed]
35. Beyersdorf, F.; Bauer, T.; Freemantle, N.; Walther, T.; Frerker, C.; Herrmann, E.; Bleiziffer, S.; Möllmann, H.; Landwehr, S.; Ensminger, S. Five-year outcome in 18 010 patients from the German Aortic Valve Registry. *Eur. J. Cardio-Thorac. Surg.* **2021**, *60*, 1139–1146. [CrossRef] [PubMed]
36. Deharo, P.; Leroux, L.; Theron, A.; Ferrara, J.; Vaillier, A.; Jaussaud, N.; Porto, A.; Morera, P.; Gariboldi, V.; Iung, B. Long-term prognosis value of paravalvular leak and patient–prosthesis mismatch following transcatheter aortic valve implantation: Insight from the France-TAVI registry. *J. Clin. Med.* **2022**, *11*, 6117. [CrossRef] [PubMed]
37. Oh, N.A.; Kampaktsis, P.N.; Gallo, M.; Guariento, A.; Weixler, V.; Staffa, S.J.; Avgerinos, D.V.; Colli, A.; Doulamis, I.P. An updated meta-analysis of MitraClip versus surgery for mitral regurgitation. *Ann. Cardiothorac. Surg.* **2021**, *10*, 1–14. [CrossRef] [PubMed]
38. Stone, G.W.; Lindenfeld, J.; Abraham, W.T.; Kar, S.; Lim, D.S.; Mishell, J.M.; Whisenant, B.; Grayburn, P.A.; Rinaldi, M.; Kapadia, S.R. Transcatheter mitral-valve repair in patients with heart failure. *N. Engl. J. Med.* **2018**, *379*, 2307–2318. [CrossRef]
39. Gerçek, M.; Goncharov, A.; Narang, A.; Körber, M.L.; Friedrichs, K.P.; Baldridge, A.S.; Meng, Z.; Puthumana, J.J.; Davidson, L.J.; Malaisrie, S.C. Characterization of screen failures among patients evaluated for transcatheter tricuspid valve repair (TriSelect-study). *Cardiovasc. Interv.* **2023**, *16*, 1579–1589. [CrossRef]
40. Barili, F.; Freemantle, N.; Casado, A.P.; Rinaldi, M.; Folliguet, T.; Musumeci, F.; Gerosa, G.; Parolari, A. Mortality in trials on transcatheter aortic valve implantation versus surgical aortic valve replacement: A pooled meta-analysis of Kaplan-Meier-derived individual patient data. *Eur. J. Cardiothorac. Surg.* **2020**, *58*, 221–229. [CrossRef]
41. Makkar, R.R.; Thourani, V.H.; Mack, M.J.; Kodali, S.K.; Kapadia, S.; Webb, J.G.; Yoon, S.-H.; Trento, A.; Svensson, L.G.; Herrmann, H.C.; et al. Five-Year Outcomes of Transcatheter or Surgical Aortic-Valve Replacement. *N. Engl. J. Med.* **2020**, *382*, 799–809. [CrossRef] [PubMed]
42. Van Mieghem, N.M.; Windecker, S.; Manoharan, G.; Bosmans, J.; Bleiziffer, S.; Modine, T.; Linke, A.; Scholtz, W.; Tchétché, D.; Finkelstein, A.; et al. Final 3-year clinical outcomes following transcatheter aortic valve implantation with a supra-annular self-expanding repositionable valve in a real-world setting: Results from the multicenter FORWARD study. *Catheter. Cardiovasc. Interv.* **2022**, *99*, 171–178. [CrossRef] [PubMed]
43. Armoiry, X.; Obadia, J.-F.; Pascal, L.; Polazzi, S.; Duclos, A. Comparison of transcatheter versus surgical aortic valve implantation in high-risk patients: A nationwide study in France. *J. Thorac. Cardiovasc. Surg.* **2018**, *156*, 1017–1025.e4. [CrossRef] [PubMed]
44. Barbanti, M.; Tamburino, C.; D'errigo, P.; Biancari, F.; Ranucci, M.; Rosato, S.; Santoro, G.; Fusco, D.; Seccareccia, F.; For the OBSERVANT Research Group. Five-Year Outcomes of Transfemoral Transcatheter Aortic Valve Replacement or Surgical Aortic Valve Replacement in a Real World Population. *Circ. Cardiovasc. Interv.* **2019**, *12*, e007825. [CrossRef] [PubMed]

45. Schaefer, A.; Schofer, N.; Goßling, A.; Seiffert, M.; Schirmer, J.; Deuschl, F.; Schneeberger, Y.; Voigtländer, L.; Detter, C.; Schaefer, U.; et al. Transcatheter aortic valve implantation versus surgical aortic valve replacement in low-risk patients: A propensity score-matched analysis. *Eur. J. Cardiothorac. Surg.* **2019**, *56*, 1131–1139. [CrossRef] [PubMed]
46. Kowalówka, A.R.; Kowalewski, M.; Wańha, W.; Kołodziejczak, M.; Mariani, S.; Li, T.; Pasierski, M.; Łoś, A.; Stefaniak, S.; Malinowski, M.; et al. Surgical and transcatheter aortic valve replacement for severe aortic stenosis in low-risk elective patients: Analysis of the Aortic Valve Replacement in Elective Patients From the Aortic Valve Multicenter Registry. *J. Thorac. Cardiovasc. Surg.* **2022**, *in press*. [CrossRef] [PubMed]
47. Jacquemyn, X.; Eynde, J.V.D.; Iwens, Q.; Billiau, J.; Jabagi, H.; Serna-Gallegos, D.; Chu, D.; Sultan, I.; Sá, M.P. Transcatheter aortic valve implantation versus surgical aortic valve replacement in chronic kidney disease: Meta-analysis of reconstructed time-to-event data. *Trends Cardiovasc. Med.* **2023**, *in press*. [CrossRef] [PubMed]
48. Doenst, T. Training in mitral valve surgery at the expense of the patient? *Z. Herz- Thorax- Gefäßchirurgie* **2012**, *26*, 298–299. [CrossRef]
49. Chikwe, J.; Toyoda, N.; Anyanwu, A.C.; Itagaki, S.; Egorova, N.N.; Boateng, P.; El-Eshmawi, A.; Adams, D.H. Relation of mitral valve surgery volume to repair rate, durability, and survival. *J. Am. Coll. Cardiol.* **2017**, *69*, 2397–2406. [CrossRef]
50. Holzhey, D.M.; Seeburger, J.; Misfeld, M.; Borger, M.A.; Mohr, F.W. Learning minimally invasive mitral valve surgery: A cumulative sum sequential probability analysis of 3895 operations from a single high-volume center. *Circulation* **2013**, *128*, 483–491. [CrossRef]
51. Berretta, P.; Kempfert, J.; Van Praet, F.; Salvador, L., Lamelas, J.; Nguyen, T.C.; Wilbring, M.; Gerdisch, M.; Rinaldi, M.; Bonaros, N.; et al. Risk-related clinical outcomes after minimally invasive mitral valve surgery: Insights from the Mini-Mitral International Registry. *Eur. J. Cardiothorac. Surg.* **2023**, *63*, ezad090. [CrossRef] [PubMed]
52. Färber, G.; Tkebuchava, S.; Dawson, R.S.; Kirov, H.; Diab, M.; Schlattmann, P.; Doenst, T. Minimally Invasive, Isolated Tricuspid Valve Redo Surgery: A Safety and Outcome Analysis. *Thorac. Cardiovasc. Surg.* **2018**, *66*, 564–571. [CrossRef] [PubMed]
53. Ökten, E.M.; Özcan, Z.S.; Arslanhan, G.; Şenay, Ş.; Güllü, A.; Koçyiğit, M.; Değirmencioğlu, A.; Alhan, C. Robotic-assisted mitral valve surgery without aortic cross-clamping: A safe and feasible technique. *Front. Cardiovasc. Med.* **2023**, *10*, 1111496. [CrossRef] [PubMed]
54. Romano, M.A.; Haft, J.W.; Pagani, F.D.; Bolling, S.F. Beating heart surgery via right thoracotomy for reoperative mitral valve surgery: A safe and effective operative alternative. *J. Thorac. Cardiovasc. Surg.* **2012**, *144*, 334–339. [CrossRef]
55. Borger, M.A.; Raschpichler, M.; Makkar, R. Repeat Aortic Valve Surgery or Transcatheter Valve-in-Valve Therapy: We Need a Randomized Trial. *J. Am. Coll. Cardiol.* **2020**, *76*, 500–502. [CrossRef]

Journal of
Cardiovascular Development and Disease

MDPI

Article

Transferring Surgical Expertise: Analyzing the Learning Curve of Robotic Cardiac Surgery Operative Time Reduction When Surgeon Moves from One Experienced Center to Another

Sherif M. Khairallah [1,2,†], Mohamed Rahouma [1,*,†] and Stephanie L. Mick [1,*]

[1] Cardiothoracic Surgery Department, Weill Cornell Medicine New York-Presbyterian Hospital (WCM), 525 East 68th Street, Suite M404, New York, NY 10065, USA; smk4005@med.cornell.edu
[2] National Cancer Institute, Cairo University, Cairo 11562, Egypt
[*] Correspondence: mmr2011@med.cornell.edu (M.R.); slmick@med.cornell.edu (S.L.M.); Tel.: +1-512-843-1515 (M.R.); +1-212-746-670 (S.L.M.)
[†] These authors contributed equally to this work.

Abstract: Background: Robotically assisted cardiac surgery is performed in a team setting and is well known to be associated with learning curves. Surgeon and operative team learning curves are distinct entities, with total operative time representing the entire operative team (surgery, anesthesia, nursing, and perfusion) and cross-clamp time representing mainly the surgical team. Little is known about how a team learning curve evolves when an experienced surgeon transitions from one surgical center to another. This study investigates the dynamics of the team learning curve expressed as total operative time in the case of a surgeon with previous experience transitioning to a new team. Methods: A retrospective analysis was conducted on robotic cardiac surgeries performed by a surgeon who transitioned from one experienced surgical center to another. Operative time data were collected and categorized to assess the evolution of the learning curve. Statistical analysis, including learning curve modeling and linear regression analysis, was used to evaluate changes in total time in the operating room per case. Results: 103 cases were included in Weill Cornell Medicine (2019–2023). The median patient age was 63 years, 68% were males, 90.3% of cases were repaired for degenerative mitral valve disease, and the median body mass index was 23.87. Operative time (ORT) decreased from a median of 5.00 h [95%CI: 4.76, 6.00] in the first 30 cases to 4.83 [95%CI: 4.10, 5.27] thereafter, with the apparent curve plateauing indicative of the adaptation period to the new surgical environment ($p = 0.01$). Subgroup analysis among mitral cases ($n = 93$) showed a decrease in ORT from 5.00 [95%CI: 4.71, 5.98] in the first 26 cases to 4.83 [95%CI: 4.14, 5.30] ($p = 0.045$). There was no difference between the initial 30 cases and subsequent cases regarding cardiopulmonary bypass time, myocardial ischemia time, reoperation for bleeding, prolonged ventilation, reintubation, renal failure, need for an intra-aortic balloon pump, readmission to the ICU, reoperation for valvular dysfunction within 30 days, pneumonia, and deep venous thrombosis. Multivariate significant predictors of longer operative time were the first 30 cases, resection-based repairs, and MAZE as a concomitant procedure. Conclusions: Total operative time can be expected to decrease after about 30 cases when an experienced robotic surgeon moves between centers. Complications and cross-clamp times are less susceptible to a learning curve phenomenon in such a circumstance, as these depend primarily on the operating surgeon's level of experience. Understanding these dynamics can inform the planning and management of surgical transitions, ensuring optimal patient care and continued improvement in surgical outcomes.

Keywords: learning curve; robotic cardiac surgery; surgeons transfer

1. Introduction

Mitral valve repair is widely recognized as being superior to replacement in terms of long-term durability and reduced complications for treating degenerative mitral regurgitation [1,2]. The choice between replacement and repair is predominantly dependent on the surgeon's experience and volume [3–6]. For instance, New York State data have demonstrated that surgeons with lower annual volumes (performing fewer than 25 operations per year) were more likely to opt for mitral replacement rather than repair in patients with degenerative disease, and patients undergoing surgery by lower-volume surgeons demonstrated worse survival rates and higher rates of reoperation in the long term compared to those undergoing surgery by higher-volume practitioners. Interestingly, this study also found that the presence of a high-volume surgeon at the same institution was linked to improved repair rates for low-volume surgeons at the same centers [7].

The use of robotics in mitral valve surgery started in 1998 [8], with the first complete repair performed by the East Carolina University group in 2000 [9]. Adoption of this new, expensive, and technically demanding procedure has been slow due to concerns about the time and effort required for efficient, safe, and effective use by both surgeons and health systems. Over the years, numerous studies have shown that robotic mitral valve surgery is equivalent in safety, outcomes, and repair rates compared to conventional sternotomy surgery. The benefits of robotic surgery included improved cosmetic results, a shorter hospital length of stay, a faster return to normal activities, reduced transfusion rates, and the ability to afford the surgeon an excellent 3D view of the mitral valve with a 10× magnification.

As with any technique, the use of robotics in mitral valve surgery is subject to a learning curve. The primary concern during this process is ensuring patient safety and maintaining clinical effectiveness during the early stages of the learning curve. Several studies have investigated the learning curve in robotic mitral surgery, but the data are limited. Some studies have reported a rapid decrease in operative time, composite complication rates, and increased efficiency as surgeons and surgical teams become more experienced [10–12].

Overall, the available evidence suggests that the learning curve in robotic mitral surgery is complex and dependent on various factors, including the surgeon's prior experience, the surgical team's experience (consisting of cardiac anesthesia, surgical assistants, surgical nurses, and technicians), the patient population, and the specific surgical techniques used. Further research is needed to fully understand the impact of experience on outcomes in robotic mitral surgery. Herein, we carried out this investigation to assess the learning curve of robotic mitral surgery at the Weill Cornell Medical Center—New York Presbyterian Hospital, a center of excellence and a leading tertiary referral center.

2. Patients and Methods

2.1. Inclusion, and Exclusion Criteria

The study included all patients between June 2019 and December 2022 who had isolated moderately severe or severe primary degenerative mitral regurgitation affecting either the anterior and posterior leaflets or bileaflet and required repair according to the patient selection protocol of Weill Cornell Medicine and underwent robotic repair. Supplementary Figure S1 showed the robotic team ergonomics at Weill Cornell Medicine. Patients with cardiac tumors who underwent robotic resection procedures were also included in the study. Additionally, patients who had concomitant cryo-ablative procedures for atrial fibrillation and/or closure of the patent foramen oval during the same procedure were included. Exclusion criteria included patients who had additional procedures (other than cryoablation and/or PFO closure) conducted during the mitral valve repair.

2.2. Study Type and Data Retrieval

This research is retrospective in nature. Weill Cornell Medicine institutional review board approval number is 1704018121. The data were gathered from the Cardio-Thoracic Information Registry of Weill Cornell Medicine New York Presbyterian Hospital (EPIC, and REDCap for the robotic mitral valve data base).

2.3. End Points and Outcomes Definition

In this study, the total operative time was defined as the duration from the initiation of the skin incision to the closure of the incision. This duration specifically excluded the time allocated for anesthesia administration and the initiation and termination of cardiopulmonary bypass (CPB) procedures. Perioperative mortality and morbidity were defined as any operative and early postoperative morbidity and/or mortality occurring within 30 days of the surgery, and all were as defined in the Society of Thoracic Surgeons National Database.

Mitral regurgitation (MR) severity was stratified based on established criteria. Grade +3 MR was categorized as moderately severe, indicating a significant but not yet severe regurgitation, while grade +4 MR was designated as severe, denoting a critical and advanced stage of mitral valve insufficiency.

Our primary outcome is an assessment of the impact of altering the ergonomics of the operating room and the cardiac team on surgeon performance (measured by assessing the operative time). Secondary outcomes include assessment of cardiopulmonary bypass (CPB) and myocardial ischemia times in addition to the rate of conversion to open, i.e., technical proficiency and operative success. Furthermore, we evaluated the effectiveness of robotic cardiac surgery when performed by an experienced surgeon (via assessing the incidence of more than +2 mitral regurgitation at the end of the case and on the predischarge echocardiography in addition to intraoperative blood loss, hospital mortality, new-onset atrial fibrillation, stroke, renal failure, sepsis, the need for ventilator support for more than 24 h, and the need for reoperation due to bleeding, i.e., Patient safety parameters).

2.4. Data Statistical Analysis

Continuous variables were presented as median and interquartile range (IQR) and compared using the Mann–Whitney U test, or as mean and standard deviation and compared using the *t* test after testing for normality, while categorical variables were presented as frequency count and percentage and compared across groups using the Chi-square or Fisher's test, as appropriate.

Learning curve analyses were performed using case sequence numbers, starting with the first robotic case performed in our institute by the index surgeon (S.L.M.). Patients were divided into 2 groups of consecutive patients based on the point of inflection/plateauing to evaluate the influence of growing surgical experience on the total operative time. To clearly identify and depict the relationship between sequence number and continuous responses, we modeled the sequence number and all other variables as additive components using spline smoothing in the semiparametric model [13].

All statistical analyses will be performed using R version 4.2.1 (R Foundation for Statistical Computing) within RStudio. Tableone and ggplot2 R packages were used.

3. Results

3.1. Patients' Demographics

Between June 2019 and December 2022, a total of 103 robotic cardiac procedures were performed by a single experienced robotic cardiac surgeon (S.M.K.). The median age of the patients enrolled in the study was 63 years, with 68% being male. The median body mass index (BMI) was 23.87. Table 1 shows the detailed demographics of the studied cohort.

Among the cases studied, 21 patients (20.4%) were identified with preoperative atrial fibrillation (A Fib). Additionally, 9 cases (8.7%) exhibited a history of prior coronary artery disease (CAD), while only one case had a previous myocardial infarction (MI). Eighty-three patients (80%) presented with New York Heart Association (NYHA) class II and III symptoms (57 patients with NYHA class II and 26 patients with NYHA class III, respectively). The median preoperative ejection fraction (EF) was 62 [IQR 55.5–65.0].

Table 1. Criteria of included patients.

	Overall	After	First 30 Cases	p
N	103	73	30	
Age (years (median [IQR])	63.00 [56.50, 69.00]	62.00 [53.00, 68.00]	65.50 [58.25, 69.00]	0.235
Gender (Males %)	70 (68.0)	52 (71.2)	18 (60.0)	0.38
Diagnosis				
• MR (%)	93 (90.3)	67 (91.8)	26 (86.7)	0.667
• TR (%)	2 (1.9)	0 (0.0)	2 (6.7)	0.149
• Cardiac Tumor (Atrial myxoma (%))	7 (6.8)	4 (5.5)	3 (10.0)	0.691
• ASD (%)	2 (1.9)	1 (1.4)	1 (3.3)	1
• Afib (%)	9 (8.7)	5 (6.8)	4 (13.3)	0.5
• Heart Failure (%)	1 (1.0)	0 (0.0)	1 (3.3)	0.644
• PFO (%)	3 (2.9)	0 (0.0)	3 (10.0)	0.036
• Other (%)	6 (5.8)	3 (4.1)	3 (10.0)	0.486
Body Mass Index (median [IQR])	23.87 [22.02, 26.49]	24.34 [22.07, 26.18]	23.77 [21.94, 26.83]	0.925
Prior HTN (%)	47 (45.6)	32 (43.8)	15 (50.0)	0.724
Prior DM (%)	3 (2.9)	3 (4.1)	0 (0.0)	0.63
Prior HLD (%)	41 (39.8)	26 (35.6)	15 (50.0)	0.257
Prior CAD (%)	9 (8.7)	7 (9.6)	2 (6.7)	0.926
Prior Peripheral artery disease (%)	1 (1.0)	1 (1.4)	0 (0.0)	1
Prior Atrial Fibrillation (%)	21 (20.4)	12 (16.4)	9 (30.0)	0.199
Prior Atrial Flutter (%)	3 (2.9)	1 (1.4)	2 (6.7)	0.419
Prior MI (%)	1 (1.0)	1 (1.4)	0 (0.0)	1
Prior Significant lung disease (%)	9 (8.7)	6 (8.2)	3 (10.0)	1
Prior Liver disease (%)	1 (1.0)	1 (1.4)	0 (0.0)	1
Prior CVA (%)	3 (2.9)	2 (2.7)	1 (3.3)	1
Prior Smoking (%)	27 (26.2)	19 (26.0)	8 (26.7)	1
NYHA class (%)				
• 1	20 (19.4)	16 (21.9)	4 (13.3)	0.507
• 2	57 (55.3)	38 (52.1)	19 (63.3)	
• 3	26 (25.2)	19 (26.0)	7 (23.3)	
Ejection fraction, __% (median [IQR])	62.00 [55.50, 65.00]	61.00 [58.00, 65.00]	65.00 [54.00, 67.00]	0.881
AI (%)				
• 0	72 (69.9)	49 (67.1)	23 (76.7)	0.428
• 1	29 (28.2)	23 (31.5)	6 (20.0)	
• 2	2 (1.9)	1 (1.4)	1 (3.3)	
MR (%)				
• 0	8 (7.8)	5 (6.8)	3 (10.0)	0.294
• 1	1 (1.0)	0 (0.0)	1 (3.3)	
• 2	1 (1.0)	1 (1.4)	0 (0.0)	
• 3	17 (16.5)	10 (13.7)	7 (23.3)	
• 4	76 (73.8)	57 (78.1)	19 (63.3)	
TR (%)				
• 0	50 (48.5)	34 (46.6)	16 (53.3)	0.224
• 1	48 (46.6)	35 (47.9)	13 (43.3)	
• 2	4 (3.9)	4 (5.5)	0 (0.0)	
• 3	1 (1.0)	0 (0.0)	1 (3.3)	

Table 1. *Cont.*

	Overall	After	First 30 Cases	p
Etiology of MV disease				
• unknown (%)	1 (1.0)	1 (1.4)	0 (0.0)	1
• degenerative (%)	91 (88.3)	65 (89.0)	26 (86.7)	0.997
• Other (%)	2 (1.9)	2 (2.7)	0 (0.0)	0.897
• Barlows Disease (%)	15 (14.6)	12 (16.4)	3 (10.0)	0.593
• Prior endocarditis with damage to MV (%)	2 (1.9)	2 (2.7)	0 (0.0)	0.897
MV lesions				
• posterior leaflet prolapse (%)	66 (64.1)	48 (65.8)	18 (60.0)	0.744
• anterior leaflet prolapse (%)	9 (8.7)	4 (5.5)	5 (16.7)	0.149
• bi-leaflet prolapse (%)	15 (14.6)	11 (15.1)	4 (13.3)	1
• elongated/ruptured chords (%)	72 (69.9)	50 (68.5)	22 (73.3)	0.802
• annular dilation (%)	30 (29.1)	27 (37.0)	3 (10.0)	0.012
• chordal thickening and shortening (%)	1 (1.0)	1 (1.4)	0 (0.0)	1
• calcified leaflets (%)	1 (1.0)	0 (0.0)	1 (3.3)	0.644
• leaflet perforation (%)	1 (1.0)	1 (1.4)	0 (0.0)	1
• None (%)	5 (4.9)	4 (5.5)	1 (3.3)	1
• Other (%)	13 (12.6)	11 (15.1)	2 (6.7)	0.401
Carpentier MR Classification (%)				
• Type I	2 (1.9)	1 (1.4)	1 (3.3)	1
• Type II	93 (90.3)	67 (91.8)	26 (86.7)	0.667
• Type IIIa	0 (0.0)	0 (0.0)	0 (0.0)	NA
• Type IIIb	0 (0.0)	0 (0.0)	0 (0.0)	NA
• N/A	6 (5.8)	3 (4.1)	3 (10.0)	0.486

No cases with MS, CRI, hemodialysis, carotid stenosis, TIA, prior cardiac surgery, Rheumatic heart disease. Regarding etiology, there were no cases with rheumatic, acute/chronic ischemic MR, acute endocarditis, rheumatic, ischemic, post-infarction, ischemic chronic endocarditis, HOCM, trauma, congenital, prior MV intervention, or SAM. No cases with pap muscle rupture, commissural fusion, Restrictive anterior/posterior leaflet.

3.2. Detailed Mitral Pathology

Out of 103 patients, a total of seven cases underwent robotic cardiac procedures for the excision of cardiac tumors, specifically cardiac myxomas. A total of 95 patients (92.2%) exhibited mitral pathology. Notably, all cases presented with either class 3 or class 4 mitral regurgitation (MR) (16.5% vs. 73.8% for class 3 and class 4, respectively). Additionally, two patients demonstrated mitral valve damage resulting from prior endocarditis (Carpentier class 1); one case featured perforation, while the other showed chordae shortening and thickening. Table 1 also showed a detailed description of the mitral pathology.

Furthermore, most cases (90.3%) experienced MR due to degenerative etiology (Carpentier class II). Within this group, 66 cases (64.1%) were attributed to posterior leaflet etiology. 15 cases (14.6%) were diagnosed with bileaflet prolapse (Barlow's disease), and a smaller subset (8.7%) exhibited anterior leaflet prolapse. The presence of annular dilatation was in 30 cases (29.1%), occurring either in isolation or in conjunction with leaflet pathology (2 cases demonstrated isolated annular dilatation, while in 28 cases, it was associated with other leaflet pathology).

In addition to mitral pathology, various associated cardiac lesions were observed within the studied cohort. Two patients (1.9%) displayed tricuspid regurgitation (TR), another two patients (1.9%) exhibited atrial septal defects (ASD), and three patients (5.8%) presented with patent foramen oval (PFO).

3.3. Details of the Used Repair Methods

The predominant repair technique employed in this study was neochordae implantation, which was utilized in 68 patients (66.1%). Within this category, posterior leaflet neochordae account for the majority (58.3%), in contrast to anterior neochordae (7.8%). The second most frequently used repair methods was resection-based techniques (33.9%). Among these, triangular resection was employed in 16.5% of cases, quadrangular resection in 8.7%, and sliding plasty in 8.7% of cases. Alfieri stitches were utilized in only 1.9% of patients. Table 2.

Table 2. Operative details and outcomes.

	Overall	After	First 30 Cases	*p*
Operative details and outcomes	103	73	30	
Operative time (mean (SD))	5.10 (1.21)	4.93 (1.15)	5.51 (1.28)	0.026
Operative time (median [IQR])	4.92 [4.26, 5.48]	4.83 [4.10, 5.27]	5.00 [4.76, 6.00]	0.01
No. of pump runs (%)				
• 1	94 (91.3)	66 (90.4)	28 (93.3)	0.656
• 2	7 (6.8)	5 (6.8)	2 (6.7)	
• 3	2 (1.9)	2 (2.7)	0 (0.0)	
Operations performed:				
• MV repair (%)	93 (90.3)	67 (91.8)	26 (86.7)	0.667
• TV repair (%)	4 (3.9)	2 (2.7)	2 (6.7)	0.707
• ASD closure (%)	3 (2.9)	2 (2.7)	1 (3.3)	1
• Pulmonary vein isolation (%)	1 (1.0)	1 (1.4)	0 (0.0)	1
• LA MAZE (%)	15 (14.6)	9 (12.3)	6 (20.0)	0.487
• LA appendage closure (%)	6 (5.8)	3 (4.1)	3 (10.0)	0.486
• PFO closure (%)	7 (6.8)	4 (5.5)	3 (10.0)	0.691
• Cardiac tumor removal (%)	7 (6.8)	4 (5.5)	3 (10.0)	0.691
• Other (%)	6 (5.8)	3 (4.1)	3 (10.0)	0.486
If MV Repair:				
• Posterior Triangular Resection (%)	17 (16.5)	12 (16.4)	5 (16.7)	1
• Posterior Quadrangular Resection (%)	9 (8.7)	8 (11.0)	1 (3.3)	0.389
• Sliding Plasty (%)	9 (8.7)	9 (12.3)	0 (0.0)	0.103
• Neochords to Posterior Leaflet (%)	60 (58.3)	43 (58.9)	17 (56.7)	1
• Anterior Leaflet Neochords (%)	8 (7.8)	5 (6.8)	3 (10.0)	0.891
• Partial Band (%)	81 (78.6)	58 (79.5)	23 (76.7)	0.961
• Complete Flexible Ring (%)	2 (1.9)	1 (1.4)	1 (3.3)	1
• Complete Rigid/Semi-Rigid Ring (%)	1 (1.0)	1 (1.4)	0 (0.0)	1
• Partial Semi-Rigid Band (%)	8 (7.8)	7 (9.6)	1 (3.3)	0.501
• Annular Reconstruction (%)	1 (1.0)	0 (0.0)	1 (3.3)	0.644
• Patch closure of perforation (%)	1 (1.0)	1 (1.4)	0 (0.0)	1
• Alfieri Stitch (%)	2 (1.9)	1 (1.4)	1 (3.3)	1
• Commisurroplasty (Magic Stitch) (%)	10 (9.7)	7 (9.6)	3 (10.0)	1
• MV cleft closure (%)	33 (32.0)	23 (31.5)	10 (33.3)	1
• Other (%)	18 (17.5)	8 (11.0)	10 (33.3)	0.015
Cardiopulmonary Bypass Time (median [IQR])	145.00 [130.00, 174.50]	144.00 [128.50, 173.00]	144.00 [128.50, 173.00]	0.255
Aortic Cross-clamp time (median [IQR])	82.00 [72.00, 95.75]	83.00 [70.75, 94.25]	81.00 [74.25, 96.00]	0.719
Did the patient receive blood products in the OR? (%)	23 (22.5)	17 (23.6)	6 (20.0)	0.891
MR grade at the end of the case (%)				
• 0	65 (63.7)	51 (69.9)	14 (48.3)	0.123
• 1	32 (31.4)	19 (26.0)	13 (44.8)	
• 2	5 (4.9)	3 (4.1)	2 (6.9)	

Table 2. *Cont.*

	Overall	After	First 30 Cases	*p*
Extubation in in the OR (%)	82 (79.6)	56 (76.7)	26 (86.7)	0.384
Conversion to open procedure (%)	1 (1.0)	1 (1.4)	0 (0.0)	1
Postoperative blood product (%)	16 (15.5)	12 (16.4)	4 (13.3)	0.924
Postoperative complications				
Return to OR for bleeding (%)	2 (1.9)	2 (2.7)	0 (0.0)	0.897
Prolonged Ventilation >24 h (%)	1 (1.0)	1 (1.4)	0 (0.0)	1
Reintubated during hospitalization (%)	3 (2.9)	1 (1.4)	2 (6.7)	0.419
New/Acute Renal Failure (%)	2 (1.9)	1 (1.4)	1 (3.3)	1
Groin Infection (%)	1 (1.0)	0 (0.0)	1 (3.3)	0.644
Groin Lymphocele (%)	4 (3.9)	2 (2.7)	2 (6.7)	0.707
Need for IABP (%)	1 (1.0)	0 (0.0)	1 (3.3)	0.644
Readmit to ICU (%)	1 (1.0)	0 (0.0)	1 (3.3)	0.644
Reoperation for valvular dysfunction within 30 days (%)	1 (1.0)	0 (0.0)	1 (3.3)	0.644
Pneumonia (%)	2 (1.9)	1 (1.4)	1 (3.3)	1
Pleural Effusion requiring drainage (%)	7 (6.8)	6 (8.2)	1 (3.3)	0.642
DVT (%)	1 (1.0)	0 (0.0)	1 (3.3)	0.644
Pneumothorax requiring intervention (%)	2 (1.9)	1 (1.4)	1 (3.3)	1
Tamponade, surgical intervention (%)	1 (1.0)	1 (1.4)	0 (0.0)	1
Aortic Dissection (%)	1 (1.0)	1 (1.4)	0 (0.0)	1
Atrial Fibrillation (%)	34 (33.0)	21 (28.8)	13 (43.3)	0.231
Uneventful post operative course (%)	36 (35.0)	25 (34.2)	11 (36.7)	0.995
If re-exploration for bleeding:				
• VATs or Robotic (%)	1 (1.0)	1 (1.4)	0 (0.0)	1
• Mini-Thoracotomy (%)	1 (1.0)	1 (1.4)	0 (0.0)	1
Anti-coagulation required in AF (%)	25 (24.3)	15 (20.5)	10 (33.3)	0.262
Did the patient survive 30 day or discharge whichever is longer? (%)	101 (99.0)	72 (100.0)	29 (96.7)	0.65
Readmitted within 30 days? (%)	13 (12.7)	9 (12.5)	4 (13.3)	1
ICU stay (days) (median [IQR])	2.00 [2.00, 3.00]	2.00 [2.00, 3.00]	2.00 [2.00, 4.00]	0.293
Last follow-up status (Alive (%))	103 (100.0)	73 (100.0)	30 (100.0)	NA
MR degree at last follow up (%)				
• no	66 (64.1)	45 (61.6)	21 (70.0)	0.082
• mild +1	12 (11.7)	7 (9.6)	5 (16.7)	
• moderate	1 (1.0)	0 (0.0)	1 (3.3)	
• severe	2 (1.9)	1 (1.4)	1 (3.3)	
• trace	22 (21.4)	20 (27.4)	2 (6.7)	

No cases underwent Anterior Leaflet Resection or Commissurotomy, Leaflet plication, Anterior or posterior Leaflet Augmentation, Folding Plasty, or Posterior Annular Decalcification. No cases had TV replacement, Bi Atrial MAZE, Stem Cell implant, VSD Repair, Septal Myectomy for HOCM, Robotic MIDCAB, TECAB, Reconstruction of Damaged Leaflet, and Complete Reconstruction of Valve with Tissue. No cases with CVA, CVA with neuro deficit >7 days), Trach during hospitalization, Renal Failure requiring New Dialysis, Chest Wall Incision Infection, Chest Wall Incision Infection, sepsis, Limb loss or Limb ischemic complications, PE, Positive blood cultures, Phrenic nerve injury, Cardiac Arrest, VA ECMO, VV ECMO, Multi-system organ failure, Hemoperitoneum, Liver injury, Diaphragm injury. No cases with re-exploration for bleeding through Sternotomy, Laparotomy, or Laparoscopy.

Additionally, nearly all cases underwent annuloplasty, either as a standalone procedure or in combination with other repair methods. The Duran annuloplasty band emerged as the most frequently utilized annuloplasty device (78.6%). Ninety-one percent of patients underwent only one CPB pump run, with only seven patients (6.8%) and two patients

(1.9%) undergoing two and three pump runs, respectively. Only 23 cases (22.5%) received an intraoperative blood transfusion, indicating minimal overall blood loss. Table 2.

3.4. Assessment of Technical Proficiency

The operative timeline observed across the study period displayed a distinct inflection point at 30 cases, followed by a plateau. There was a significant reduction from a median of 5.00 h [95% CI: 4.76–6.00] in the initial 30 cases to 4.83 h [4.10–5.27] thereafter, indicating an apparent plateau in the curve ($p = 0.01$). Figure 1A. This trend is suggestive of an adaptation period to the new surgical environment. Subgroup analysis on mitral cases (n = 93) further supported this finding, demonstrating a decrease in ORT from 5.00 h [4.71–5.98] in the first 26 cases to 4.83 h [CI = 4.14–5.30, $p = p = 0.04$]. In multivariate analysis, the first 30 cases, resection-based repair techniques, and the inclusion of the LA MAZE procedure as a concomitant surgical intervention emerged as influential factors associated with prolonged ORT. Figure 1B.

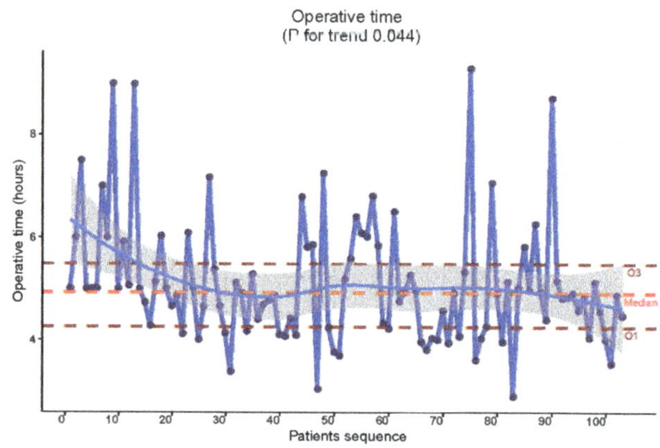

(A)

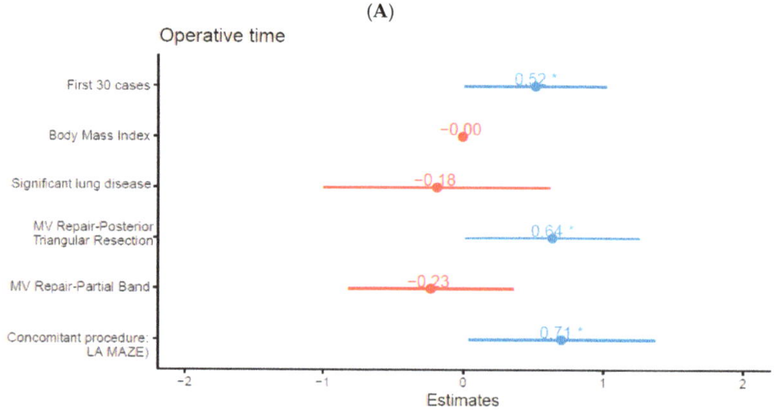

(B)

Figure 1. (**A**) operative time trend throughout the study period. (**B**) factors associated with longer operative time on multivariate analysis. Asterix represent the significant p-value. Number reflects regression coefficient (Beta). Beta <= 0 was colored in red while beta > 0 was colored in blue.

In contrast, cardiopulmonary bypass time (CBP) and myocardial ischemia time were not affected by the learning curve phenomenon in this context. Throughout the study timeline, there were no discernible differences in these metrics. CBP time remained consistent at 144.00 min [CI = 128.50, 173.00] in both the initial 30 cases and the subsequent cases ($p = 0.255$). Table 2, Figure 2. Similarly, myocardial ischemia time showed uniformity: 83.00 min [CI = 70.75, 94.25] for the first 30 cases and 81.00 min [CI = 74.25, 96.00] for the subsequent cases ($p = 0.719$). Table 2, Figure 3.

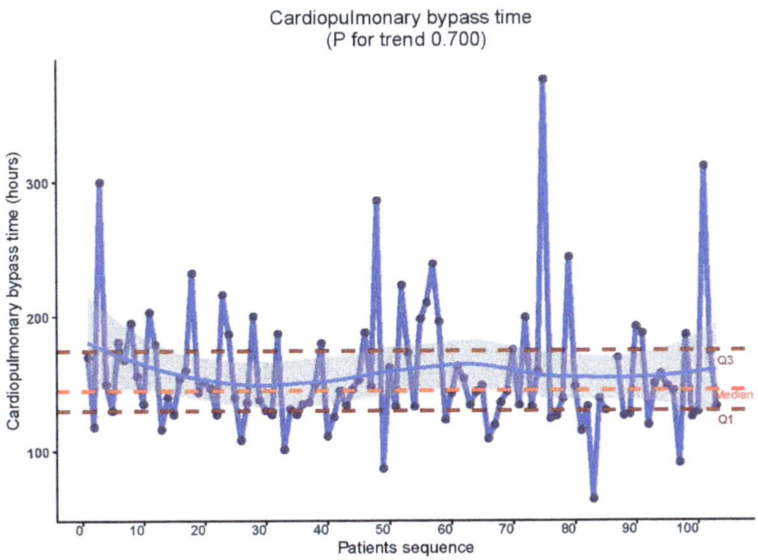

Figure 2. Cardiopulmonary bypass time trend throughout the study period.

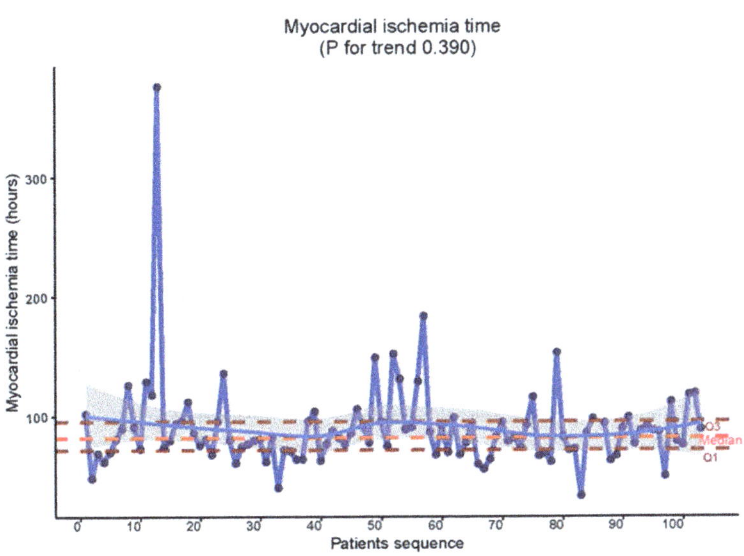

Figure 3. Myocardial ischemia time trend throughout the study period.

3.5. Assessment of Operative Success

Ninety-nine percent of cases (102 patients) were successfully completed as intended, while 1% (1 case) necessitated conversion to an open sternotomy procedure. At the completion of the repair, 95% of cases (97 patients) exhibited either grade +0 or +1 MR, and only 5% of cases (5 patients) had grade +2 MR. Table 2.

3.6. Assessment of Patient Safety

Analysis of postoperative complications revealed no significant disparities between the first 30 cases and subsequent cases, indicating that they are not subject to a learning curve phenomenon when surgeons transition between different practice settings. Supplementary Figure S2.

For the overall cohort, 36 cases (35%) experienced an uneventful postoperative course. Eighty-two cases (79.6%) were successfully extubated in the operating room. Only one case (1%) necessitated prolonged ventilatory support exceeding 24 h, while three cases (2.9%) required reintubation during their hospitalization period. The mean duration of the Intensive Care Unit (ICU) stay was 2 days [CI = 2.00, 3.00], with only one case experiencing ICU readmission.

There was no perioperative mortality. Two cases were returned to the operating room due to postoperative bleeding issues. Moreover, only one case required a salvage operation due to valvular dysfunction within the initial 30 days.

In terms of specific complications, 34 cases (33%) developed postoperative A fib, with 25 of them necessitating anticoagulation therapy. Additionally, 13 cases (12.7%) required hospital readmission within 30 days.

During the six-month follow-up period, only two cases developed severe MR, necessitating further intervention.

4. Discussion

The healthcare industry operates within a highly intricate ecosystem where expertise and seamless coordination among medical professionals are of utmost importance [14,15]. Within this dynamic environment, a notable phenomenon is the transfer of doctors from one team to another, driven by factors such as professional growth, staffing needs, and advancements in medical technology.

It is well recognized that in medicine, transitions or adaptations can affect health care practitioners' performance and even patient outcomes. For instance, Scarponi et al. [16] reported a decreased compliance rate when pediatric renal failure patients were transitioned to adult services at the age of 18, and this was notably improved by adopting a model that specifically took into account the additional needs specific to a time of transition. Another study reported that social processes, including alignment professionals working together as cohesive groups, were key factors in establishing well-functioning, successful healthcare endeavors [17]. In Canada, Behruzi et al. reported that lack of interpersonal communication skills among healthcare providers and differences in philosophy and scope of practice affected the quality of patient care [18] and noted that healthcare provider transition is a time associated with risks to that provider, including risks of encountering different goals, changes in work ergonomics, and scopes of practice.

During the transition of healthcare providers, a crucial adjustment period occurs, requiring both the team and the new member (in this situation, the surgeon) to acclimate to each other's working dynamics [19]. The team must familiarize themselves with the surgeon's unique approach, preferences, and specialized knowledge. Simultaneously, the transferred surgeon should invest time in understanding the intricacies of the hospital's protocols, equipment, and procedures. This mutual adaptation process is essential for maintaining the high standards of care and efficiency that patients expect and deserve [20,21].

In this study, our investigation centered around the followings: the impact of altering the ergonomics of the operating room and the cardiac team on surgeon performance, in addition to the evaluation of the effectiveness of robotic cardiac surgery when performed by an experienced surgeon.

Our findings revealed a noteworthy declining trend, followed by a plateau in operative time. After the initial 30 cases, an adaptation period was observed, leading to a plateau in operative time (p = 0.01). While this trend was statistically significant, it held limited clinical significance, with operative time reducing marginally from 5.0 [IQR: 4.8–6.0] hours to 4.83 [IQR: 4.1–5.3] hours between the first 30 cases and subsequent cases, respectively.

This observation indicates that altering the surgical environment exerts a minimal impact on surgeon performance and operative time, provided both the cardiac team and the surgeon possess adequate experience [22]. Many studies have documented that changing the operating room characteristics might affect overall surgical performance [21,23]. This might also raise the crucial insight that high-volume centers, characterized by standardized protocols, advanced equipment, and consistent operational standards, exhibit striking similarities, shortening the adaptation period. This uniformity in operational procedures across high-volume centers further emphasizes the minimal influence of changes in the surgical environment on surgeon performance when both the team and surgeon have attained the requisite level of proficiency.

Operative success, assessed at the end of MR repair and lack of/minimal conversion to open, along with evaluation of perioperative complications, did not exhibit a learning curve plateau effect. Instead, these outcomes were primarily contingent upon the patient's performance status and the extensive experience of the surgeon involved.

Several studies have corroborated that the critical decision-making process regarding mitral valve replacement or repair and patients' outcomes were substantially influenced by the surgeon's proficiency and their annual caseload [3–6]. Specifically, it has been established that a reference surgeon should ideally undertake a minimum of 25 index mitral valve procedures within a single calendar year [24]. Moreover, medical centers performing a minimum of 50 index mitral procedures annually are designated as reference centers [24]. This standardized approach has demonstrated a significant impact on the rate of successful repairs and overall perioperative outcomes in national-based (STS-ACS) studies [4,25] and/or institutional-based studies [7,26–28].

Our study result reflects the previously mentioned evidence-based facts related to both the surgeon's and the center's volume. Notably, we ensured the elimination of bias related to the heterogeneity of surgeons' experiences and their potential impact on perioperative outcomes. To achieve this, all surgical interventions in our study were exclusively conducted by a single experienced cardiac surgeon, thereby enhancing the reliability and integrity of our study's results.

Our study possesses inherent limitations, primarily due to its retrospective nature and the utilization of a relatively small sample size within a specific patient group, rendering it susceptible to biases and confounding variables, diminishing its statistical power, and limiting its generalizability to broader populations. However, the study also exhibits a notable strength (the mitigation of bias from heterogeneity in surgeons' experiences) as all cases were performed by a single experienced surgeon, enhancing the internal validity of the study.

5. Conclusions

In this study, total operative time can be expected to decrease after about 30 cases when an experienced robotic surgeon moves between centers. Complications and cross-clamp times are less susceptible to a learning curve phenomenon in such a circumstance, as these depend primarily on the operating surgeon's level of experience. Patients' safety was not affected during this transition period. Understanding these dynamics can inform the planning and management of surgical transitions, ensuring optimal patient care and continued improvement in surgical outcomes.

Supplementary Materials: The following supporting information can be downloaded at: https://www.mdpi.com/article/10.3390/jcdd11030081/s1, Figure S1: The robotic team ergonomics at Weill Cornell Medicine; Figure S2: Postoperative outcomes.

Author Contributions: Conceptualization, S.L.M.; methodology, S.L.M. and M.R.; software, M.R. and S.M.K.; validation, S.L.M.; formal analysis, M.R.; investigation, S.M.K.; data curation, S.M.K.; writing—original draft preparation, S.M.K.; writing—review and editing, M.R. and S.L.M.; visualization, M.R.; supervision, M.R. and S.L.M.; project administration, S.M.K. All authors have read and agreed to the published version of the manuscript.

Funding: This research received no external funding.

Institutional Review Board Statement: The study was conducted according to the guidelines of the Declaration of Helsinki and approved by the Institutional Review Board (Ethics Committee) of Weill Cornell medicine, New York presbyterian hospital (protocol number 1704018121).

Informed Consent Statement: Informed consent was obtained from all subjects involved in the study.

Data Availability Statement: The data are not publicly available due to commercial confidentiality, as they contain information that could compromise the privacy of research participants.

Acknowledgments: This study was supported by charitable research gift of Charles and Irene Hamm.

Conflicts of Interest: The authors declare no conflicts of interest.

References

1. Nishimura, R.A.; Otto, C.M.; Bonow, R.O.; Carabello, B.A.; Erwin, J.P., III; Fleisher, L.A.; Jneid, H.; Mack, M.J.; McLeod, C.J.; O'Gara, P.T. 2017 AHA/ACC focused update of the 2014 AHA/ACC guideline for the management of patients with valvular heart disease: A report of the American College of Cardiology/American Heart Association Task Force on Clinical Practice Guidelines. *Circulation* **2017**, *135*, e1159–e1195. [CrossRef]
2. Members, A.T.F.; Vahanian, A.; Alfieri, O.; Andreotti, F.; Antunes, M.J.; Barón-Esquivias, G.; Baumgartner, H.; Borger, M.A.; Carrel, T.P.; De Bonis, M. Guidelines on the management of valvular heart disease (version 2012) The Joint Task Force on the Management of Valvular Heart Disease of the European Society of Cardiology (ESC) and the European Association for Cardio-Thoracic Surgery (EACTS). *Eur. Heart J.* **2012**, *33*, 2451–2496.
3. Bolling, S.F.; Li, S.; O'Brien, S.M.; Brennan, J.M.; Prager, R.L.; Gammie, J.S. Predictors of mitral valve repair: Clinical and surgeon factors. *Ann. Thorac. Surg.* **2010**, *90*, 1904–1912. [CrossRef]
4. Gammie, J.S.; O'Brien, S.M.; Griffith, B.P.; Ferguson, T.B.; Peterson, E.D. Influence of hospital procedural volume on care process and mortality for patients undergoing elective surgery for mitral regurgitation. *Circulation* **2007**, *115*, 881–887. [CrossRef]
5. LaPar, D.J.; Ailawadi, G.; Isbell, J.M.; Crosby, I.K.; Kern, J.A.; Rich, J.B.; Speir, A.M.; Kron, I.L.; Investigators for the Virginia Cardiac Surgery Quality Initiative. Mitral valve repair rates correlate with surgeon and institutional experience. *J. Thorac. Cardiovasc. Surg.* **2014**, *148*, 995–1004. [CrossRef]
6. Kilic, A.; Shah, A.S.; Conte, J.V.; Baumgartner, W.A.; Yuh, D.D. Operative outcomes in mitral valve surgery: Combined effect of surgeon and hospital volume in a population-based analysis. *J. Thorac. Cardiovasc. Surg.* **2013**, *146*, 638–646. [CrossRef] [PubMed]
7. Chikwe, J.; Toyoda, N.; Anyanwu, A.C.; Itagaki, S.; Egorova, N.N.; Boateng, P.; El-Eshmawi, A.; Adams, D.H. Relation of mitral valve surgery volume to repair rate, durability, and survival. *J. Am. Coll. Cardiol.* **2017**, *69*, 2397–2406. [CrossRef] [PubMed]
8. Carpentier, A.; Loulmet, D.; Aupecle, B.; Kieffer, J.; Tournay, D.; Guibourt, P.; Fiemeyer, A.; Méléard, D.; Richomme, P.; Cardon, C. Computer assisted open heart surgery. First case operated on with success. *Comptes Rendus L'academie Des. Sci. Ser. III Sci. Vie* **1998**, *321*, 437–442.
9. Chitwood, W.R.; Nifong, L.W.; Elbeery, J.E.; Chapman, W.H.; Albrecht, R.; Kim, V.; Young, J.A. Robotic mitral valve repair: Trapezoidal resection and prosthetic annuloplasty with the da Vinci surgical system. *J. Thorac. Cardiovasc. Surg.* **2000**, *120*, 1171–1172. [CrossRef] [PubMed]
10. Goodman, A.; Koprivanac, M.; Kelava, M.; Mick, S.L.; Gillinov, A.M.; Rajeswaran, J.; Brzezinski, A.; Blackstone, E.H.; Mihaljevic, T. Robotic mitral valve repair: The learning curve. *Innovations* **2017**, *12*, 390–397. [PubMed]
11. Seo, Y.J.; Sanaiha, Y.; Bailey, K.L.; Aguayo, E.; Chao, A.; Shemin, R.J.; Benharash, P. Outcomes and resource utilization in robotic mitral valve repair: Beyond the learning curve. *J. Surg. Res.* **2019**, *235*, 258–263. [CrossRef] [PubMed]
12. Yaffee, D.W.; Loulmet, D.F.; Kelly, L.A.; Ward, A.F.; Ursomanno, P.A.; Rabinovich, A.E.; Neuburger, P.J.; Krishnan, S.; Hill, F.T.; Grossi, E.A. Can the learning curve of totally endoscopic robotic mitral valve repair be short-circuited? *Innovations* **2014**, *9*, 43–48. [PubMed]
13. Ruppert, D.; Wand, M.P.; Carroll, R.J. *Semiparametric Regression*; Cambridge University Press: Cambridge, UK, 2003.
14. Singhal, S.; Kayyali, B.; Levin, R.; Greenberg, Z. *The Next Wave of Healthcare Innovation: The Evolution of Ecosystems*; McKinsey & Company: Chicago, IL, USA, 2020.
15. Laihonen, H. Knowledge structures of a health ecosystem. *J. Health Organ. Manag.* **2012**, *26*, 542–558. [CrossRef] [PubMed]
16. Scarponi, D.; Cangini, G.; Pasini, A.; La Scola, C.; Mencarelli, F.; Bertulli, C.; Amabile, D.; Busutti, M.; La Manna, G.; Pession, A. The process of transition from pediatric to adult healthcare services for nephrological patients: Recommendations vs. reality—A single center experience. *Front. Pediatr.* **2022**, *10*, 954641. [CrossRef] [PubMed]
17. Kjellström, S.; Avby, G.; Areskoug-Josefsson, K.; Andersson Gäre, B.; Andersson Bäck, M. Work motivation among healthcare professionals: A study of well-functioning primary healthcare centers in Sweden. *J. Health Organ. Manag.* **2017**, *31*, 487–502. [CrossRef] [PubMed]
18. Behruzi, R.; Klam, S.; Dehertog, M.; Jimenez, V.; Hatem, M. Understanding factors affecting collaboration between midwives and other health care professionals in a birth center and its affiliated Quebec hospital: A case study. *BMC Pregnancy Childbirth* **2017**, *17*, 200. [CrossRef] [PubMed]

19. Arrow, H.; McGrath, J.E.; Staw, B.; Cummings, L. Membership dynamics in groups at work: A theoretical framework. *Res. Organ. Behav.* **1995**, *17*, 373.
20. Levi, D.; Askay, D.A. *Group Dynamics for Teams*; Sage Publications: Thousand Oaks, CA, USA, 2020.
21. Wong, S.W.; Smith, R.; Crowe, P. Optimizing the operating theatre environment. *ANZ J. Surg.* **2010**, *80*, 917–924. [CrossRef]
22. Arora, S.; Sevdalis, N.; Nestel, D.; Woloshynowych, M.; Darzi, A.; Kneebone, R. The impact of stress on surgical performance: A systematic review of the literature. *Surgery* **2010**, *147*, 318–330.e6. [CrossRef]
23. Helmreich, R.L.; Schaefer, H.-G. Team performance in the operating room. *Hum. Error Med.* **1994**, *225*, 253.
24. Adams, D.; Swain, J.; Accola, K. Standards and Best Practices for Mitral Valve Repair Reference Centers. *Mitral Found.* **2020**.
25. Gammie, J.S.; Chikwe, J.; Badhwar, V.; Thibault, D.P.; Vemulapalli, S.; Thourani, V.H.; Gillinov, M.; Adams, D.H.; Rankin, J.S.; Ghoreishi, M. Isolated mitral valve surgery: The society of thoracic surgeons adult cardiac surgery database analysis. *Ann. Thorac. Surg.* **2018**, *106*, 716–727. [CrossRef] [PubMed]
26. Gillinov, A.M.; Blackstone, E.H.; Alaulaqi, A.; Sabik, J.F., III; Mihaljevic, T.; Svensson, L.G.; Houghtaling, P.L.; Salemi, A.; Johnston, D.R.; Lytle, B.W. Outcomes after repair of the anterior mitral leaflet for degenerative disease. *Ann. Thorac. Surg.* **2008**, *86*, 708–717. [CrossRef] [PubMed]
27. Goldstone, A.B.; Cohen, J.E.; Howard, J.L.; Edwards, B.B.; Acker, A.L.; Hiesinger, W.; MacArthur, J.W., Jr.; Atluri, P.; Woo, Y.J. A "repair-all" strategy for degenerative mitral valve disease safely minimizes unnecessary replacement. *Ann. Thorac. Surg.* **2015**, *99*, 1983–1991. [CrossRef]
28. Chikwe, J.; Goldstone, A.B.; Passage, J.; Anyanwu, A.C.; Seeburger, J.; Castillo, J.G.; Filsoufi, F.; Mohr, F.W.; Adams, D.H. A propensity score-adjusted retrospective comparison of early and mid-term results of mitral valve repair versus replacement in octogenarians. *Eur. Heart J.* **2011**, *32*, 618–626. [CrossRef]

Journal of
Cardiovascular Development and Disease

MDPI

Review

Anaesthesia for Minimally Invasive Cardiac Surgery

Daniel Aston *, Daniel Zeloof and Florian Falter

Department of Anaesthesia and Critical Care, Royal Papworth NHS Foundation Trust, Cambridge Biomedical Campus, Papworth Road, Cambridge CB2 0AY, UK; dzeloof@gmail.com (D.Z.); florian.falter@gmail.com (F.F.)
* Correspondence: daniel.aston@nhs.net

Abstract: Minimally invasive cardiac surgery (MICS) has been used since the 1990s and encompasses a wide range of techniques that lack full sternotomy, including valve and coronary artery graft surgery as well as transcatheter procedures. Due to the potential benefits offered to patients by MICS, these procedures are becoming more common. Unique anaesthetic knowledge and skills are required to overcome the specific challenges presented by MICS, including mastery of transoesophageal echocardiography (TOE) and the provision of thoracic regional analgesia. This review evaluates the relevance of MICS to the anaesthetist and discusses pre-operative assessment, the relevant adjustments to intra-operative conduct that are necessary for these techniques, as well as post-operative care and what is known about outcomes.

Keywords: cardiac surgery; minimally invasive; minimal access; anaesthesiology

1. Introduction

While cardiac surgery is still predominantly performed via median sternotomy, a growing number of procedures are being performed that fall under the umbrella of minimally invasive cardiac surgery (MICS). First performed in the mid-1990s [1], MICS does not have a universally agreed definition. The Society of Thoracic Surgeons (STS) defines minimally invasive surgery as 'any procedure not performed with a full sternotomy and cardiopulmonary bypass (CPB)' [2], although some procedures (particularly some types of minimally invasive valve surgery) are performed using CPB. The American Heart Association (AHA) gives the definition of minimally invasive cardiac surgery as any procedure performed via a "small chest wall incision that does not include the conventional full sternotomy" [3]. A variety of different techniques are employed [4] with the unifying hallmark of a lack of full sternotomy [5]. Cardiopulmonary bypass is utilised for some procedures and avoided for others. Examples range from Minimally Invasive Direct Coronary Artery Bypass (MIDCAB) and Minimally Invasive Mitral Valve Surgery (MIMVS) to procedures carried out in the cardiac catheter laboratory ('cath lab') such as Transcatheter Aortic Valve Replacement (TAVR) and Transcatheter Edge-to-Edge Repair (TEER) of the mitral valve.

MICS is an attractive option for many patients, in part offering advantages over traditional surgery such as reduced post-operative pain, shorter hospital stay, and earlier return to normal life. There is also a smaller risk of wound infection, bleeding, respiratory complications, and atrial fibrillation [5,6]. Younger patients are especially keen on superior cosmetic outcomes [7]. However, there are drawbacks of MICS including procedure-specific complications, the considerable surgical training, and skill required, and the need for careful patient selection as minimally invasive procedures are not appropriate for all.

2. Pre-Operative Assessment and Patient Selection

The pre-operative anaesthetic assessment of a patient presenting for MICS includes the standard history, examination and investigations obtained prior to any cardiac surgery. Some areas require enhanced attention or special emphasis when a minimally invasive technique is to be used. A history of previous thoracic surgery, chest wall or rib abnormalities or some inflammatory disease processes may lead to the development of adhesions and make the minimally invasive approach to the heart difficult or impossible. Table 1 shows a list of conditions where alternatives to MICS should be considered carefully. Severe aortic regurgitation is listed as a contraindication to MIMVS; some techniques used for minimally invasive aortic valve replacement can be used in the presence of aortic incompetence, such as the use of rapid-deployment valve prostheses and in TAVR. Effective cardioplegia may sometimes be possible in MICS using retrograde delivery when aortic regurgitation renders the antegrade route ineffectual.

Table 1. Contraindications to minimally invasive valve surgery (adapted from [8,9]).

Aortic Surgery	Mitral Surgery
Severe calcification of the aortic root and/or ascending aorta	Severe aortic regurgitation
	Severe mitral annular calcification
Significant tortuosity of iliac or femoral arteries if femoral access for CPB planned	
Morbid obesity	
Severe chest wall deformities or previous radiotherapy to the chest	
Mobile aortic atheroma	
Absolute contraindication to TOE	

Symptoms and signs of the surgical cardiac lesion should be elicited, along with those of any other cardiac problems that may be additional surgical targets; the presence of multiple cardiac pathologies that all require surgical intervention is likely to make minimally invasive surgery a less feasible option. Echocardiographic assessment should pay particular attention to excluding the presence of poor ventricular function, aortic valve incompetence, mitral annular calcification, patent foramen ovale (PFO), and persistent left superior vena cava—all of which may make MICS significantly more challenging.

Evaluation of the vascular system as a whole is essential, especially if peripheral cannulation is planned for CPB [4]. CT angiography is often included as part of the standard pre-operative assessment for MICS [10]; aneurysm, significant tortuosity or atheroma, dissection or the presence of stents, grafts or other previous surgical repairs must be carefully assessed.

Some MICS procedures are performed via a small thoracotomy and many of these require one-lung ventilation (OLV) to give adequate surgical access to the heart. The patient may be supine or in a semi-lateral position. All these factors predispose to hypoxia and a history of chronic respiratory disease may compound this. Therefore, the threshold for performing Pulmonary Function Tests (PFTs) should be low. In patients presenting for thoracic surgery, a finding of a Forced Expiratory Volume in 1 s (FEV-1) and transfer factor (TLCO), both of which are greater than 40% of what was predicted, suggest the patient is at low risk of post-operative pulmonary complications, although patients with values below this should not necessarily be denied surgery as there may still be a significant chance of an acceptable outcome [11]. One small retrospective trial of patients with chronic obstructive pulmonary disease (COPD) undergoing cardiac valve surgery suggested more favourable outcomes in the group undergoing surgery using a minimally invasive technique, despite the use of OLV in this group [12].

The presence of pulmonary hypertension and right ventricular dysfunction needs to be assessed, as it is possible that the use of OLV may occasionally lead to complications including further increased pulmonary arterial pressure, raised right ventricular afterload, and cardiac failure in these patients [13].

The use of transoesophageal echocardiography (TOE) is widely regarded as essential for some MICS procedures (especially MIMVS) to the extent that a contraindication to TOE is often considered a contraindication to a minimal access approach [6,14]. Any suggestion of upper gastrointestinal pathologies such as known oesophageal webs, pouches or varices, active peptic ulcer disease, hiatus hernia, or previous surgery or radiotherapy to the neck and chest should be carefully reviewed and risks evaluated appropriately.

The planned position of the patient on the operating table should be considered, and it is likely to be challenging to place patients with chest wall deformities, kyphoscoliosis, or other significant musculoskeletal pathology into a posture that offers sufficient surgical access. Orthopaedic problems with the ipsilateral upper limb that preclude a position allowing access to the hemithorax may make the surgical approach difficult. Some positions may predispose to brachial plexus injury due to tension on the arm, and measures should be taken to minimise this risk.

Patients with significant obesity present particular challenges for the surgeon and anaesthetist. In addition to the difficulty in positioning these patients, it may be difficult to properly site a double-lumen endotracheal tube, they may tolerate OLV less well and they may require an additional venous drainage cannula to allow adequate flow during CPB.

3. Relevant Surgical Principles and Techniques

The surgical principles clearly depend largely on the procedure to be performed, as does the surgical approach. Aortic valve surgery is usually approached via a ministernotomy or right anterior thoracotomy, while the mitral valve is accessed using the right mid-axillary approach.

TOE-guided positioning of cannulae inserted via the femoral artery and veins is the most common strategy to facilitate CPB. In contrast to conventional cardiac surgery via full sternotomy, the venous cannula is inserted first in MICS [6]. If right atriotomy is required, two drainage cannulae will be required; the inferior vena cava (IVC) cannula is inserted via the femoral vein as discussed above, but the superior vena cava (SVC) cannula may need to be sited percutaneously via the right internal jugular (RIJ) vein. This can be alongside the central venous catheters, or these can be sited in the left internal jugular vein instead.

Arterial return flow is usually achieved using a cannula inserted using the Seldinger technique via the femoral artery. However, end-to-side grafting of a dacron graft to the femoral artery, or direct cut down onto the artery are alternative techniques.

Cross-clamping the aorta can be achieved in a similar way to open surgery, under direct vision using a transthoracic Chitwood aortic clamp or via an endoaortic balloon-tipped catheter (endoballoon) [15]. The former is the technique more familiar to most surgeons, allows the use of reusable clamps and is inexpensive. However, the presence of the clamp clutters the already small surgical field further and the technique necessitates a puncture in the aortic wall for infusion of cardioplegia. This must then be closed at the end of surgery and carries a risk of bleeding.

The endoballoon occludes the ascending aorta and simultaneously allows an infusion of cardioplegia, root venting, and pressure monitoring through a central lumen in the catheter, which opens proximal to the balloon. This reduces the number of instruments in the surgical field and eliminates the need for a cardioplegia cannulation site in the aorta. Disadvantages of the endoballoon include its single-use (and therefore expensive) nature, and the fact that it can migrate both proximally and distally during the procedure to obscure the surgical field or occlude arterial flow via the innominate artery to the upper body and head, respectively. Additionally, the endoballoon is usually passed through the arterial cannula which can reduce flow and lead to high line pressures. If the aortic line pressure is higher than 300 mmHg, the endoballoon is usually inserted via separate cannulation of the contralateral femoral artery [15].

There have been no prospective randomised controlled trials comparing the use of endoballoon with traditional cross-clamping, but retrospective data does not demonstrate an advantage of one technique over the other in terms of the degree of cardioprotection or incidence of bleeding [16,17]. There is some evidence that the use of the endoballon carries a higher risk of aortic dissection [18,19]. The use of retrograde cardioplegia is unusual in MICS due to the technical difficulty in siting a coronary sinus (CS) catheter through the small surgical field. That said, a catheter can be placed either via the right internal jugular vein when using the HeartPort, or via the right atrium in other cases. The technique is the same in both cases and relies on guidance from the TOE the pressure waveform transduced from the catheter tip. The limiting factor in both cases is the lack of a stabilising hand behind the heart and it can on occasion be impossible to place the CS catheter in an appropriate position.

Management of CPB follows the same principles as those used in conventional cardiac surgery.

4. Intra-Operative Anaesthetic Management

Differences from standard cardiac surgical setup include the use of a double-lumen endotracheal tube, and the mandatory placement of external defibrillator pads as internal cardioversion is often not possible during MICS.

4.1. Monitoring

Monitoring standards are not dissimilar to those for standard cardiac surgery.

The planned use of an endoballoon mandates the use of bilateral radial arterial pressure monitoring, as the loss of perfusion to the right side suggests distal migration of the balloon and allows prompt correction. The pressure at the distal tip of the endoballoon is also monitored.

The use of cerebral oximetry may also allow the detection of poor perfusion of one or both sides of the upper body. This may occur if the endoballoon migrates but can also be seen if the heart is allowed to eject blood while there is no ventilation and the CPB return flow is distal to the innominate artery. The perfusion of the upper body with deoxygenated blood while the lower body enjoys oxygenated perfusion is known as Harlequin syndrome and may lead to life-threatening cerebral hypoxia [20].

The use of OLV and lung isolation may lead to high impedance of cardiac electrical signals to the skin surface and a poor electrocardiograph trace. Modification of the standard ECG electrode positions may be required to avoid this problem.

4.2. Induction and Maintenance

Anaesthetic induction proceeds as for any cardiac surgery. The patient is intubated with a double-lumen endotracheal tube (DLT), and the position is checked—usually using a bronchoscope. Alternatively, a single-lumen tube is used with a bronchial blocker used to isolate the lung. Prophylactic antibiotics are given. Maintenance of anaesthesia is commonly achieved using an intravenous agent.

4.3. Positioning

The majority of procedures are performed through a mini-thoracotomy, often requiring OLV to facilitate access to the heart, or through a partial sternotomy [21]. For the former, the patient is positioned with one hemithorax raised by a gel pad or inflatable bag to open the anterior intercostal spaces while the arm is secured away from the surgical site and pressure points must be carefully padded to avoid tension on the brachial plexus. The latter is performed in the supine position.

As for any anaesthetic, routine care must be taken to ensure that the cervical spine and upper and lower limb joints are in a neutral position and that the eyes and other pressure points are adequately protected.

4.4. TOE

The TOE is used to perform a comprehensive study at the beginning of the case. In particular, the diagnosis and surgical target should be confirmed, and aortic regurgitation excluded or quantified. The diameter of the ascending aorta and aortic root should also be measured if using the endoballoon. The integrity of the interatrial septum should be assessed.

During cannulation for CPB, TOE is used to help guide the position of the cannulae. Venous cannulation is best seen in the bicaval view, and guidance of the cannula position helps to reduce the risk of complications such as malposition in the hepatic vein or interatrial septum perforation. Unless right atriotomy is required during surgery, the tip of the venous drainage cannula should be in the proximal SVC. If there is a need to open the atrium, then the IVC cannula should be positioned at the cavoatrial junction and a separate SVC cannula must be sited.

If an endoballoon is to be used, TOE can be used to guide its position. The tip should be placed in the ascending aorta. As the balloon is inflated the pressure causes an indentation on the aortic wall. The flow of cardioplegia into the aortic root can be seen using TOE and can be followed into the coronary ostia. Lack of regurgitation of cardioplegia into the left ventricle (LV) can also be confirmed. It is important to visualise the LV while cardioplegia is given. Application of the endoballoon can lead to distortion of aortic valve anatomy and subsequent ventricular distention should the valve become incompetent. Venting of the aortic root is also possible using the endoballoon.

Finally, since it is not possible for the anaesthetist or surgeon to easily see the right ventricle—as it is during conventional cardiac surgery—TOE provides information regarding volume status and right ventricular (RV) function. This is particularly useful during the process of separation from CPB.

4.5. Separation from CPB

Separation from CPB is not significantly different to the process that occurs during conventional cardiac surgery. There are several reasons why it may be beneficial to temporarily ventilate using both lungs during weaning from CPB:

1. Two-lung ventilation will allow superior gas exchange; normoxia and the absence of respiratory acidosis will promote better cardiac function;
2. The isolated and collapsed lung presents a higher pulmonary vascular resistance (PVR) to the RV than a normally ventilated lung, while ventilating both lungs is likely to improve right ventricular function by optimising PVR;
3. Ventilation of both lungs will enhance the mobilisation of air collections in the pulmonary veins and aid with deairing the heart. As is the case with conventional cardiac surgery, TOE can be used to guide deairing.

Following successful separation, it is often necessary to isolate the lung again so that surgical haemostasis can be ensured.

4.6. Analgesia

Like conventional cardiac surgery, intraoperative analgesia for MICS relies heavily on opioids, although opioid-sparing and opioid-free approaches have been described [22]. In light of modern approaches such as Enhanced Recovery after Surgery (ERAS), the side effects of opioids and their effect on recovery [23] should be considered and the doses used moderated [24]. Other available modalities of analgesia should also be considered. These include non-opioid pharmacological agents such as ketamine and clonidine and specific local anaesthetic nerve blockade. The latter is particularly useful in MICS and may aid in achieving intra-operative haemodynamic stability. In selected cases, good regional analgesia may allow extubation of patients in the operating room at the end of surgery and therefore lead to a significantly reduced length of stay in intensive care.

Thoracic wall regional nerve blockade can be provided both pre or post-operatively with paravertebral, serratus anterior plane, erector spinae and Pectoralis (PEC) I + II blocks. In some instances, a local anaesthetic can be placed under direct vision by the surgeon (e.g., intercostal nerve blockade) [10]. Analgesia using local anaesthetic can also be provided with continuous infusions, and catheters may be placed using ultrasound guidance (e.g., for paravertebral block [25]) or under direct vision by the surgeon (e.g., intrapleural block [26]).

It is important to consider that in patients with ongoing infusions of local anaesthetic, pain that would otherwise indicate the presence of a significant surgical complication may be masked and therefore a high index of suspicion is required.

5. Post-Operative Management

In selected cases, it may be appropriate to extubate patients who have had MICS before leaving the operating theatre. In most cases, however, admission to a cardiothoracic intensive care unit will be required. If a DLT has been used for OLV during surgery, this should be exchanged for a standard single-lumen tube.

Post-operative monitoring post MICS follows the same principles as following conventional cardiac surgery, with some important caveats. The first is that bleeding may be more concealed in MICS than following full sternotomy, and the development of haemodynamic instability should prompt early investigation to rule out tamponade or the development of other covert haemorrhages. If cannulation for CPB has been performed peripherally, there should be vigilance against haematoma formation and development of peripheral limb ischaemia.

6. Redo Surgery

Minimally invasive approaches to cardiac valve surgery are increasingly being used where reoperation is required as an alternative to resternotomy. Resternotomy carries an increased risk of damage to structures such as patent coronary grafts due to distorted anatomy caused by adhesions and scarring [27]. It is also associated with prolonged CPB and cross-clamp times as well as higher transfusion requirements compared to first-time cardiac surgery. The theoretical appeal of minimally invasive redo surgery is therefore the minimisation of trauma and avoidance of the challenging dissection planes. This needs to be carefully balanced with the concern over suboptimal myocardial protection due to the smaller surgical field and the difficulty of successfully isolating any internal mammary artery grafts during aortic cross-clamping and myocardial ischaemia [28].

Despite these concerns, one meta-analysis comparing minimally invasive redo aortic valve replacement (MIrAVR) with conventional redo surgery has shown no significant difference in mortality, risk of stroke, rates of permanent pacemaker implantation, renal failure, re-operation for bleeding, or length of hospital stay [29]. Perhaps unexpectedly, cross-clamp and CPB times were similar in this study too. Reassuringly, in this review, myocardial protection was achieved without occlusion of the IMA and by utilising deeper hypothermia and there were subsequently no reported post-operative myocardial infarctions.

Two recent meta-analyses comparing MIMVS vs. conventional resternotomy for redo mitral valve surgery showed an improved mortality rate in patients who had a minimally invasive approach rather than resternotomy [30,31]. A recent analysis of patients having mitral surgery after a previous sternotomy in the national Netherlands heart registry showed no difference in thirty-day mortality or five-year survival, although there was a lower incidence of prolonged intubation and new-onset arrhythmia in the minimally invasive group [32]. There have so far been no large randomised controlled trials and therefore these meta-analyses were only able to use retrospective non-randomised data.

7. TAVR

MICS includes many percutaneous cardiac interventions that are less invasive than surgery and can be performed in the cath lab without CPB. The most commonly performed of these is transcatheter aortic valve replacement (TAVR).

TAVR via the transfemoral approach is the most frequently used technique. However, in some patients, other approaches may be utilised, including trans-axillary (TAX) and, less commonly, trans-carotid (TC), trans-apical (TA), and trans-caval (TCV). Factors that are associated with increased vascular complications, and therefore favour a non-femoral approach, include small iliofemoral artery calibre or the presence of vessel aneurysm or severe atheroma, significant arterial wall calcification and degree of tortuosity [33]. TAX is usually the second most preferred approach.

The approach to TAVR is one of the principal factors used to decide on the anaesthetic technique. In a high proportion of cases, transfemoral TAVR may be achieved with local anaesthesia and conscious sedation while other approaches will often require a general anaesthetic.

One important consideration is the proximity of the surgical field to the airway. For this reason alone, TAX and TC approaches are likely to warrant general anaesthesia. The ability of the patient to tolerate the procedure under sedation must also be taken into consideration. Emergent conversion to general anaesthetic can be challenging even for the experienced anaesthetist due to the ergonomics of the cath lab and the physiology of the patient with severe aortic valve disease. If TOE is likely to offer significant advantages over transthoracic echo (which is the mainstay of ultrasound imaging used during TAVR) for a particular patient, general anaesthesia facilitates this.

Routine monitoring for TAVR is not dissimilar to that used for standard cardiac surgery if the procedure is being performed under general anaesthesia. Invasive arterial pressure monitoring is usually established using a left-sided arterial line although the laterality of lines should be discussed, as the cardiologist may need to insert an angiography catheter into a radial artery. In cases where TAVR is being performed under conscious sedation, invasive monitoring may be established by the cardiologist. Central venous pressure monitoring is not commonly used, although central venous access should be available regardless of the anaesthetic technique so that vasoactive medications may be administered if required.

Recognised complications that the anaesthetist should be aware of include those due to poor positioning of the valve that may lead to haemodynamic compromise, such as para-valvular regurgitation (3–4%) [34] or due to occlusion of a coronary ostium (<1%) [35] and myocardial ischaemia [36]. Self-expanding TAVR valves (e.g., Edwards Core-valve) can be captured and redeployed in the event of suboptimal positioning. Patients with a pre-existing poor LV function are particularly susceptible to haemodynamic compromise that may persist beyond valve deployment. Major vascular complications occur in 2–3% [34]. Very rarely, the valve may embolise leading to distal ischaemic consequences. Approximately 9% of patients will require a permanent pacemaker [34], particularly if there is a pre-existing right bundle branch block [37]. Neurological complications such as stroke are a recognised risk of TAVR, occurring in approximately 2% of patients [38]. The BHF PROTECT-TAVI study is a large ongoing randomised controlled trial studying whether the use of cerebral embolic protection (CEP) devices during the procedure will reduce this risk [39].

Transcatheter procedures are significantly less painful than open procedures and often require little more than local infiltration, ultrashort-acting opioids, and paracetamol. An exception to this is the TA TAVR as this relies on a mini-thoracotomy [40]. Paravertebral blocks have been shown to provide effective analgesia for this procedure and at the authors' institution PECS and serratus anterior blockade are routinely utilised to augment general anaesthesia [41].

Post-operative pain can be managed with supplemental oral or IV analgesia. It is prudent to consider the probability of the pain being the first presentation of a hitherto unrecognised occult complication (e.g., tamponade, bleeding, etc.) before prescribing patient-controlled analgesia.

8. Outcomes

The outcomes of MICS compared with conventional cardiac surgery performed via a full median sternotomy have been studied, although in some cases more randomised data are needed. In general, the overall surgical, bypass and cross-clamp times tend to be longer with MICS [42–44]. However, rates of mortality, kidney injury, post-op atrial fibrillation, and stroke are generally not significantly different [42,45–48], while pain scores, patient satisfaction, and ICU length of stay have been reported as improved when compared with conventional surgery [42,43,45,49].

8.1. Mitral Valve

There has been a lack of high-quality randomised trials comparing outcomes of MIMVS with conventional sternotomy for mitral valve surgery (CMVS), especially in the longer term. A recent systematic review and meta-analysis comparing 119 studies showed a reduced requirement for blood transfusion and a shorter length of hospital stay associated with MIMVS compared with CMVS. Some non-randomised retrospective studies suggested a lower mortality associated with MIMVS, but this finding was not supported by randomised prospective trials [50]. Earlier meta-analyses showed similar findings and suggested reduced pain and faster recovery following MIMVS, despite longer cardiopulmonary bypass and cross-clamp times [44,45,51,52].

A recent analysis of the Mini-mitral International Registry separated patients having MIMVS by surgical risk according to their EuroSCORE-II (ESII). Operative results were considered excellent in all categories except those whose ESII was 12% or over. Overall, the observed mortality was found to be lower than expected in all risk groups [53].

8.2. Aortic Valve

A plethora of studies have compared traditional surgical aortic valve replacement (SAVR) with TAVR. A 2019 meta-analysis [54] included seven trials with over 8000 patients comparing TAVR with SAVR for severe aortic stenosis. When transfemoral TAVR was used, a relative reduction in all-cause mortality of 17% was seen up to two years post procedure. Additionally, those undergoing TAVR had a lower risk of stroke, acute kidney injury, major bleeding and new-onset atrial fibrillation when compared with those having a SAVR. These advantages were seen regardless of the type of TAVR used and of the surgical risk cohort.

However, indications for SAVR remain [55]. Patients with bicuspid aortic valves, unfavourable aortic root anatomy, significant subannular calcification or peripheral vascular disease are still thought to be more suited to SAVR than TAVR, as are patients with or post-endocarditis and those who require multiple valve procedures. Questions also remain regarding how appropriate TAVR is for younger patients in whom the durability of the valve replacement is of increased importance.

High-quality studies comparing conventional SAVR with other minimally invasive techniques such as mini-sternotomy or anterior right thoracotomy for aortic valve procedures have generally been lacking and there has been slow surgical uptake of these techniques, being used in only 12% of SAVRs in the UK and the US in the 12 years to 2018 [56]. However, there is some evidence to suggest they carry some advantages. In one meta-analysis including data from 50 studies and more than 12,000 patients, minimally invasive AVR (MIAVR) was associated with reduced requirement for blood transfusion, shorter length of intensive care stay, less pain and lower incidence of renal failure compared with conventional SAVR. On closer analysis, the study demonstrated that these advantages tend to be a feature of the mini-sternotomy but not the mini-thoracotomy approach to AVR. There was no difference in rates of mortality, stroke, respiratory failure, and re-look surgery for bleeding or deep wound infection when compared with conventional SAVR [57]. Similarly, a small study comparing MIAVR with full sternotomy in patients over 80 years of age who required redo aortic valve surgery demonstrated improved survival at 5 and 8 years [27]. A larger subsequent meta-analysis of patients having redo aortic valve surgery could not confirm a difference in in-hospital mortality, but did not have sufficient data to compare outcomes for a longer period of time after surgery [29].

9. Future Directions and Emerging Applications of MICS

Mechanical support is another area of cardiac surgery where a minimally invasive approach is showing increasing promise. A small non-randomised prospective study [58] of patients over 60 years of age with congestive cardiac failure had a left ventricular assist device (LVAD) implanted as destination therapy either using a conventional open surgical technique or using a minimally invasive technique. There was no difference in 2-year survival, but the latter group had a lower incidence of post-op bleeding and lower rates of post-operative extended inotropic support. One hypothesis proposed as an explanation for this latter finding was that the minimally invasive approach allowed LVAD implantation while preserving the majority of the pericardium and therefore maintaining the natural limits of the right ventricle. This avoided over-distension and better safeguarded right ventricular function [58].

10. Conclusions

In summary, MICS is a diverse range of techniques that in many cases are closely aligned with the principles of enhanced recovery. Post-operative pain and recovery times are reduced, which translates into reduced length of intensive care and hospital stay. Patient satisfaction is therefore increased. Success depends upon careful patient selection and an institutional learning curve is to be expected. However, many aspects of these techniques remain to be proven and high-quality randomised trials are still needed to better delineate which approaches offer the best outcomes for patients.

It is essential that anaesthetists are familiar with minimally invasive cardiac surgical techniques, along with the challenges they present and the changes to practice that they demand. Anaesthetists must have the skills to carry out a thorough pre-operative assessment, maintain a high degree of attentiveness and communicate clearly with the surgical team. They must be able to perform high-quality TOE and be prepared to provide multi-modal analgesia. These skills will help to ensure that the best surgical results are obtained while risks are minimised.

Funding: This article received no external funding.

Institutional Review Board Statement: Not applicable.

Informed Consent Statement: Not applicable.

Data Availability Statement: Data sharing not applicable.

Conflicts of Interest: The authors declare no conflict of interest.

References

1. Cosgrove, D.M.; Sabik, J.F., 3rd; Navia, J.L. Minimally invasive valve operations. *Ann. Thorac. Surg.* **1998**, *65*, 1535–1538; discussion 8–9. [CrossRef] [PubMed]
2. Schmitto, J.D.; Mokashi, S.A.; Cohn, L.H. Minimally-invasive valve surgery. *J. Am. Coll. Cardiol.* **2010**, *56*, 455–462. [CrossRef] [PubMed]
3. Di Bacco, L.; Miceli, A.; Glauber, M. Minimally invasive aortic valve surgery. *J. Thorac. Dis.* **2021**, *13*, 1945–1959. [CrossRef] [PubMed]
4. Malik, V.; Jha, A.K.; Kapoor, P.M. Anesthetic challenges in minimally invasive cardiac surgery: Are we moving in a right direction? *Ann. Card. Anaesth.* **2016**, *19*, 489–497. [PubMed]
5. Rosengart, T.K.; Feldman, T.; Borger, M.A.; Vassiliades, T.A., Jr.; Gillinov, A.M.; Hoercher, K.J.; Vahanian, A.; Bonow, R.O.; O'Neill, W. Percutaneous and minimally invasive valve procedures: A scientific statement from the American Heart Association Council on Cardiovascular Surgery and Anesthesia, Council on Clinical Cardiology, Functional Genomics and Translational Biology Interdisciplinary Working Group, and Quality of Care and Outcomes Research Interdisciplinary Working Group. *Circulation* **2008**, *117*, 1750–1767.
6. Parnell, A.; Prince, M. Anaesthesia for minimally invasive cardiac surgery. *BJA Educ.* **2018**, *18*, 323–330. [CrossRef]
7. Iyigun, T.; Kaya, M.; Gulbeyaz, S.O.; Fistikci, N.; Uyanik, G.; Yilmaz, B.; Onan, B.; Erkanli, K. Patient body image, self-esteem, and cosmetic results of minimally invasive robotic cardiac surgery. *Int. J. Surg.* **2017**, *39*, 88–94. [CrossRef]
8. Klein, P.; Klop, I.D.G.; Kloppenburg, G.L.T.; van Putte, B.P. Planning for minimally invasive aortic valve replacement: Key steps for patient assessment. *Eur. J. Cardio-Thorac. Surg.* **2018**, *53* (Suppl. S2), ii3–ii8. [CrossRef]
9. Zaky, A.; Meers, B. Anesthetic Management for Minimally Invasive Cardiac Surgery. In *Cardiac Anesthesia: The Basics of Evaluation and Management*; Awad, A.S., Ed.; Springer International Publishing: Cham, Switzerland, 2021; pp. 405–417.
10. White, A.; Patvardhan, C.; Falter, F. Anesthesia for minimally invasive cardiac surgery. *J. Thorac. Dis.* **2021**, *13*, 1886–1898. [CrossRef]
11. Keogh, B.F.; Alexander, D. Preoperative assessment for thoracic surgery. *Anaesth. Intensive Care Med.* **2015**, *16*, 59–62. [CrossRef]

12. Santana, O.; Reyna, J.; Benjo, A.M.; Lamas, G.A.; Lamelas, J. Outcomes of minimally invasive valve surgery in patients with chronic obstructive pulmonary disease. *Eur. J. Cardio-Thorac. Surg.* **2012**, *42*, 648–652. [CrossRef]
13. Ross, A.F.; Ueda, K. Pulmonary hypertension in thoracic surgical patients. *Curr. Opin. Anaesthesiol.* **2010**, *23*, 25–33. [CrossRef] [PubMed]
14. Aybek, T.; Doss, M.; Abdel-Rahman, U.; Simon, A.; Miskovic, A.; Risteski, P.S.; Dogan, S.; Moritz, A. Echocardiographic assessment in minimally invasive mitral valve surgery. *Med. Sci. Monit.* **2005**, *11*, MT27–MT32. [PubMed]
15. Ailawadi, G.; Agnihotri, A.K.; Mehall, J.R.; Wolfe, J.A.; Hummel, B.W.; Fayers, T.M.; Farivar, R.S.; Grossi, E.A.; Guy, T.S.; Hargrove, W.C.; et al. Minimally Invasive Mitral Valve Surgery I: Patient Selection, Evaluation, and Planning. *Innovations* **2016**, *11*, 243–250.
16. Gammie, J.S.; Zhao, Y.; Peterson, E.D.; O'Brien, S.M.; Rankin, J.S.; Griffith, B.P.; Maxwell, J. Chamberlain Memorial Paper for adult cardiac surgery. Less-invasive mitral valve operations: Trends and outcomes from the Society of Thoracic Surgeons Adult Cardiac Surgery Database. *Ann. Thorac. Surg.* **2010**, *90*, 1401–1410.e1; discussion 8–10. [CrossRef]
17. Mazine, A.; Pellerin, M.; Lebon, J.S.; Dionne, P.O.; Jeanmart, H.; Bouchard, D. Minimally invasive mitral valve surgery: Influence of aortic clamping technique on early outcomes. *Ann. Thorac. Surg.* **2013**, *96*, 2116–2122. [CrossRef] [PubMed]
18. Khan, H.; Hadjittofi, C.; Uzzaman, M.; Salhiyyah, K.; Garg, S.; Butt, S.; Aya, H.; Chaubey, S. External aortic clamping versus endoaortic balloon occlusion in minimally invasive cardiac surgery: A systematic review and meta-analysis. *Interact. Cardiovasc. Thorac. Surg.* **2018**, *27*, 208–214. [CrossRef]
19. Rival, P.M.; Moore, T.H.M.; McAleenan, A.; Hamilton, H.; Du Toit, Z.; Akowuah, E.; Angelini, G.D.; Vohra, H.A. Transthoracic clamp versus endoaortic balloon occlusion in minimally invasive mitral valve surgery: A systematic review and meta-analysis. *Eur. J. Cardio-Thorac. Surg.* **2019**, *56*, 643–653. [CrossRef]
20. Kanda, H.; Kunisawa, T.; Kitahara, H.; Iida, T.; Toyama, Y.; Kanao-Kanda, M.; Mori, C.; Kamiya, H. Cerebral Hypoxia Caused by Flow Confliction During Minimally Invasive Cardiac Surgery with Retrograde Perfusion: A Word of Caution. *J. Cardiothorac. Vasc. Anesth.* **2018**, *32*, 1838–1840. [CrossRef]
21. Wolfe, J.A.; Malaisrie, S.C.; Farivar, R.S.; Khan, J.H.; Hargrove, W.C.; Moront, M.G.; Ryan, W.H.; Ailawadi, G.; Agnihotri, A.K.; Hummel, B.W.; et al. Minimally Invasive Mitral Valve Surgery II: Surgical Technique and Postoperative Management. *Innovations* **2016**, *11*, 251–259.
22. Lavand'homme, P.; Steyaert, A. Opioid-free anesthesia opioid side effects: Tolerance and hyperalgesia. *Best. Pract. Res. Clin. Anaesthesiol.* **2017**, *31*, 487–498. [CrossRef] [PubMed]
23. Forget, P. Opioid-free anaesthesia. Why and how? A contextual analysis. *Anaesth. Crit. Care Pain. Med.* **2019**, *38*, 169–172. [CrossRef] [PubMed]
24. Rong, L.Q.; Kamel, M.K.; Rahouma, M.; Naik, A.; Mehta, K.; Abouarab, A.A.; Di Franco, A.; Demetres, M.; Mustapich, T.L.; Fitzgerald, M.M.; et al. High-dose versus low-dose opioid anesthesia in adult cardiac surgery: A meta-analysis. *J. Clin. Anesth.* **2019**, *57*, 57–62. [CrossRef] [PubMed]
25. Yu, S.; Valencia, M.B.; Roques, V.; Aljure, O.D. Regional analgesia for minimally invasive cardiac surgery. *J. Card. Surg.* **2019**, *34*, 1289–1296. [CrossRef]
26. Mehta, Y.; Swaminathan, M.; Mishra, Y.; Trehan, N. A comparative evaluation of intrapleural and thoracic epidural analgesia for postoperative pain relief after minimally invasive direct coronary artery bypass surgery. *J. Cardiothorac. Vasc. Anesth.* **1998**, *12*, 162–165. [CrossRef]
27. Kaneko, T.; Loberman, D.; Gosev, I.; Rassam, F.; McGurk, S.; Leacche, M.; Cohn, L. Reoperative aortic valve replacement in the octogenarians-minimally invasive technique in the era of transcatheter valve replacement. *J. Thorac. Cardiovasc. Surg.* **2014**, *147*, 155–162. [CrossRef]
28. Kaneko, T.; Nauta, F.; Borstlap, W.; McGurk, S.; Rawn, J.D.; Cohn, L.H. The "no-dissection" technique is safe for reoperative aortic valve replacement with a patent left internal thoracic artery graft. *J. Thorac. Cardiovasc. Surg.* **2012**, *144*, 1036–1040. [CrossRef]
29. Phan, K.; Zhou, J.J.; Niranjan, N.; Di Eusanio, M.; Yan, T.D. Minimally invasive reoperative aortic valve replacement: A systematic review and meta-analysis. *Ann. Cardiothorac. Surg.* **2015**, *4*, 15–25. [CrossRef]
30. Hanafy, D.A.; Melisa, S.; Andrianto, G.A.; Suwatri, W.T.; Sugisman. Outcomes of minimally invasive versus conventional sternotomy for redo mitral valve surgery according to Mitral Valve Academic Research Consortium: A systematic review and meta-analysis. *Asian J. Surg.* **2023**, *in press*. [CrossRef]
31. Hussain, A.; Chacko, J.; Uzzaman, M.; Hamid, O.; Butt, S.; Zakai, S.B.; Khan, H. Minimally invasive (mini-thoracotomy) versus median sternotomy in redo mitral valve surgery: A meta-analysis of observational studies. *Asian Cardiovasc. Thorac. Ann.* **2021**, *29*, 893–902. [CrossRef]
32. Olsthoorn, J.R.; Heuts, S.; Houterman, S.; Maessen, J.G.; Sardari Nia, P.; Cardiothoracic Surgery Registration Committee of the Netherlands Heart Registration. Minimally invasive approach compared to resternotomy for mitral valve surgery in patients with prior cardiac surgery: Retrospective multicentre study based on the Netherlands Heart Registration. *Eur. J. Cardio-Thorac. Surg.* **2022**, *62*, ezac420. [CrossRef] [PubMed]
33. Steinvil, A.; Leshem-Rubinow, E.; Halkin, A.; Abramowitz, Y.; Ben-Assa, E.; Shacham, Y.; Bar-Dayan, A.; Keren, G.; Banai, S.; Finkelstein, A. Vascular complications after transcatheter aortic valve implantation and their association with mortality reevaluated by the valve academic research consortium definitions. *Am. J. Cardiol.* **2015**, *115*, 100–106. [CrossRef] [PubMed]
34. Ludman, P.F. UK TAVI registry. *Heart* **2019**, *105* (Suppl. S2), s2–s5. [CrossRef] [PubMed]

35. Ribeiro, H.B.; Webb, J.G.; Makkar, R.R.; Cohen, M.G.; Kapadia, S.R.; Kodali, S.; Tamburino, C.; Barbanti, M.; Chakravarty, T.; Jilaihawi, H.; et al. Predictive factors, management, and clinical outcomes of coronary obstruction following transcatheter aortic valve implantation: Insights from a large multicenter registry. *J. Am. Coll. Cardiol.* **2013**, *62*, 1552–1562. [CrossRef]
36. Genereux, P.; Head, S.J.; Van Mieghem, N.M.; Kodali, S.; Kirtane, A.J.; Xu, K.; Smith, C.; Serruys, P.W.; Kappetein, A.P.; Leon, M.B. Clinical outcomes after transcatheter aortic valve replacement using valve academic research consortium definitions: A weighted meta-analysis of 3,519 patients from 16 studies. *J. Am. Coll. Cardiol.* **2012**, *59*, 2317–2326. [CrossRef]
37. Chacko, M.; Weinberg, L. Aortic valve stenosis: Perioperative anaesthetic implications of surgical replacement and minimally invasive interventions. *BJA* **2012**, *12*, 295–301. [CrossRef]
38. Myat, A.; Buckner, L.; Mouy, F.; Cockburn, J.; Baumbach, A.; Banning, A.P.; Blackman, D.J.; Curzen, N.; MacCarthy, P.; Mullen, M.; et al. In-hospital stroke after transcatheter aortic valve implantation: A UK observational cohort analysis. *Catheter. Cardiovasc. Interv.* **2021**, *97*, E552–E559. [CrossRef]
39. Kharbanda, R.K.; Perkins, A.D.; Kennedy, J.; Banning, A.P.; Baumbach, A.; Blackman, D.J.; Dodd, M.; Evans, R.; Hildick-Smith, D.; Jamal, Z.; et al. Routine cerebral embolic protection in transcatheter aortic valve implantation: Rationale and design of the randomised British Heart Foundation PROTECT-TAVI trial. *EuroIntervention* **2023**, *18*, 1428–1435. [CrossRef]
40. Mittnacht, A.J.C.; Shariat, A.; Weiner, M.M.; Malhotra, A.; Miller, M.A.; Mahajan, A.; Bhatt, H.V. Regional Techniques for Cardiac and Cardiac-Related Procedures. *J. Cardiothorac. Vasc. Anesth.* **2019**, *33*, 532–546. [CrossRef]
41. Berthoud, V.; Ellouze, O.; Bievre, T.; Konstantinou, M.; Jazayeri, S.; Bouchot, O.; Girard, C.; Bouhemad, B. Serratus Anterior Plane Block for Apical TAVR in an Awake Patient. *J. Cardiothorac. Vasc. Anesth.* **2018**, *32*, 2275–2277. [CrossRef]
42. Cao, C.; Gupta, S.; Chandrakumar, D.; Nienaber, T.A.; Indraratna, P.; Ang, S.C.; Phan, K.; Yan, T.D. A meta-analysis of minimally invasive versus conventional mitral valve repair for patients with degenerative mitral disease. *Ann. Cardiothorac. Surg.* **2013**, *2*, 693–703. [PubMed]
43. Nair, S.K.; Sudarshan, C.D.; Thorpe, B.S.; Singh, J.; Pillay, T.; Catarino, P.; Valchanov, K.; Codispoti, M.; Dunning, J.; Abu-Omar, Y.; et al. Mini-Stern Trial: A randomized trial comparing mini-sternotomy to full median sternotomy for aortic valve replacement. *J. Thorac. Cardiovasc. Surg.* **2018**, *156*, 2124–2132.e31. [CrossRef] [PubMed]
44. Moscarelli, M.; Fattouch, K.; Casula, R.; Speziale, G.; Lancellotti, P.; Athanasiou, T. What Is the Role of Minimally Invasive Mitral Valve Surgery in High-Risk Patients? A Meta-Analysis of Observational Studies. *Ann. Thorac. Surg.* **2016**, *101*, 981–989. [CrossRef] [PubMed]
45. Modi, P.; Hassan, A.; Chitwood, W.R., Jr. Minimally invasive mitral valve surgery: A systematic review and meta-analysis. *Eur. J. Cardio-Thorac. Surg.* **2008**, *34*, 943–952. [CrossRef]
46. Galloway, A.C.; Schwartz, C.F.; Ribakove, G.H.; Crooke, G.A.; Gogoladze, G.; Ursomanno, P.; Mirabella, M.; Culliford, A.T.; Grossi, E.A. A decade of minimally invasive mitral repair: Long-term outcomes. *Ann. Thorac. Surg.* **2009**, *88*, 1180–1184. [CrossRef]
47. Mohr, F.W.; Falk, V.; Diegeler, A.; Walther, T.; Gummert, J.F.; Bucerius, J.; Jacobs, S.; Autschbach, R. Computer-enhanced "robotic" cardiac surgery: Experience in 148 patients. *J. Thorac. Cardiovasc. Surg.* **2001**, *121*, 842–853. [CrossRef]
48. Suri, R.M.; Taggarse, A.; Burkhart, H.M.; Daly, R.C.; Mauermann, W.; Nishimura, R.A.; Li, Z.; Dearani, J.A.; Michelena, H.I.; Enriquez-Sarano, M. Robotic Mitral Valve Repair for Simple and Complex Degenerative Disease: Midterm Clinical and Echocardiographic Quality Outcomes. *Circulation* **2015**, *132*, 1961–1968. [CrossRef]
49. Kirmani, B.H.; Jones, S.G.; Malaisrie, S.C.; Chung, D.A.; Williams, R.J. Limited versus full sternotomy for aortic valve replacement. *Cochrane Database Syst. Rev.* **2017**, *4*, CD011793. [CrossRef] [PubMed]
50. Eqbal, A.J.; Gupta, S.; Basha, A.; Qiu, Y.; Wu, N.; Rega, F.; Chu, F.V.; Belley-Cote, E.P.; Whitlock, R.P. Minimally invasive mitral valve surgery versus conventional sternotomy mitral valve surgery: A systematic review and meta-analysis of 119 studies. *J. Card. Surg.* **2022**, *37*, 1319–1327. [CrossRef]
51. Sa, M.; Van den Eynde, J.; Cavalcanti, L.R.P.; Kadyraliev, B.; Enginoev, S.; Zhigalov, K.; Ruhparwar, A.; Weymann, A.; Dreyfus, G. Mitral valve repair with minimally invasive approaches vs sternotomy: A meta-analysis of early and late results in randomized and matched observational studies. *J. Card. Surg.* **2020**, *35*, 2307–2323. [CrossRef]
52. Hage, A.; Hage, F.; Al-Amodi, H.; Gupta, S.; Papatheodorou, S.I.; Hawkins, R.; Ailawadi, G.; Mittleman, M.A.; Chu, M.W.A. Minimally Invasive Versus Sternotomy for Mitral Surgery in the Elderly: A Systematic Review and Meta-Analysis. *Innovations* **2021**, *16*, 310–316. [CrossRef] [PubMed]
53. Berretta, P.; Kempfert, J.; Van Praet, F.; Salvador, L.; Lamelas, J.; Nguyen, T.C.; Wilbring, M.; Gerdisch, M.; Rinaldi, M.; Bonaros, N.; et al. Risk-related clinical outcomes after minimally invasive mitral valve surgery: Insights from the Mini-Mitral International Registry. *Eur. J. Cardio-Thorac. Surg.* **2023**, *63*, ezad090. [CrossRef] [PubMed]
54. Siontis, G.C.M.; Overtchouk, P.; Cahill, T.J.; Modine, T.; Prendergast, B.; Praz, F.; Pilgrim, T.; Petrinic, T.; Nikolakopoulou, A.; Salanti, G.; et al. Transcatheter aortic valve implantation vs. surgical aortic valve replacement for treatment of symptomatic severe aortic stenosis: An updated meta-analysis. *Eur. Heart J.* **2019**, *40*, 3143–3153. [CrossRef] [PubMed]
55. Webb, J.G.; Landes, U. The final meta-analysis? *Eur. Heart J.* **2019**, *40*, 3154–3155. [CrossRef] [PubMed]
56. Young, C.P.; Sinha, S.; Vohra, H.A. Outcomes of minimally invasive aortic valve replacement surgery. *Eur. J. Cardio-Thorac. Surg.* **2018**, *53* (Suppl. S2), ii19–ii23. [CrossRef]

57. Phan, K.; Xie, A.; Di Eusanio, M.; Yan, T.D. A meta-analysis of minimally invasive versus conventional sternotomy for aortic valve replacement. *Ann. Thorac. Surg.* **2014**, *98*, 1499–1511. [CrossRef]
58. Rojas, S.V.; Hanke, J.S.; Avsar, M.; Ahrens, P.R.; Deutschmann, O.; Tumler, K.A.; Uribarri, A.; Rojas-Hernandez, S.; Sanchez, P.L.; Gonzalez-Santos, J.M.; et al. Left Ventricular Assist Device Therapy for Destination Therapy: Is Less Invasive Surgery a Safe Alternative? *Rev. Esp. Cardiol.* **2018**, *71*, 13–17. [CrossRef]

Journal of
Cardiovascular
Development and Disease

MDPI

Opinion

Reduced Invasiveness of Cardiopulmonary Bypass: The Mini-Circuit and the Micro-Cardioplegia

Thierry Carrel [1,2]

[1] Departement of Cardiac Surgery, University of Zürich, CH-8006 Zürich, Switzerland; thierry.carrel@gmail.com
[2] Department of Cardiac Surgery, University Hospital Basel, CH-4052 Basel, Switzerland

Abstract: The aim of cardiopulmonary bypass is the maintenance of a sufficient whole body perfusion and gas exchange during open or closed heart surgery procedure (coronary artery bypass grafting, valve repair and replacement, surgical intervention on the ascending aorta and/or aortic arch, repair of congenital malformations, and finally implantation of ventricular assist devices or cardiac transplantation). The main components of cardiopulmonary bypass are the pump that supplies the circulation and the oxygenator that regulates gas exchange. However, even though this technology has been extensively developed and improved over the last decades, one of the major drawbacks—which is the fact that blood has to flow through tubing systems with foreign surfaces—persists so far. Nevertheless, interesting innovations have been made more recently in order to better control the side-effects that culminate into a major activation of the coagulation and inflammatory systems: among them, miniaturization of the circuits, together with reduction of the priming volume and a simplified cardioplegia concept. All of these lead to a significant decrease of hemodilution and thereby a significant reduction of volume overload during surgery. In this brief review we will present some of these most interesting topics around minimized circuits and the simplified low-volume cardioplegia and discuss their potential benefits on the clinical outcome.

Keywords: cardiopulmonary bypass; minimal invasive; cardioplegia; systemic inflammation

1. Introduction

Cardiopulmonary bypass (CPB) support is required when the heart has to be empty for an intracardiac repair, when a mechanical arrest is required or when manipulations on the heart (luxation) need support for the systemic circulation. Another condition is the case where moderate or deep hypothermia is necessary to allow circulatory arrest, for instance when the aortic arch has to be repaired and complex congenital surgeries performed. Although it has been introduced in the late fifties and further developed in the sixties and seventies to repair congenital heart diseases, to bypass coronary arteries, to repair or replace heart valves, to treat aortic pathologies and last but not least to transplant hearts, CPB technology did not receive too much attention to reduce unintended adverse effects, often referred to as the postperfusion syndrome, or the whole body inflammatory response. These adverse effects may result in different degrees of organ dysfunction and therefore in the need for prolonged intensive care treatment and longer hospital stay.

To allow work on or into the heart, deoxygenated blood is drained into an extracorporeal reservoir, usually made of compressible polyvinyl bags or hard-shell plastic, which results in blood-air interface. Once it enters into the extracorporeal bypass circuit, the blood encounters a number of abnormal elements, like air bubbles, fibrin, tissue debris, platelets thrombi and defoaming agents. From the reservoir, the blood is directed to the oxygenator and runs thereafter into a heat exchanger that regulates the blood temperature into the circuit (and therefore also in the body). Finally, the blood is filtered through nylon or polyester screens and pumped back into the patient at a controlled flow rate either by a roller pump or a centrifugal impeller.

2. From Conventional to Miniaturized Cardiopulmonary Bypass Circuits

Two of the major innovations in CPB technology were the introduction of membrane instead of bubble oxygenators and later the use of centrifugal instead of roller pumps. In the nineties, off-pump coronary artery bypass grafting was promoted in order to avoid some of the side effects of extracorporeal circulation (ECC) and to become more competitive with the rising number of percutaneous coronary procedures. At this time only a small number of multidisciplinary teams, including surgeons, anesthesiologists and perfusionists performed "off-pump" coronary artery bypass grafting (CABG) and slightly thereafter other teams started to develop what was called a minimally invasive CPB system [1,2]. The initial concept was based on a closed-loop perfusion circuit with a non-occlusive pump. These systems have considerably developed since then and the first clinical observations were encouraging, in terms of favorable overall morbidity and reduced mortality but also because of the clinical benefits due to less microcirculatory alterations because of improved microcirculation, reduced hemodilution, better preservation of the immune reactions and less coagulation disorders [3–6].

These advances in surgical technique and in CPB technology have allowed to minimize the invasiveness of surgery and—together with improved perioperative care—made it acceptable for high-risk and aging patients, suffering often from multiple and/or severe comorbidities.

Additional technical innovations in the field of the ECC included the better biocompatibility of CPB circuits, for instance by heparin coating of the tubing systems and by reduction of the amount of foreign surfaces (shorter tubes, elimination of unnecessary components). These options helped to reduce the adverse effects generated by the plasma protein defense system and the cellular-based cytokine-mediated responses. Thereby they significantly contribute to improve clinical results.

3. Definition and Potential Benefits a Minimally Invasive Perfusion Systems

In the 1990'ies, discussion emerged about the potentials for reduction of the side-effects caused by ECC and the possibility to perfuse with a reduced equipment partially because off-pump surgery could not convince the entire cardiosurgical community. These discussions constituted a boost for what is called nowadays miniaturized extracorporeal systems. Nevertheless, it was rapidly shown that a miniaturized circuit is not only a reduced size system but a completely new concept of ECC. The overall goal is a constant volume perfusion with minimized blood trauma, reduced hemodilution and therefore less inflammatory response; in addition, lower transfusion requirements and accelerated early postoperative recovery are targeted.

The original miniaturized CPB systems were simplified heart-lung machines where the venous reservoir and the suckers were left off and the tubing system was significantly shortened. Heparin-coating of the tubing and the compounds is optional. A separate heat exchanger is futile since it is incorporated in the oxygenator.

Nowadays a true minimally invasive extracorporeal perfusion system consists of a closed CPB circuit that can be transformed immediately in an open circuit in case of unexpected event (massive bleeding requiring rapid re-transfusion as an example): this type of system includes as a minimal option a centrifugal pump and a membrane oxygenator. Therefore, the priming volume is significantly reduced to 300–500 mL. All other components are optional: the heat exchanger, an additional pump for cardioplegia, a venous bubble trap/venous air removing device and finally a shed blood management system. Depending on the adopted strategy, the inclusion or not of such compounds may differ from system to system [7,8].

One of the most interesting observation made when using a minimal invasive CPB circuit is the beneficial effects on the activation of the inflammatory cascade, both directly (through a blunting of the contact-phase activation) and indirectly (through a limited thrombin generation, platelet activation, and consequent lower release of pro-inflammatory cytokines). From the clinical point of view, we have observed a considerably lower rate of postoperative atrial fibrillation and need for blood transfusion while the incidence of pulmonary and renal complications was significantly decreased when a minimal invasive CPB system was used [9].

Another interesting aspect of minimally invasive CPB is its influence on the microcirculation, especially when some remnants of pulsatility (through a roller pump) are lost in favor of non-pulsatile perfusion as observed when a centrifugal pump is used in such systems. Near infrared reflectance spectroscopy (NIRS) and sublingual microscopy may be used to explore alterations in microcirculation. There is some evidence that microcirculation remains more physiological during perfusion through a minimal invasive CPB system [3,10].

In addition to all mechanical methods of reducing CPB-induced inflammation, several pharmacological approaches have been tested, including steroids, aprotinin, anticomplement strategies as well as other options to better control endothelial cell activation [11].

The main indication for miniaturized CPB system was originally coronary artery bypass grafting, where the cardiac cavities remain closed. With increasing experience, valve repair and replacement, excision of right and left atrial myxoma and simple ascending aortic replacement could be performed but required additional refinements, like introduction of a pulmonary vent that is connected to the venous return line and a smart sucker that enters in function only through an infrared light signal, which activates vacuum only once the tip enters in contact with blood in the operative field. This allows to reduce the blood-air contact even in a semi-open system [12,13].

4. Application in Pediatric and More Complex Adult Surgery

Based on the improved perioperative outcomes observed in adult cardiac patients, minimal invasive perfusion appears particularly attractive for smaller patients (pediatric cardiac surgery), since this particular group may significantly suffer from hemodilution.

Our initial experience with a pilot group of 38 patients in 2017–2018 using a type I circuit for closed and a type III perfusion circuits for open heart procedures was very encouraging [14]. Minimal invasive perfusion was successfully performed in all patients without technical complications nor any need for conversion. No cardiac nor neurological complication did occur in this group of patients.

Despite a clear evidence of clinical advantages in coronary surgery, the use of such systems for more complex open-heart procedures remains low [15–17]. Some concerns have been raised by surgeons and perfusionists regarding safety of perfusion in situations when the heart is opened and air may enter the closed system. Moreover, issues of blood and volume management have been found by some as not really practicable without having a reservoir. In the evolution of minimal invasive CPB technologies, safety aspects concerning air and volume management have been addressed by the integration of active air removal devices, and the possibility of venting and volume buffering. This has made the minimal invasive circuits suitable for valvular or even more complex aortic surgery. However, typical clinical benefits found in coronary artery bypass grafting surgery, in particular blood sparing effects, were not always reproducible. With the introduction of modular (type IV) minimally invasive systems containing a second, accessory circuit for immediate conversion to open cardiopulmonary bypass, the last obstacles have been cleared [8,18,19].

5. Different Types of Minimally Invasive Circuits

Over time, different types of minimally invasive cardiopulmonary circuits have been developed and are usually classified into 4 types, mainly depending from the components they include (Figure 1) [8,19].

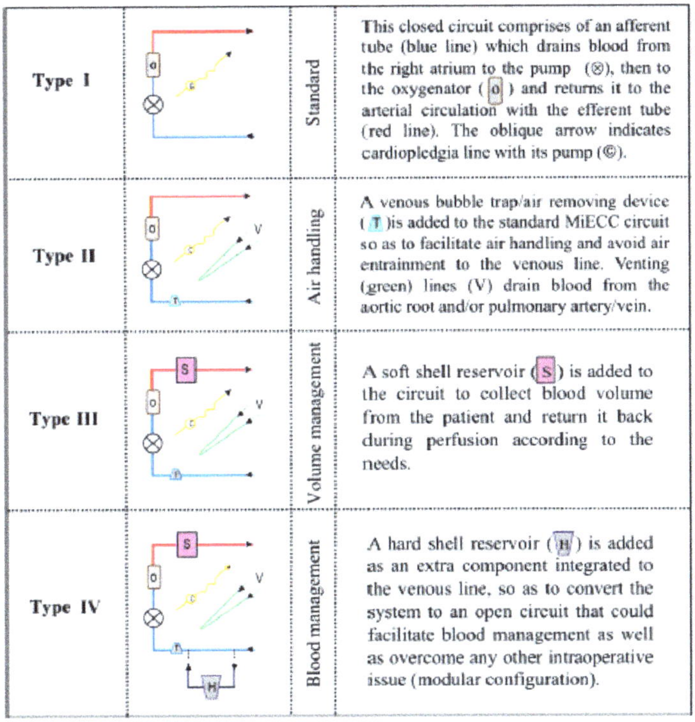

Figure 1. Different types of minimally invasive extracorporeal circulation systems (reproduced with permission from ref. [8]).

Type I is the simplest one and consists of a closed circuit, which includes the oxygenator and the pump. There is no open venous reservoir. All components are coated with heparin and the tubing system is significantly reduced in length. This type of circuit is nowadays not frequently used but represents an ideal concept for patients requiring extracorporeal life support (ECLS) and for isolated coronary bypass grafting procedure. The absence of a venous bubble trap and venting lines in the original MECC system from Maquet® (Rastatt, Germany) and the fact that removal or re-transfusion of shed blood is only possible with an external cardiotomy sucker is considered by some as a drawback of such a simplified system (Figure 2).

The latter constitutes the main difference between type I and type II, since type II includes a venous bubble trap or a venous air removing device (for instance the Resting Heart System® from Medtronic, Minneapolis, MN, USA). With the help of ultrasound detectors, air bubbles can be recognized and automatically removed, which makes the system much safer. If necessary, a left ventricular vent can be integrated but this makes the system semi-closed. Finally shed blood can be separated and processed. In such closed circuits no shift of volume between the patient and the system is possible while the patient's own venous capacitance serves as a volume compensation system. This means that positioning of the patient (Trendelenburg or anti-Trendelenburg) is the most efficient method to shift volume within the patient. The characteristics of type I and II circuits allow a reduction of the priming volume of between 400 and 650 mL. Anticoagulation is monitored using the activated clotting time, with a targeted value around 300–400 s. Initial heparin administration consists of 150 IE/kg.

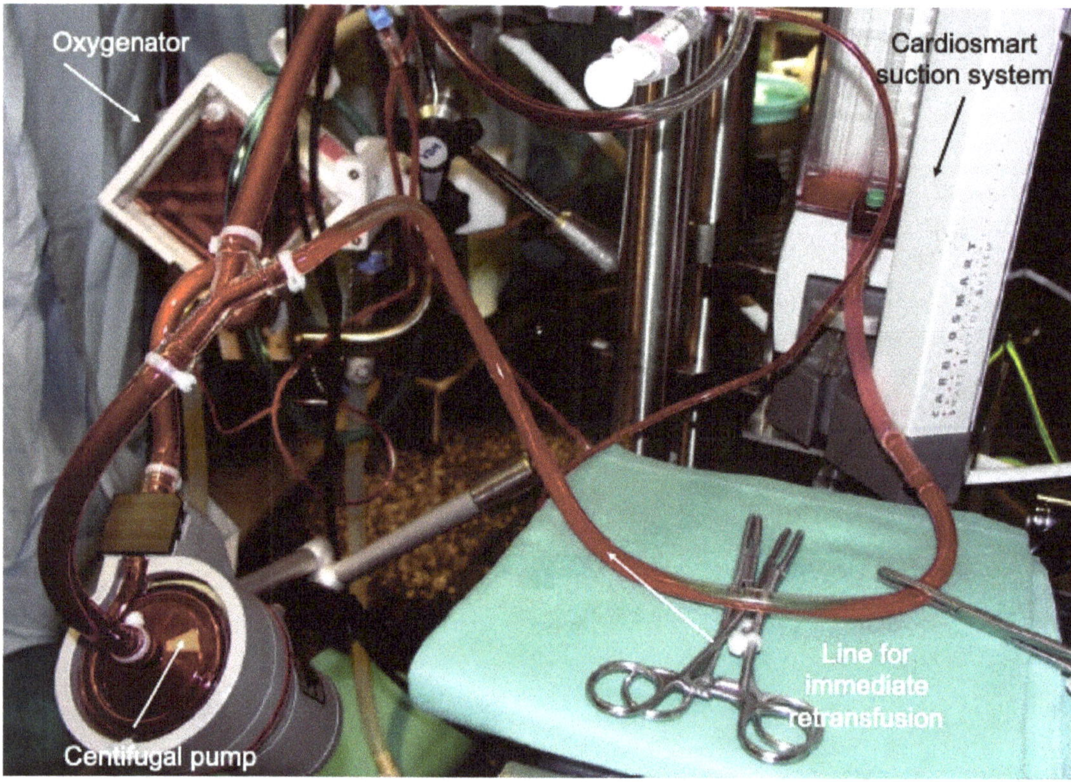

Figure 2. Type I mini-ECC system, including a centrifugal pump and the oxygenator. Integrated vacuum suction system (Cardiosmart©) (on the right) allowing a maintenance of a constant volume and whole blood transfusion in case of bleeding. Air removal through active handling.

During a true open-heart procedure like valve surgery, left ventricular venting is usually required as blood-air interaction is usual. The main additional characteristic of a type III (Figure 3) circuit is the ability to control volume shifts and variations more efficiently. This is achieved through the inclusion of a volume collection bag into the circuit and a bubble trap. In addition, one or more of the following components are usually included: a pulmonary artery vent, an aortic root vent or a left ventricular venting. This helps to operate in a blood free surgical field.

The main advantage of a pulmonary artery vent is the possibility to connect it directly with the venous return line. With this, the vent is directly dependent on the negative pressure of the centrifugal pump. However, this is also the limiting factor for vent performance. However, the speed of the centrifugal pumps has to be adjusted to the venous return, otherwise venous vascular collapse may happen and lead to unstable perfusion. In addition, the pulmonary artery vent is not a true left ventricular vent and thereby cannot properly de-air the left heart cavities during reperfusion. Immediate re-transfusion of the volume drained by pulmonary artery vent into the circuit without blood-air contact is one of the major advantages of type III. When a left ventricular vent is introduced, the drainage of the left heart cavities will be more effective but this happens with the loss of one of the major advantages of a true minimally invasive circuit, namely, the avoidance of blood-air contact. Consequently, the shed blood collected by the left ventricular vent cannot be drained directly into the circuit without the risk of risking air trapping into the system. This can be avoided by using a venous bubble trap which is introduced in the line to the soft bag reservoir for direct blood re-transfusion. Another option might be the direct but manually cross-clamped connection to a hard-shell reservoir where the volume can be intermittently re-transfused into the circuit by manual de-clamping the connection line [19].

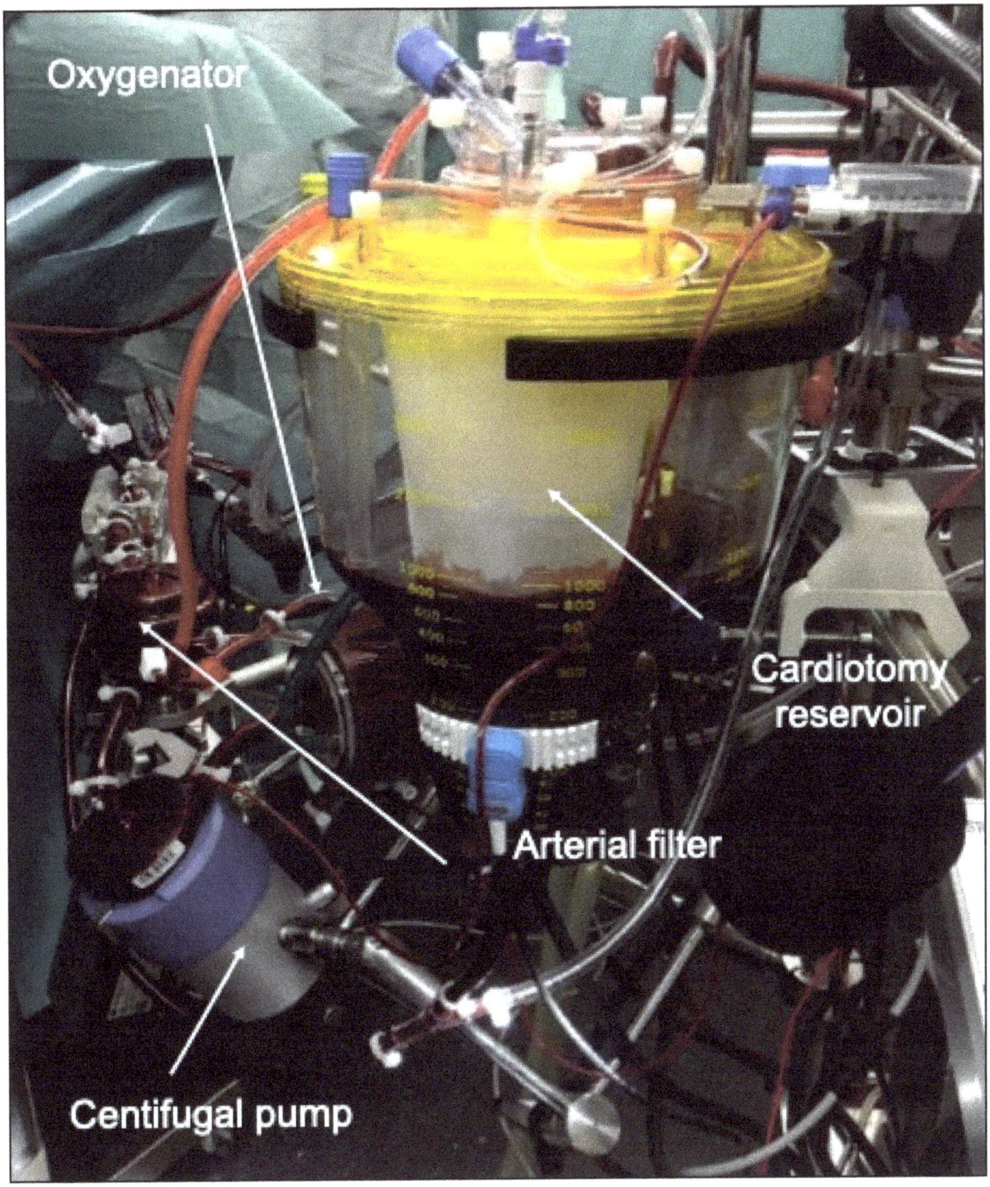

Figure 3. Type III mini-ECC system with a priming volume of 700 mL (not completely closed system with remaining blood/air contact).

Type IV is the most versatile type that is still considered by some as a minimized circuit; the major advantage is the possibility to convert it very instantaneously in a fully conventional CPB circuit in case of any technical trouble (for instance massive bleeding and need for immediate major re-transfusion). Critically thinking, the types III and IV diverge somewhat from the original "reductionistic" concept of what a minimally invasive cardiopulmonary circuit should be. On the other side, most recent developments in the field of ECC have led to the construction of minimized conventional circuits that also allow a significant reduction of the foreign surfaces and a minimization of the priming volume of the circuit (Figure 4).

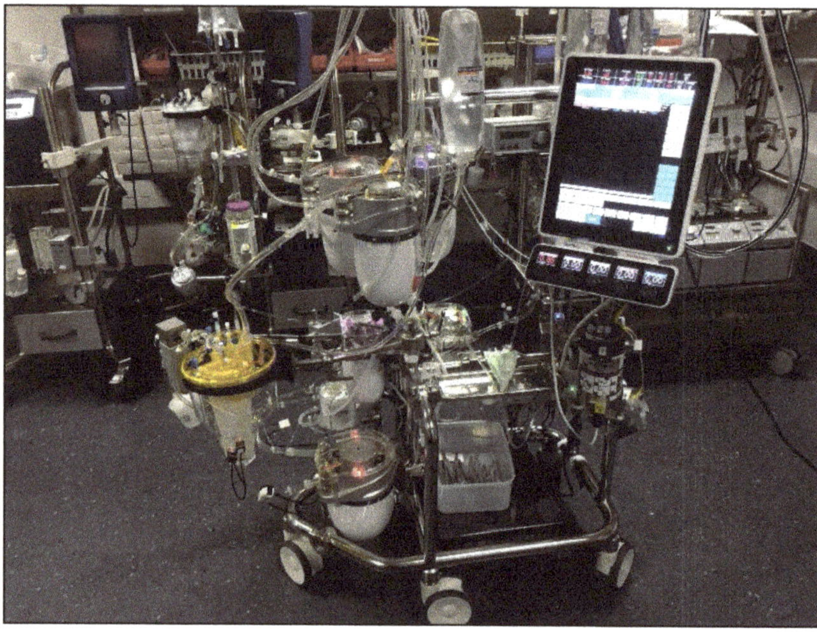

Figure 4. The most modern conventional ECC system with compact arrangements of all compounds.

A specific aspect of the use of minimally invasive CPB systems is the need for more intensive communication that is required between the perfusionist, the cardiac surgeon and the anesthesiologist. Since the tubing system is significantly shortened, the console of the CPB has to be placed much closer to the operating table.

6. Micro-Cardioplegia

One of the most interesting aspects when performing cardiac procedures using a minimal invasive perfusion system is the administration of cardioplegia. Basically, the aim of myocardial protection is to create conditions that permit a cardiac surgery procedure while myocardial integrity and function are preserved. This goal is realized by lowering the metabolic rate during cardiac arrest, creating a favorable milieu that may provide safety during arrest and finally by a controlled reperfusion to decrease structural and/or functional damage. Over the years, a multitude of strategies for myocardial protection has been used, both with crystalloid or blood cardioplegia. In addition, the technique of delivery (antegrade or retrograde) and the amount of administered volume varies considerably. Because no superiority of either delivery technique could be proven, cardioplegia administration is far from being standardized among institutions.

In patients operated with a miniaturized CPB system, there is usually no additional pump for cardioplegia. Therefore, the majority of teams have used a conventional crystalloid cardioplegia (Bretschneider, St-Thomas or Del Nido) but this usually means that 1 to 2 L of volume are infused following aortic cross-clamping. Therefore, some advantages of the mini-circuits to decreased hemodilution are lost during cardioplegia application [20–22].

Alternatively, cardioplegia is administered with low volume, according to the Calafiore technique: arterial blood is deviated from the main line, enriched with potassium and then returned to the venous line. To maintain the system closed, a sucker is not part of the system and the collected blood is washed through a cell saver and re-transfused by the anesthesiologist.

With increasing experience using mini-CPB circuits, we developed our own low volume cardioplegia solution, Cardioplexol™ (Bichsel, Interlaken, Switzerland. The latter is composed of potassium, magnesium and xylitol (solution A, 95 mL) and procain (solution B, 5 mL). Immediately before administration, solutions A and B are mixed (total = 100 mL) and are ready for use. Cardioplexol™ has been introduced in 2003 at the University Hospital in Bern (Switzerland), and then slightly modified [18,19]. Practical advantages including the easy and rapid administration by the surgeon him/herself, the almost immediate cardiac arrest and a protection time of 50 to 60 min have been observed. In a single centre, retrospective observational analysis of 7447 adult cardiac operations prospectively collected, 2416 were isolated coronary bypass operations performed with a miniaturized circuit. Patients were 81.3% males, 66.2 ± 9.7 years old and had a median logistic EuroSCORE of 3.2. Median cross-clamp time was 45 min and more than 75% of the patients received only one dose of Cardioplexol™ (100 mL). Following opening of the aortic crossclamp, more than 90% of the hearts spontaneously recovered a rhythmic activity [23].

Maximal value of troponin T during the first hours following myocardial reperfusion was 0.9 ± 4.5 ng/mL (median = 0.4 ng/mL). Mortality at 30 days was 0.9%. In this study Cardioplexol™ was found to be promising, because it appeared efficient and safe. In case the ischemic time is estimated to be far over 60 min, a second dose of 50–100 mL Cardioplexol™ (depending on the estimated remaining ischemic period) must be administered. The same applies if the ischemic time will be over 90 min, and so on.

During an extended period of observation, no adverse event could be directly related to the use of this cardioplegic solution. Cardioplegia with Cardioplexol™ was in our eyes particularly beneficial when minimally invasive system was used. Its application, although very simple, requires however a few words of caution: since it is often used once only, it is obvious that the solution must be administered perfectly. For this, the aortic valve should be checked for significant regurgitation since the latter would preclude the correct perfusion of the coronary arteries. In that case, selective administration should be performed directly into the coronary ostia. The presence of a ventricular hypertrophy must also be checked as a higher initial dose may then provide a better protection [24].

7. Coagulation Management

Point of care testing of the anticoagulation has been proposed to facilitate assessment of intraoperative patient's coagulation status and to make subsequent adaptation more expedient. In previous works, we have advocated individualized heparin and protamine management. Low anticoagulation protocols are routinely followed when a minimally invasive circuit is used while continuous intravenous heparin infusion is preferred instead of intermittent heparin bolus administration [25]. A heparin-protamine ratio of 0.7 is used. Residual heparin levels are excluded before the patient leaves from the operating theater. Point of care coagulation management is especially helpful when diffuse nonsurgical bleeding is observed in the surgical field after heparin reversal because it allows expedient correction in the operating theater.

In cases with severely impaired coagulation because of hypothermia or any other adverse condition (emergency, preoperative anticoagulation or anti-aggregation), thromboelastometry allows for precise assessment of a patient's coagulation status even in the presence of full heparinization before weaning from CPB. This will significantly reduce the so-called bleed-to-treat time. In case of fibrinogen deficiency, fibrinogen concentrate or an appropriate amount of fresh-frozen plasma (FFP) or cryoprecipitate is administered. Prothrombin complex concentrates are administered in case of a significantly prolonged clotting time without evidence of residual heparin or fibrinogen deficiency, or as a second line in the case of a prolonged clotting time after fibrinogen/FFP supplementation. If nonsurgical bleeding after heparin reversal is observed despite adequate fibrinogen levels, aggregometry should be evaluated. In case of low values ADP and TRAP tests, platelet transfusion should be considered. Minimally invasive perfusion systems should make possible to adopt a more restrictive policy of foreign blood transfusion anyway [26].

8. Clinical Experience

Several studies have described the advantages of minimally invasive extracorporeal perfusion [15–17,26,27]. One of the rare prospective randomized multicenter trial hypothesized that minimally invasive extracorporeal circulation would reduce the risk of serious adverse events after cardiac surgery operations [28].

The study was conducted in patients undergoing elective or urgent isolated coronary artery bypass grafting, isolated aortic valve replacement surgery, or combined coronary and aortic valve surgery [29]. The primary outcome was a composite of 12 post-operative significant adverse events up to 30 days after surgery, the risk of which minimized circuits was hypothesized to reduce. Unfortunately, the trial was terminated early due to the COVID-19 pandemic [24]. 1071 participants with median Euroscore II 1.24 were randomized. 50 of 517 (9.7%) randomized to minimized circuits and 69/522 (13.2%) randomized to conventional CPB experienced the primary outcome (risk ratio = 0.732, p = 0.025). The risk of any significant adverse event not contributing to the primary outcome was similarly reduced (risk ratio = 0.791, p = 0.250). The potential benefits of minimally invasive cardiopulmonary bypass remained uncertain because the trial did not achieve the target sample size (29).

Nevertheless, the most recent developments in CPB technology go in direction of improving and simplifying the conventional circuits as well; in that term, the differences between a type III or IV minimally invasive circuit and the most modern conventional CPB (Figure 4) circuit are continuously shrinking.

Although there are several differences between miniaturized and conventional CPB circuits, potential advantages and disadvantages are difficult to be detected; in addition, the large heterogenicity of the systems used in clinical practice makes comparison difficult.

The foundation of the multidisciplinary Minimal Invasive Extracorporeal Technologies International Society (MiECTiS) in 2014, constituted a new era in perfusion with the aim to build up a group of experts interested in refining the technology and implementing it into clinical practice. Another important aspect was to promote a common language between all specialties involved, such as cardiac surgeons, anesthesiologists and perfusionists. The position paper published in 2016 and updated in 2022 was a collaborative effort to set standards for definition of mini-CPB systems and to provide evidence-based recommendations for the major European scientific societies in the field of cardiovascular surgery (8,19). This group of experts also designed the randomized controlled trial to evaluate minimal invasive versus conventional ECC [28]. The results of this study will be published soon (29).

Funding: This ressearch received no external funding.

Institutional Review Board Statement: Not applicable.

Informed Consent Statement: Not applicable.

Data Availability Statement: Not applicable.

Conflicts of Interest: TC was co-founder of SwissCardioTechnologies that developed Cardioplexol® cardioplegia.

References

1. Fromes, Y.; Gaillard, D.; Ponzio, O.; Chauffert, M.; Gerhardt, M.-F.; Deleuze, P.; Bical, O.M. Reduction of the inflammatory response following coronary artery bypass grafting with total minimal extracorporeal circulation. *Eur. J. Cardio-Thorac. Surg.* **2002**, *22*, 527–533. [CrossRef]
2. Wiesenack, C.; Liebold, A.; Philipp, A.; Ritzka, M.; Koppenberg, J.; Birnbaum, D.E.; Keyl, C. Four years' experience with a miniaturized extracorporeal circulation system and its influence on clinical outcome. *Artif. Organs* **2004**, *28*, 1082–1088. [CrossRef]
3. De Backer, D.; Dubois, M.-J.; Schmartz, D.; Koch, M.; Ducart, A.; Barvais, L.; Vincent, J.-L. Microcirculatory alterations in cardiac surgery: Effects of cardiopulmonary bypass and anesthesia. *Ann. Thorac. Surg.* **2009**, *88*, 1396–1403. [CrossRef] [PubMed]
4. Anastasiadis, K.; Antonitsis, P.; Haidich, A.-B.; Argiriadou, H.; Deliopoulos, A.; Papakonstantinou, C. Use of minimal extracorporeal circulation improves outcome after heart surgery: A systematic review and meta-analysis of randomized controlled trials. *Int. J. Cardiol.* **2013**, *164*, 158–169. [CrossRef]
5. Anastasiadis, K.; Antonitsis, P.; Argiriadou, H.; Deliopoulos, A.; Grosomanidis, V.; Tossios, P. Modular minimally invasive extracorporeal circulation systems; can they become the standard practice for performing cardiac surgery. *Perfusion* **2015**, *30*, 195–200. [CrossRef] [PubMed]
6. Mehta, R.L.; Kellum, J.A.; Shah, S.V.; Molitoris, B.A.; Ronco, C.; Warnock, D.G.; Levin, A. Acute Kidney Injury Network: Report of an Initiative to Improve Outcomes in Acute Kidney Injury. *Crit. Care* **2007**, *11*, R31. [CrossRef] [PubMed]
7. Jenni, H.; Heinisch, P.P.; Eberle, B.; Gisler, F.; Kadner, A.; Carrel, T. From minimal invasive extracorporeal circulation type I to type III: The perfusionist's view. *J. Thorac. Dis.* **2019**, *11*, S1515–S1518. [CrossRef] [PubMed]
8. Anastasiadis, K.; Murkin, J.; Antonitsis, P.; Bauer, A.; Ranucci, M.; Gygax, E.; Schaarschmidt, J.; Fromes, Y.; Philipp, A.; Eberle, B.; et al. Use of minimal invasive extracorporeal circulation in cardiac surgery: Principles, definitions and potential benefits. A position paper from the Minimal invasive Extra-Corporeal Technologies international Society (MiECTiS). *Interact. Cardiovasc. Thorac. Surg.* **2016**, *22*, 647–662. [CrossRef]
9. Immer, F.F.; Pirovino, C.; Gygax Englberger, L.; Tevaearai, H.; Carrel, T. Minimal versus conventional cardiopulmonary bypass: Assessment of intraoperative myocardial damage in coronary bypass surgery. *Eur. J. Cardio-Thorac. Surg.* **2005**, *28*, 701–704. [CrossRef]
10. Skrabal, C.; Choi, Y.H.; Kaminski, A.; Steiner, M.; Kundt, G.; Steinhoff, G.; Liebold, A. Circulating endothelial cells demonstrate an attenuation of endothelial damage by minimizing the extracorporeal circulation. *J. Thorac. Cardiovasc. Surg.* **2006**, *132*, 291–296. [CrossRef]
11. Liebold, A.; Khosravi, A.; Westphal, B.; Skrabal, C.; Choi, Y.; Stamm, C.; Kaminski, A.; Alms, A.; Birken, T.; Zurakowski, D.; et al. Effect of closed minimized cardiopulmonary bypass on cerebral tissue oxygenation and microembolization. *J. Thorac. Cardiovasc. Surg.* **2006**, *131*, 268–276. [CrossRef] [PubMed]
12. Winkler, B.; Heinisch, P.P.; Zuk, G.; Zuk, K.; Gahl, B.; Jenni, H.-J.; Kadner, A.; Huber, C.; Carrel, T. Minimally invasive extracorporeal circulation: Excellent outcome and life expectancy after coronay artery bypass grafting surgery. *Swiss Med. Wkly.* **2017**, *147*, w14474. [CrossRef] [PubMed]
13. Stalder, M.; Gygax, E.; Immer, F.F.; Englberger, L.; Tevaearai, H.; Carrel, T.P. Minimized cardiopulmonary bypass combined with a smart suction device: The future of cardiopulmonary bypass? *Heart Surg. Forum.* **2007**, *10*, E235–E238. [CrossRef]
14. Kadner, A.; Heinisch, P.P.; Bartkevics, M.; Wyss, S.; Jenni, H.-J.; Erdoes, G.; Eberle, B.; Carrel, T. Initial experiences with a centrifugal-pump based minimal invasive extracorporeal circulation system in pediatric congenital cardiac surgery. *J. Thorac. Dis.* **2019**, *11*, S1446–S1452. [CrossRef]
15. Kowalewski, M.; Pawliszak, W.; Kołodziejczak, M.; Navarese, E.; Anisimowicz, L. 30-day mortality reduction with miniaturized extracorporeal circulation as compared to conventional cardiopulmonary bypass for coronary revascularization. Meta-analysis of randomized controlled trials. *Int. J. Cardiol.* **2015**, *198*, 63–65. [CrossRef] [PubMed]
16. Kowalewski, M.; Pawliszak, W.; Raffac, G.M.; Malvindi, P.G.; Kowalkowska, M.E.; Zaborowska, K.; Kowalewski, J.; Tarelli, G.; Taggart, D.P.; Anisimowicz, L. Safety and efficacy of miniaturized extracorporeal circulation when compared with off-pump and conventional coronary artery bypass grafting: Evidence synthesis from a comprehensive Bayesian-framework network meta-analysis of 134 randomized controlled trials involving 22,778 patients. *Eur. J. Cardiothorac. Surg.* **2016**, *49*, 1428–1440.
17. Benedetto, U.; Ng, C.; Frati, G.; Biondi-Zoccai, G.; Vitulli, P.; Zeinah, M.; Raja, S.G.; Cardiac Outcomes METa-analysis (COMET) group. Miniaturized extracorporeal circulation versus off-pump coronary artery bypass grafting: A meta-analysis of randomized controlled trials. *Int. J. Surg.* **2015**, *14*, 96–104. [CrossRef]
18. Anastasiadis, K.; Argiriadou, H.; Deliopoulos, A.; Antonitsis, P. Minimal invasive extracorporeal circulation (MiECC): The state-of-the-art in perfusion. *J. Thorac. Dis.* **2019**, *11*, S1507–S1514. [CrossRef]
19. Anastasiadis, K.; Murkin, J.; Antonitsis, P.; Bauer, A.; Ranucci, M.; Gygax, E.; Schaarschmidt, J.; Fromes, Y.; Philipp, A.; Eberle, B.; et al. Use of minimal invasive extracorporeal circulation in cardiac surgery: Principles, definitions and potential benefits. A position paper from the minimal invasive extra-corporeal technologies international society (MiECTiS). *Perfusion*, 2022; Aug 12:2676591221119002, *in press*.
20. Takeuchi, K.; Maida, K.; Tanaka, S.; Yoshida, S.; McGowan, X., Jr.; del Nido, P.J. Superior myocardila protection with a new histidine-buffered crystalloid cardioplegic solution in clinical trial. *Thorac. Cardiovasc. Surg.* **1999**, *47*, 148–152. [CrossRef]

21. Fresilli, S.; Labanca, R.; Monaco, F.; Belletti, A.; D'Amico, F.; Blasio, A.; Kotani, Y.; Landoni, G.; Del Nido Study Group. Del Nido cardioplegia in adult ischemic myocardium: Meta-analysis of randomized clinical trials. *J. Cardiothorac. Vasc. Anesth.* **2023**, *37*, 1152–1159. [CrossRef]
22. Zhang, X.; Du, Y.; Wang, A. Protective efficacy on adult ischemic myocardium under Bypass: Del Nido versus St. Thomas blood cardioplegia. *Ann. Thorac. Cardiovasc. Surg.* **2023**, *29*, 125–132. [CrossRef] [PubMed]
23. Tevaearai Stahel, H.; Barandun, S.; Kaufmann, E.; Gahl, B.; Englberger, L.; Jenni, H.; Weber, A.; Aymard, T.; Gygax, E.; Carrel, T. Single-center experience with the combination of Cardioplexol™ cardioplegia and MiECC for isolated coronary artery bypass graft procedures. *J. Thorac. Dis.* **2019**, *11*, S1471–S1479. [CrossRef] [PubMed]
24. Matt, P.; Arbeleaz, E.; Schwirtz, G.; Doebele, T.; Eckstein, F. Low volume, single-shot crystalloid cardioplegia is safe for isolated aortic valve replacement. *Thorac. Cardiovasc. Surg.* **2012**, *60*, 360–362. [CrossRef] [PubMed]
25. Nydegger, U.E.; Gygax, E.; Carrel, T. Point-of-care testing in the cardiovascular operating theatre. *Clin. Chem. Lab. Med.* **2006**, *44*, 1060–1065. [CrossRef] [PubMed]
26. Murphy, G.J.; Pike, K.; Rogers, C.A.; Wordsworth, S.; Stokes, E.A.; Angelini, G.D.; Reeves, B.C. Liberal or restrictive transfusion after cardiac surgery. *N. Engl. J. Med.* **2015**, *372*, 997–1008. [CrossRef]
27. Biancari, F.; Rimpilainen, R. Meta-analysis of randomized trials comparing the effectiveness of miniaturised versus conventional cardiopulmonary bypass in adult cardiac surgery. *Heart* **2009**, *95*, 964–969. [CrossRef]
28. COMICS Investigators. Conventional versus minimally invasive extracorporeal circulation in patients undergoing cardiac surgery: Protocol for a randomised controlled trial (COMICS). *Perfusion* **2021**, *36*, 388–394. [CrossRef]
29. Angelini, G.D.; Reeves, B.C.; Evans, J.; Culliford, L.A.; Collett, L.; Rogers, C.A.; Stokes, E.; Anastasiadis, K.; Antonitsis, P.; Carrel, T.; et al. Conventional versus Minimally Invasive extra-corporeal circulation in patients undergoing Cardiac Surgery: A randomized controlled trial (COMICS). *Eur. J. Cardio-Thorac. Surg.* 2023; *submitted*.

Journal of
Cardiovascular
Development and Disease

MDPI

Perspective

The Current Status of Minimally Invasive Conduit Harvesting for Coronary Artery Bypass Grafting

Devon Anderson *, Bob Kiaii and Jorge Catrip

Division of Cardiac Surgery, Department of Surgery, University of California Davis Medical Center, Sacramento, CA 95817, USA; bkiaii@ucdavis.edu (B.K.); jcatrip@ucdavis.edu (J.C.)
* Correspondence: daanderson@ucdavis.edu

Abstract: The harvesting of conduits for coronary artery bypass surgery has evolved over the last decade to include endoscopic approaches to access the saphenous vein, radial artery, and internal mammary artery. These minimally invasive techniques reduce the morbidity associated with open procedures by decreasing pain and recovery time and increasing mobility post operatively. This review highlights the differences in morbidity, quality, and patency between the most common conduits that are harvested minimally invasively for coronary artery bypass grafting surgery.

Keywords: coronary artery bypass grafting surgery; minimally invasive; conduit; cardiac surgery

1. Introduction

Coronary artery disease remains the most common heart disease in the United States and continues to impact the lives of millions of American yearly [1,2]. Coronary artery bypass grafting (CABG) surgery is the surgical revascularization procedure used to address this condition and is the most common cardiac surgical procedure performed in the world [1]. Traditionally, the harvesting of conduits for this procedure has been performed using an open technique; however, over the last two decades there has been an increased adoption of minimally invasive and endoscopic approaches to obtain the various conduits for coronary artery bypass grafts. The goal of this transition has been to reduce the morbidity of open procedures by decreasing pain and recovery time and increasing mobility post operatively, all of which has ultimately led to increased patient satisfaction [1,3,4]. This review highlights the differences in morbidity, quality, and patency in conduits that are harvested minimally invasively for coronary artery bypass grafting surgery.

2. Endoscopic Saphenous Vein Harvesting

The greater saphenous vein is the second most widely harvested conduit used during coronary artery bypass surgery, which can be attributed to its accessibility and the ability to harvest long segments [5]. These conduits can be anastomosed to coronary arteries with a lesser degree of native artery stenosis, which ideally would be avoided if utilizing arterial conduits. Despite these positive features, the greater saphenous vein's durability and patency has been shown to be inferior compared to arterial conduits, which can be attributed to endothelial hyperplasia or damage to the endothelial lining during the harvesting technique or during reperfusion with higher arterial pressure [6,7].

Greater saphenous vein grafts were originally harvested through a long skin incision, which contributed to longer hospital stays due to the increased incidence of wound infections and pain and subsequently decreased patient satisfaction [5]. Endoscopic subcutaneous greater saphenous vein harvesting was first described in 1996 in response to the increased interest in minimally invasive surgery at the time [8]. The ROOBY randomized trial in 2010 performed a sub-analysis on the graft patency of endoscopic vein harvesting versus open vein harvesting in patients undergoing on- and off-pump CABG and found that saphenous veins that were endoscopically harvested had a statistically significant lower patency rate than the veins that were harvested openly; 74.5% vs. 85.2%, $p < 0.0001$ [9]. They also found a higher 1-year revascularization rate in the group of patients who had endoscopic harvesting of their saphenous vein versus open harvesting (6.7% vs. 3.4%, $p < 0.05$) [9]. The outcomes of this particular study could be secondary to the method by which the greater saphenous vein grafts were harvested endoscopically, by utilizing carbon dioxide to insufflate the subcutaneous cavity, to the use of bipolar cautery with potential thermal injury, or to the longer manipulation times with the rigid scope [9,10].

Later in 2019, the REGROUP trial, a randomized controlled trial, evaluated clinical outcomes in 1150 patients who were randomized to either endoscopic or open vein harvesting and did not show a significant difference in the rate of major adverse cardiac events amongst the two groups [10]. In addition, this trial showed a decreased incidence of leg infections in the endoscopic harvesting group (1.4%) vs. the open harvesting group (3.1%) [10]. The ISMICS systematic review and consensus paper on the endoscopic harvesting of conduits for CABG by Ferdinand et al. found that wound complications and wound infections were significantly reduced with endoscopic harvesting versus the traditional open harvesting of vein conduits after performing a pooled analysis that included over 1300 patients [1]. Based on their findings, they also recommended endoscopic saphenous vein and radial artery harvesting as the standard of care over open harvesting due to noninferiority in respect to patency rates, the quality of the conduit, and major adverse cardiac events [1]. Thus, the comparable long-term outcomes, in conjunction with decreased harvesting site complications, contributed to the adoption of the endoscopic harvesting technique for the saphenous vein grafts, despite concerns regarding increased costs [1,10,11]. However, cost analyses have shown that the cumulative costs are not statistically different between the open and endoscopic harvesting technique, as the higher equipment-related costs in the operating room associated with endoscopic harvesting are outbalanced by the costs associated with managing harvest site complications with the open harvesting technique [11–13].

Advancements in endoscopic harvesting have led to the "no touch" technique, which decreases the manipulation of the graft by harvesting the saphenous vein with a pedicle of surrounding perivascular tissue [14,15]. Studies have also shown that saphenous vein grafts with perivascular tissue left intact have superior levels of nitric oxide production, which may contribute to improved patency rates due to the protective features of nitric oxide [16,17]. The retrospective review by Sakurai et al. found that early outcomes of saphenous vein grafts harvested with the "no touch" technique had similar pathological characteristics to grafts harvested with the original open technique, with a preservation of the wall structure, normal architecture, and smooth muscle cells [18]. A randomized longitudinal trial by Souza et al. showed statistically significant improvement in patency rates in the group who underwent the "no touch" technique compared to the traditional method of harvesting saphenous vein grafts (90% and 76%, $p = 0.01$) [14,15]. As mentioned above, all of these features provide protection against the distention of the graft once it is placed under arterial pressure, and the endothelial nitric oxide activity decreases intimal hyperplasia and atherosclerosis [15–18]. The "no touch" technique also utilizes the ultrasonic scalpel, which has been reported to reduce thermal injury and subsequent injury to the graft [18]. A table of key trials and studies can be seen in Table 1.

Despite the earlier trials showing decreased patency and increased revascularization with endoscopic saphenous vein harvesting, the ultimate key to providing the best results with this procedure is to harvest the saphenous vein atraumatically. Decreasing endothelial damage and its potential downstream consequences is highly dependent on the skill level of the operator. The comprehensive review by Krishnamoorthy et al. highlights the important aspects and features that a standardized training program should encompass in order to harvest the best quality vein, as it has been shown that the number of conduit repairs is inversely proportional to the level of expertise of the harvester [17,19]. In addition, a structured and standardized training program with a set surgical skill curriculum provides consistent training and reproducible results across all of the harvesters [17,20].

Table 1. Results of key trials and studies for endoscopic saphenous vein harvesting.

Author	Year	Type of Study	Results
Zenati et al. [9] (ROOBY Trial)	2010	Randomized controlled trial	• Statistically significant lower patency rate in endoscopically harvested veins than veins that were harvested open; 74.5% vs. 85.2%, $p < 0.0001$ • Higher 1-year revascularization rate in the group of patients who had endoscopic harvesting of their saphenous vein versus open harvesting (6.7% vs. 3.4%, $p < 0.05$)
Zenati et al. [10] (REGROUP Trial)	2019	Randomized controlled trial	• No significant difference in the rate of major adverse cardiac events • Leg infections occurred in 3.1% of patients in the open harvesting group and 1.4% of patients in the endoscopic harvesting group (relative risk, 2.26; 95% CI, 0.99 to 5.15)
Ferdinand et al. [1]	2017	Systematic review and meta-analysis	• Odds of a wound infection were significantly reduced with endoscopic harvesting (OR = 0.28, 95% CI = 0.13 to 0.63, $p = 0.002$)
Souza et al. [14]	2006	Randomized longitudinal trial	• Angiographic assessment at 18 months postoperatively showed 89% conventional versus 95% no-touch grafts were patent. Repeated angiography at 8.5 years showed a patency rate for the conventional group of 76% and 90% for the no-touch group ($p = 0.01$)
Sakurai et al. [18]	2022	Retrospective review	• Similar pathological characteristics as grafts harvested with the original and no-touch technique

3. Radial Artery Endoscopic Harvesting

The known disadvantages of endothelial and medial hyperplasia that contribute to the reduction in patency of greater saphenous vein grafts, as previously described above, have paved the way for investigations into other conduit options [21]. Total arterial myocardial revascularization is a technique utilizing all arterial grafts during coronary artery bypass surgery and includes the internal thoracic artery, radial arteries, gastroepiploic arteries, and inferior epigastric arteries. There are pros and cons to each arterial conduit that are well known and have been previously described in the literature [21]. However, this section focuses on the radial artery and the endoscopic harvesting technique.

The path for endoscopic radial artery harvesting was paved by the success noted with endoscopic greater saphenous vein harvesting over the years [3]. According to the most recent 2021 ACC/AHA/SCAI guidelines for coronary artery revascularization, the current recommendation for bypass conduits in patients undergoing CABG is for the preferential use of the radial artery over the greater saphenous vein, as the conduit to the second most important, significantly stenosed, non-left anterior-descending coronary artery to improve long-term cardiac outcomes [2]. Observational studies have shown radial artery patency rates of 92% at 1 year and 80% at 5 years when the bypassed targeted vessel has over 90% native stenosis [21].

In the systematic review and ISMICS consensus statement regarding endoscopic conduit harvesting, there is a significant reduction in wound infections with endoscopic radial artery harvesting versus open radial artery harvesting, which led to a Class I recommendation for the use of endoscopic radial artery harvesting to reduce wound-related complications [1,2,22]. Although the time to harvest the radial artery endoscopically was significantly increased compared to open harvesting, the overall operative time was not statistically different [1].

Endoscopic radial artery harvesting is also associated with increased patient satisfaction compared with the open technique with regard to cosmesis and postoperative pain, again contributing to the Class I recommendation for an endoscopic approach for radial artery harvesting [1,2,21]. In addition, the length of stay was reduced with endoscopic radial artery harvesting; however, these findings were not statistically significant [1].

A known complication associated with utilizing the radial artery as a graft during CABG is that it is prone to vasospasm, especially when exposed to competitive flow. This highlights the previously mentioned point above about the careful selection of the targeted coronary vessel with severely stenotic lesions (>90%) prior to harvesting in order to mitigate competitive flow and subsequent vasospasm [3].

Additional complications that have been noted with the use of radial artery grafts are the postoperative neurologic deficits due to injury to the superficial radial or lateral antebrachial cutaneous nerves. Sensory disturbances and neurological complications have been reported at as high as 30–67% [3,23]. These symptoms are transient and self-limiting and will usually resolve with time; however, permanent neurologic impairment was quoted to be 7.4% in one study [3,24].

Overall, endoscopically harvesting the radial artery has significant benefits when compared to open harvesting of the radial artery, as reported in the literature. The radial artery is not always available for use or the most appropriate conduit for all patients; however, it is an excellent option if the patient meets all the criteria and is amenable to endoscopic harvesting.

4. Endoscopic Internal Mammary Artery Harvesting

Endoscopic harvesting of the internal mammary artery has also gained popularity after advancements in minimally invasive cardiac surgery. This approach is used not only in patients with single-vessel disease, but also in patients undergoing hybrid treatment with stents to non-LAD vessels [25]. Minimally invasive CABG via anterolateral thoracotomy was first described by Dr. Kolessov in 1967 [26]. Endoscopic harvesting of the internal mammary artery with a sternal sparing mini thoracotomy approach and endoscopic camera, trocars, and instruments has been defined in the literature by Hrapkowicz et al. [25]. The benefits of this type of harvesting are the improved visualization of the artery and the ability to perform a full-length dissection of the internal mammary artery proximally, which is traditionally difficult with the conventional approach. The incomplete dissection of the proximal portion of the internal mammary artery can lead to "steal syndrome" [25].

In addition to improved visualization with the endoscopic approach, there is decreased postoperative pain. Statistically significant lower pain scores and decreased requirements for opioids postoperatively have been reported in patients undergoing endoscopic harvesting of the internal mammary artery versus conventional harvesting [27]. This can be attributed to the increased pain associated with rib retraction, which is required in the conventional method for harvesting the internal mammary artery [27].

An important aspect of totally endoscopic coronary artery bypass surgery is robot-assisted left internal mammary artery harvesting. As with all endoscopic harvesting techniques, there is a tremendous learning curve that needs to be overcome prior to achieving results comparable to the standard method of harvesting. The retrospective review by Oehlinger et al. found that the time to harvest the internal mammary artery decreased from 140 min in the first 10 cases to 34 min in the last 10 cases [28]. Other studies have shown decreased average IMA harvesting times, ranging from 57.8 ± 23.2 min in one study to 64.1 min in another, with the early postoperative angiogram showing patent grafts [29,30]. The utilization of devices such as the harmonic scalpel and increased experience demonstrated a 10% improvement in performance for each doubling of cases completed, which was seen in the first 20 cases [30,31].

Nonetheless, endoscopic harvesting of the internal mammary artery provides comparable results to open internal mammary artery harvesting and carries many benefits that outweigh the longer harvesting time.

5. Conclusions

Minimally invasive conduit harvesting for coronary artery bypass surgery has evolved over the last decade and continues to be modified with advancements in technology. With the more widespread adoption of the various minimally invasive techniques and increased operator expertise, the current cons associated with minimally invasive harvesting can be investigated and improved over time. It is also of paramount importance for continued institutional support to provide the necessary resources to encourage the adoption and evolution of minimally invasive approaches.

Author Contributions: Conceptualization, D.A., B.K. and J.C.; writing—original draft preparation, D.A.; writing—review and editing, D.A., B.K. and J.C.; visualization, D.A., B.K. and J.C.; supervision, B.K. and J.C. All authors have read and agreed to the published version of the manuscript.

Funding: This research did not receive any specific grants from funding agencies in the public, commercial or not-for-profit sectors.

Institutional Review Board Statement: Not applicable.

Informed Consent Statement: Not applicable.

Data Availability Statement: No new data were created.

Conflicts of Interest: Bob Kiaii is a consultant/speaker with Medtronic, a consultant with Johnson and Johnson, a speaker with Corcym and a consultant with Abbott.

References

1. Ferdinand, F.D.; MacDonald, J.K.; Balkhy, H.H.; Bisleri, G.; Hwang, H.Y.; Northrup, P.; Trimlett, R.H.J.; Wei, L.; Kiaii, B.B. Endoscopic conduit harvest in coronary artery bypass grafting surgery an ISMICS Systematic Review and Consensus Conference Statements. *Innov. Technol. Tech. Cardiothorac. Vasc. Surg.* **2017**, *12*, 301–319. [CrossRef] [PubMed]
2. Lawton, J.S.; Tamis-Holland, J.E.; Bangalore, S.; Bates, E.R.; Beckie, T.M.; Zwischenberger, B.A. 2021 ACC/AHA/SCAI Guideline for Coronary Artery Revascularization: A Report of the American College of Cardiology/American Heart Association Joint Committee on Clinical Practice Guidelines. *Circulation* **2022**, *145*, e18–e114. [CrossRef] [PubMed]
3. Aziz, O.; Athanasiou, T.; Darzi, A. Minimally invasive Conduit harvesting: A systematic review. *Eur. J. Cardio-Thorac. Surg.* **2006**, *29*, 324–333. [CrossRef] [PubMed]
4. Akowuah, E.; Burns, D.; Zacharias, J.; Kirmani, B.H. Endoscopic vein harvesting. *J. Thorac. Dis.* **2021**, *13*, 1899–1908. [CrossRef] [PubMed]
5. Mahmood, D.; Rosati, F.; Petsikas, D.; Payne, D.; Torkan, L.; Bisleri, G. Endoscopic saphenous vein harvesting with a non-sealed approach. *Multimed. Man. Cardio-Thorac. Surg.* **2019**, *2019*. [CrossRef]
6. Campeau, L.; Lespérance, J.; Hermann, J.; Corbara, F.; Grondin, C.M.; Bourassa, M.G. Loss of the improvement of angina between 1 and 7 years after aortocoronary bypass surgery: Correlations with changes in vein grafts and in coronary arteries. *Circulation* **1979**, *60*, 1–5. [CrossRef] [PubMed]
7. Raza, S.; Chang, C.; Deo, S.V.; Sabik, J.F. Current role of saphenous vein graft in coronary artery bypass grafting. *Indian J. Thorac. Cardiovasc. Surg.* **2018**, *34* (Suppl. S3), 245–250. [CrossRef] [PubMed]
8. Lumsden, A. Subcutaneous, video-assisted saphenous vein harvest: Report of the first 30 cases. *Cardiovasc. Surg.* **1996**, *4*, 771–776. [CrossRef]
9. Zenati, M.A.; Shroyer, A.L.; Collins, J.F.; Hattler, B.; Ota, T.; Almassi, G.H.; Amidi, M.; Novitzky, D.; Grover, F.L.; Sonel, A.F. Impact of endoscopic versus open saphenous vein harvest technique on late coronary artery bypass grafting patient outcomes in the ROOBY (Randomized on/off Bypass) Trial. *J. Thorac. Cardiovasc. Surg.* **2011**, *141*, 338–344. [CrossRef]
10. Zenati, M.A.; Bhatt, D.L.; Bakaeen, F.G.; Stock, E.M.; Biswas, K.; Gaziano, J.M.; Kelly, R.F.; Tseng, E.E.; Bitondo, J.; Quin, J.A.; et al. Randomized Trial of Endoscopic or Open Vein-Graft Harvesting for Coronary-Artery Bypass. *N. Engl. J. Med.* **2019**, *380*, 132–141. [CrossRef]
11. Rosati, F.; Bin Pervez, M.; Palacios, C.M.; Tomasi, C.; Mastroiacovo, G.; Pirola, S.; Bonomi, A.; Polvani, G.; Bisleri, G. Cost Analysis of Endoscopic Conduit Harvesting Technique Using a Non-Sealed System for Coronary Artery Bypass Surgery. *Innov. Technol. Tech. Cardiothorac. Vasc. Surg.* **2022**, *17*, 310–316. [CrossRef] [PubMed]
12. Eckey, H.; Heseler, S.; Hiligsmann, M. Economic Evaluation of Endoscopic vs. Open Vein Harvesting. *Ann. Thorac. Surg.* **2023**, *115*, 1144–1150. [CrossRef] [PubMed]
13. Rao, C.; Aziz, O.; Deeba, S.; Chow, A.; Jones, C.; Ni, Z.; Papastavrou, L.; Rahman, S.; Darzi, A.; Athanasiou, T. Is minimally invasive harvesting of the great saphenous vein for coronary artery bypass surgery a cost-effective technique? *J. Thorac. Cardiovasc. Surg.* **2008**, *135*, 809–815. [CrossRef] [PubMed]

14. Souza, D.S.; Johansson, B.; Bojö, L.; Karlsson, R.; Geijer, H.; Filbey, D.; Bodin, L.; Arbeus, M.; Dashwood, M.R. Harvesting the saphenous vein with surrounding tissue for CABG provides long-term graft patency comparable to the left internal thoracic artery: Results of a randomized longitudinal trial. *J. Thorac. Cardiovasc. Surg.* **2006**, *132*, 373–378.e5. [CrossRef] [PubMed]
15. Sepehripour, A.H.; Jarral, O.A.; Shipolini, A.R.; McCormack, D.J. Does a "no-touch" technique result in better vein patency? *Interact. Cardio Vasc. Thorac. Surg.* **2011**, *13*, 626–630. [CrossRef]
16. Saito, T.; Kurazumi, H.; Suzuki, R.; Matsunaga, K.; Tsubone, S.; Lv, B.; Kobayashi, S.; Nagase, T.; Mizoguchi, T.; Samura, M.; et al. Perivascular Adipose Tissue Is a Major Source of Nitric Oxide in Saphenous Vein Grafts Harvested via the No-Touch Technique. *JAHA* **2022**, *11*, e020637. [CrossRef] [PubMed]
17. Krishnamoorthy, B.; Critchley, W.R.; Venkateswaran, R.V.; Barnard, J.; Caress, A.; Fildes, J.E.; Yonan, N. A comprehensive review on learning curve associated problems in endoscopic vein harvesting and the requirement for a standardised training programme. *J. Cardiothorac. Surg.* **2016**, *11*, 45. [CrossRef] [PubMed]
18. Sakurai, H.; Someya, T.; Yamamoto, S.; Kasahara, I.; Kuroki, H.; Shirai, T. Short-Term Evaluation of a Novel No-Touch Technique for Harvesting Saphenous Veins With Long-Shafted Ultrasonic Scalpel. *Innov. Technol. Tech. Cardiothorac. Vasc. Surg.* **2022**, *17*, 56–63. [CrossRef]
19. Pagni, S.; A Ulfe, E.; Montgomery, W.D.; VanHimbergen, D.J.; Fisher, D.J.; A Gray, L.; A Spence, P. Clinical experience with the video-assisted saphenectomy procedure for coronary bypass operations. *Ann. Thorac. Surg.* **1998**, *66*, 1626–1631. [CrossRef]
20. Xue, A.; Chen, S.; Ranade, A.; Smith, K.; Kasten, J.; Catrip, J.; Kiaii, B. How to implement a clinical robotic mitral valve surgery program. *Ann. Cardiothorac. Surg.* **2022**, *11*, 504–509. [CrossRef]
21. Maestri, F.; Formica, F.; Gallingani, A.; Gripshi, F.; Nicolini, F. Radial Artery Versus Saphenous Vein as Third Conduit in Coronary Artery Bypass Graft Surgery for Multivessel Coronary Artery Disease: A Ten-Year Literature Review. *Acta Biomed.* **2022**, *93*, e2022049. [CrossRef] [PubMed]
22. Patel, A.N.; Henry, A.C.; Hunnicutt, C.; Cockerham, C.A.; Willey, B.; Urschel, H.C., Jr. Endoscopic radial artery harvesting is better than the open technique. *Ann. Thorac. Surg.* **2004**, *78*, 149–153, discussion 149–153. [CrossRef]
23. Saeed, I.; Anyanwu, A.C.; Yacoub, M.H.; Amrani, M. Subjective patient outcomes following coronary artery bypass using the radial artery: Results of a crosssectional survey of harvest site complications and quality of life. *Eur. J. Cardiothorac. Surg.* **2001**, *20*, 1142–1146. [CrossRef]
24. Casselman, F.P.; La Meir, M.; Cammu, G.; Wellens, F.; De Geest, R.; Degrieck, I.; Van Praet, F.; Vermeulen, Y.; Vanermen, H. Initial experience with an endoscopic radial artery harvesting technique. *J. Thorac. Cardiovasc. Surg.* **2004**, *128*, 463–466. [CrossRef]
25. Hrapkowicz, T.; Bisleri, G. Endoscopic harvesting of the left internal mammary artery. *Ann. Cardiothorac. Surg.* **2013**, *2*, 565–569. [CrossRef]
26. Kolessov, V.I. Mammary artery-coronary artery anastomosis as method of treatment for angina pectoris. *J. Thorac. Cardiovasc. Surg.* **1967**, *54*, 535–544. [CrossRef]
27. Bucerius, J.; Metz, S.; Walther, T.; Falk, V.; Doll, N.; Noack, F.; Holzhey, D.; Diegeler, A.; Mohr, F.W. Endoscopic internal thoracic artery dissection leads to significant reduction of pain after minimally invasive direct coronary artery bypass graft surgery. *Ann. Thorac. Surg.* **2002**, *73*, 1180–1184. [CrossRef]
28. Oehlinger, A.; Bonaros, N.; Schachner, T.; Ruetzler, E.; Friedrich, G.; Laufer, G.; Bonatti, J. Robotic Endoscopic Left Internal Mammary Artery Harvesting: What Have We Learned After 100 Cases? *Ann. Thorac. Surg.* **2007**, *83*, 1030–1034. [CrossRef] [PubMed]
29. Kodera, K.; Boyd, W.D.; Kiaii, B.; Novik, R.J.; Rayman, R.; Ganapathy, S.; Dobkowski, W.B.; McKenzie, N.F.; Menkis, A.H.; Otsuka, T.; et al. Clinical experience in thoracoscopic left internal mammary artery harvesting with voice activated robotic assistance. *Kyobu Geka* **2001**, *54*, 987–991, discussion 991–994. [PubMed]
30. Boyd, W.D.; Kiaii, B.; Novick, R.J.; Rayman, R.; Ganapathy, S.; Dobkowski, W.B.; Menkis, A.H. RAVECAB: Improving outcome in off-pump minimal access surgery with robotic assistance and video enhancement. *Can. J. Surg.* **2001**, *44*, 45–50. [PubMed]
31. Hemli, J.M.; Henn, L.W.; Panetta, C.R.; Suh, J.S.; Shukri, S.R.; Jennings, J.M.; Fontana, G.P.; Patel, N.C. Defining the Learning Curve for Robotic-Assisted Endoscopic Harvesting of the Left Internal Mammary Artery. *Innov. Technol. Tech. Cardiothorac. Vasc. Surg.* **2013**, *8*, 353–358. [CrossRef]

Journal of
Cardiovascular Development and Disease

MDPI

Review

Minimal-Access Coronary Revascularization: Past, Present, and Future

Rushmi Purmessur *, Tharushi Wijesena and Jason Ali

Department of Cardiothoracic Surgery, Royal Papworth Hospital NHS Foundation Trust, Cambridge CB2 0AY, UK; rtw27@cam.ac.uk (T.W.); jason.ali@nhs.net (J.A.)
* Correspondence: rushmi.purmessur@nhs.net

Abstract: Minimal-access cardiac surgery appears to be the future. It is increasingly desired by cardiologists and demanded by patients who perceive superiority. Minimal-access coronary artery revascularisation has been increasingly adopted throughout the world. Here, we review the history of minimal-access coronary revascularization and see that it is almost as old as the history of cardiac surgery. Modern minimal-access coronary revascularization takes a variety of forms—namely minimal-access direct coronary artery bypass grafting (MIDCAB), hybrid coronary revascularisation (HCR), and totally endoscopic coronary artery bypass grafting (TECAB). It is noteworthy that there is significant variation in the nomenclature and approaches for minimal-access coronary surgery, and this truly presents a challenge for comparing the different methods. However, these approaches are increasing in frequency, and proponents demonstrate clear advantages for their patients. The challenge that remains, as for all areas of surgery, is demonstrating the superiority of these techniques over tried and tested open techniques, which is very difficult. There is a paucity of randomised controlled trials to help answer this question, and the future of minimal-access coronary revascularisation, to some extent, is dependent on such trials. Thankfully, some are underway, and the results are eagerly anticipated.

Keywords: minimal access; coronary artery; revascularisation; MIDCAB; TECAB; HCR

1. Introduction

Coronary artery revascularisation has become the most common cardiac surgical procedure performed worldwide. Interestingly, coronary artery bypass grafting as we know it finds its roots in minimal-access approaches when the first coronary artery bypass grafts were performed by left anterolateral mini-thoracotomies without cardiopulmonary bypass (CPB).

Minimal-access cardiac surgery is becoming fashionable, and as more surgeons adopt minimal-access techniques, there is a need for all cardiac surgeons to be aware of what is becoming available so that they can offer their patients the best treatment. However, many remain sceptical about minimal-access techniques in cardiac surgery and highlight the concerns surrounding these approaches and, in many cases, there remains a paucity of evidence demonstrating clear benefits over traditional median sternotomy, which remains the commonest approach to performing cardiac surgery.

In this review, we aim to focus on the history of minimal-access coronary artery revascularisation and move to discuss the patient selection and the techniques and evidence supporting the common minimal-access approaches to coronary artery revascularisation. These approaches include minimally invasive direct coronary artery bypass grafting (MIDCAB), totally endoscopic coronary artery bypass grafting (TECAB), and hybrid coronary revascularisation (HCR).

2. Materials and Methods

A search was conducted in the PUBMED online database using the following search terms: "minimally invasive coronary artery revascularisation", "minimal access coronary artery revascularisation", "minimally invasive cardiac surgery coronary artery bypass grafting", "robotic assisted cardiac surgery", "endoscopic cardiac surgery", "robotic assisted thoracoscopic surgery coronary artery bypass graft surgery" "minimally invasive direct coronary artery bypass graft", "total endoscopic coronary artery bypass grafting", and "hybrid coronary revascularisation". The search was limited to reviews, meta-analyses, and randomised controlled trials (RCT) from January 1997 to December 2022.

3. History of Coronary Artery Bypass Grafting

The history and evolution of coronary artery bypass grafting (CABG) has been rife with successes and failures. The first CABG was performed by Alexis Carrel [1,2] in 1910 in dogs before the advent of coronary angiography or cardiopulmonary bypass (CPB). In the 1930s, John Gibbon invented the CPB machine, which revolutionised cardiac surgery [3]. Later, in 1946, Arthur Vineburg [4,5] pioneered the Vineburg technique, whereby he implanted the left internal mammary artery (LIMA) directly onto the left ventricular myocardium, which led to symptomatic relief of angina and was shown to still provide good cardiac function 30 years later [6]. The first LIMA to left anterior descending artery (LAD) anastomosis using a non-suture technique with tantalum rings appeared a few years later, in 1952, when Demikhov showed graft patency in the LIMA to LAD anastomosis at 2 years, a practice that was also adopted by others in Canada [7] and the US [8]. In 1956, Charles Bailey successfully performed coronary artery endarterectomies as a way to treat coronary artery atherosclerosis [9].

The issue, however, remained that the arteries could not be imaged and, therefore, the uncertainty of which arteries caused the symptoms persisted. This changed in 1958, when Mason Sones [10] inadvertently performed the first coronary angiogram by accidentally injecting dye in the right coronary artery when attempting to image a patient with rheumatic heart disease. He then went on to further develop coronary angiography—an achievement that changed the history of cardiovascular medicine.

In 1962, Sabiston [7] performed the first hand-sewn coronary anastomosis by suturing a saphenous vein graft to the right coronary artery—a procedure performed without CPB—but it was not reported until 1974. Garrett [11] and DeBakey in Houston also performed hand-sutured coronary anastomoses in 1964 but did not report it until 1973 when the grafts remained patent 7 years later. Kolessov, on the other hand, reported his first few CABGs with hand-sutured coronary anastomoses early in 1967—all procedures were performed without CPB in 1964 [12]. Despite being heavily involved in pioneering CPB as an artificial circulation for open-heart surgery, Kolessov was a great proponent of off-pump CABG owing to the large inflammatory response that CPB generated at the time. It was not till 1968 that Green [13] in New York performed the first hand-sutured LIMA to LAD anastomosis, which has since become the cornerstone of coronary artery revascularisation.

Moving on to the late 1960s and early 1970s, Favoloro [14] in the Cleveland Clinic really pushed forward the use of saphenous vein grafts as a conduit during coronary artery revascularisation. However, it was realised early on that owing to intimal [15,16] and medial thickening and graft thrombosis secondary to intimal hyperplasia and premature atherosclerosis of the vessel, saphenous vein grafts were prone to stenosis and occlusion. Carpentier [17] started using radial arteries as a conduit—the early experience of which was not as successful as it is today. The introduction of the no-touch technique of vein and radial artery harvesting in the early 1990s by Acar [18,19], as well as the use of vasodilators for radial artery grafts significantly, improved the long-term patency of veins and radial arteries as conduits for coronary artery revascularisation and revived the interest in using radial arteries as a conduit. It was only in the 1980s that the LIMA to LAD anastomosis was proven beyond doubt to have a prognostic benefit when Loop et al. in Cleveland clinic reported their ten-year outcomes [20].

Meanwhile, in the late 1970s, cardiologists started developing percutaneous catheter-based interventions (PCIs), initially with balloon angioplasty [21] but progressing to stenting and then more recently using drug-eluting stents to overcome the complications of in-stent restenosis observed in early versions of bare metal stents. PCIs had the overwhelming advantage of being less painful, with a shorter recovery and smaller risk of stroke.

To potentially challenge these advantages of PCIs but still obtain the higher survival rates that surgery conferred, the surgical community began to turn to minimal-access coronary surgery. In the mid-1990s, Calafiore reported isolated LIMA to LAD anastomoses performed through an anterior thoracotomy [22]. At the same, Peters described what was later renamed "The HeartPort technique", after the company Heartport developed a three-lumen catheter to be placed through the groin into the aorta, where one lumen would endovascularly occlude the aorta, the second lumen would be used to deliver cardioplegia, and the third lumen used as a root vent [23]. This has since progressed more recently to coronary revascularisation performed with fully thoracoscopic and robotic methods, with the first TECABG being performed by Loulmet [24] in 1998. Now, many centres around the world have introduced minimal-access coronary surgery with varying permutations, from mini-thoracotomy off-pump LIMA to LAD anastomosis in MIDCAB to fully robotic complete revascularisation.

A timeline summarising major events in coronary artery revascularisation has been summarised in Figure 1.

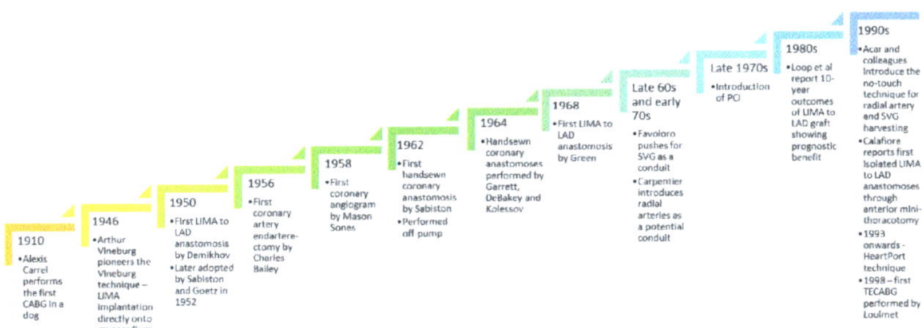

Figure 1. History of minimal-access coronary artery surgery.

4. Minimal-Access Coronary Revascularisation—International Guidelines Perspective

The 2018 EACTS/ESC guidelines on myocardial revascularisation do not make any formal recommendation regarding minimal-access surgery, but they do mention that it is an attractive alternative to conventional approaches for CABG surgery [25].

The guidelines highlight HCR to be an appealing management strategy, whether performed sequentially, i.e., minimal-access LIMA to LAD anastomosis followed by PCIs to the non-LAD vessels in another setting or performed in a hybrid theatre in one session, quoting the POL-MIDES RCT [26,27] where, in a small group of 200 patients, conventional surgery and HCR had similar outcomes at 5 years. Of course, it is important to consider if 5-year outcomes are long-term enough to justify the non-inferiority of HCR compared to more traditional approaches.

Similarly, the 2021 ACC/AHA/SCAI guidelines on coronary artery revascularisation comment that the role of HCR remains unclear and do not make any formal recommendation as to when it can or should be used [28]. They, however, do not comment on any other method of minimal-access coronary artery revascularisation surgery.

5. Patient Selection and Rationale for Minimal-Access Coronary Intervention

The surgical indication for minimal-access coronary revascularisation remains unclear in the literature. Some small studies in the early 1990s and 2000s [29] report the use of minimal-access coronary artery revascularisation surgery for patients with isolated coronary artery disease, isolated LAD lesions, or proximal right coronary artery disease. However, the conduct of minimal-access coronary artery revascularisation surgery, from patient selection, the use of CPB or lack thereof, to even conduit selection for different lesion sets, is too varied to make any reasonable conclusion as to where the actual benefit of minimal-access CABG lies. The advantage of minimal-access coronary artery revascularisation presumably is more apparent in patients with uncontrolled diabetes or multiple co-morbidities, which confer a higher risk of sternal wound non-healing, breakdown, and infection. In addition, in those performing minimal-access CABG off-pump, there are added benefits such as a reduced stroke [30] rate from the absence of aortic manipulation and cross-clamping, decreased inflammatory [31] response from the bypass circuit leading to lower rates of acute kidney injury [32], and fewer blood transfusions. Moreover, if a mini-thoracotomy is performed, no bone healing is required post-operatively, allowing patients to return to their normal lifestyle more rapidly. With the smaller incisions, patients can be extubated faster and there are fewer complications of respiratory failure. Diegeler et al. in a small prospective trial suggested that after post-operative day 4, MIDCABG had lower rates of pain compared to conventional CABG [33].

There are some patient features that are favourable for minimal-access CABG, including being slim and having a thin, tubular, and vertically positioned heart. LAD lesions that tend themselves to minimal-access surgery are those with a non-calcified distal segment (approximately 2–4 cm distal to the second diagonal branch), those with an arterial diameter greater than 1.75 mm, and total occlusion of the LAD with good collateral circulation [34].

However, it should be kept in mind that while some centres consider multivessel disease a contraindication to minimal-access coronary revascularisation, others regularly perform multi-vessel grafting using minimal-access methods.

6. Contraindications to Minimal-Access Coronary Revascularisation

The only absolute contraindications to using a minimal-access approach are an occluded left subclavian artery, which prevents the use of the LIMA, particularly in hybrid procedures where the benefit is a LIMA to LAD anastomoses, and patients in cardiogenic shock require emergent LAD revascularisation due to the longer LIMA harvesting time and the longer setup time for certain methods of minimal-access surgery [35].

Relative contraindications depend on the surgeon and their experience and the institution. These include extreme obesity, which makes access and LIMA harvesting more challenging, deep intramural and calcified LAD grafting sites, which are more challenging to identify in a minimal-access setting, previous thoracotomy, re-do surgeries, and the presence of dense adhesions, which all restrict exposure and distort the anatomy, and the presence of severe pulmonary hypertension with a large left ventricle, making the minimal-access approach higher risk and more technically challenging. While some co-morbidities would lend themselves for patients to have better outcomes with minimal-access surgery, they can often be prohibitive as well. For example, patients who are unable to tolerate single lung ventilation might not be able to undergo minimal-access surgery despite potentially benefitting greatly from the early extubation and reduced rates of respiratory failure observed with minimal-access surgical coronary revascularisations. In addition, the presence of significant peripheral vascular disease may mean that going onto peripheral cardiopulmonary bypass via the femoral vessels may not be an option intra-operatively if cardiopulmonary bypass were required—such patients should be treated with caution [34–36].

7. Techniques of Minimal-Access Coronary Artery Revascularisation

In this section, we will describe the common approaches to minimal-access coronary revascularisation surgery. We will describe patient positioning, as well as some technical considerations. The advantages and disadvantages of the different techniques are summarised in Table 1.

Table 1. Comparing the different modalities of minimal-access coronary artery surgery [37–42].

	MIDCABG	MICS CABG	TECABG/RACABG	HCR
Contra-indications	Absolute: Emergency surgery with haemodynamic compromise Severe pectus excavatum Severe pulmonary disease In TECABG/RACABG, the presence of severe left pleural scarring Relative: Left subclavian artery stenosis Haemodialysis arteriovenous fistula on the patient's left side Re-do surgery Morbid obesity Severe LV dysfunction Need for right coronary artery graft with no posterior descending or left ventricular branch target Need for circumflex coronary artery graft with no adequate marginal branch target and absence of femoral pulses bilaterally			
Advantages	Avoids the use of CPB	Allows complete revascularization in the presence of three-vessel or diffuse coronary artery disease Allows complete harvest of the LIMA, whether skeletonised or not Allows access to all coronary arteries and their territories Allows proximal anastomoses to be routinely performed	Transthoracic assistance may not be necessary for RACABG if a fourth robotic arm is available Minimal surgical trauma Allows multivessel revascularization Smaller incisions Less pain because no retractor is required for LIMA harvest	Avoids the use of CPB Still obtains the prognostic benefit of LIMA to LAD graft but complete revascularisation of other territories as well through PCIs
Dis-advantages	Restricted to single LIMA to LAD graft Cannot access all coronary artery territories Still requires a thoracotomy, which can be painful Does not lend itself to intramyocardial targets	Difficult to harvest RIMA Reasonable patency rate at 6 months	A long learning curve with higher initial rates of LIMA to LAD anastomosis failure, LIMA injuries, and longer bypass times Access depends on the port position	LIMA to LAD anastomosis failure more common than with standard CABG The use of antithrombotic medications and contrast are required for PCIs very soon before or after a major cardiac procedure More than one major intervention within days of each other

7.1. MIDCABG

7.1.1. Description

MIDCABG has been described using multiple methods and approaches in the literature. The first few descriptions of MIDCABG surgery were purely describing a LIMA–LAD anastomosis. The surgical technique has now evolved to include multivessel grafting. While most commonly performed via a left anterior mini-thoracotomy in the fourth intercostal space in the infra-mammary fold underneath the nipple with 2/3 of the incision being medial and 1/3 lateral to the nipple [36], some centres also describe accessing the chest via an upper partial sternotomy or inferior partial sternotomy. MIDCABG started as being a way of performing open-heart coronary artery revascularisation with no sternotomy but has gradually evolved to using endoscopic instruments to facilitate the process.

7.1.2. Positioning and Monitoring

The patient should be placed in an anterolateral decubitus position with the left chest and left buttock elevated by approximately 20–30 degrees using a bolster if the approach is to be through a left anterolateral mini-thoracotomy. If a partial superior or partial inferior sternotomy is to be used, then the patient can be in a supine position. The arms of the patient should be tucked at the sides. Regardless of whether peripheral CPB is used routinely or as a safety measure for emergent situations, the left groin should be prepared and draped. A guidewire is sometimes inserted under ultrasound guidance into the left femoral artery prior to prepping and draping to facilitate the emergent institution of CPB if required. External pacing and defibrillator pads, as well as warming blankets, should also be routinely placed and connected. Each institution will have its own monitoring protocols. However, it is advisable to use a pulmonary artery catheter in patients with a left ventricular ejection fraction of <30%, ECG monitoring for ischaemia, urinary bladder catheterisation, and temperature probe insertion. Transoesophageal echocardiography is used in patients with poor ventricular function or who are at higher risk of becoming haemodynamically unstable.

7.1.3. Operative Steps

The most common approach is through a 5–6 cm left anterolateral muscle-sparing mini-thoracotomy in the fourth or fifth intercostal space, 2–3 cm inferior to the nipple (Figure 2) [36]. One-lung ventilation is used to facilitate exposure. A retractor is used for LIMA harvesting, either skeletonised or pedicled, as per the surgeon's preference. In cases where bilateral IMAs will be used, bilateral mini-thoracotomies can be performed. After harvesting the LIMA, before dividing, the patient is heparinised, the pericardium opened longitudinally, usually 1–2 fingerbreadths lateral to the LIMA pedicle and suspended with traction sutures, and the LAD is identified. The lateral traction sutures are pulled upward to the upper part of the wound, which rotates the heart, exposing the LAD and facilitating anastomosis [36]. The distal end of the LIMA is then divided and prepared for anastomosis. The edges of the pericardium and selective lung inflation can be used to improve the visualisation of the LAD. A suction stabiliser is used to stabilise the LAD for anastomosis. Either a pledgeted tourniquet can be applied around the LAD proximal to the anastomosis or a soft vascular clamp used to occlude the LAD to allow for a bloodless field. Alternatively, a shunt can also be used. Once anastomosis is performed, the flow can be verified, following the restoration of blood flows through the LAD and removal of the pledgeted tourniquet or vascular clamp, for example using transit time flow measurement. Haemostasis is performed and heparin is reversed. The pericardium is closed around the apex, and a chest drain is inserted into the left pleura. The thoracotomy is then closed as per usual [34,43].

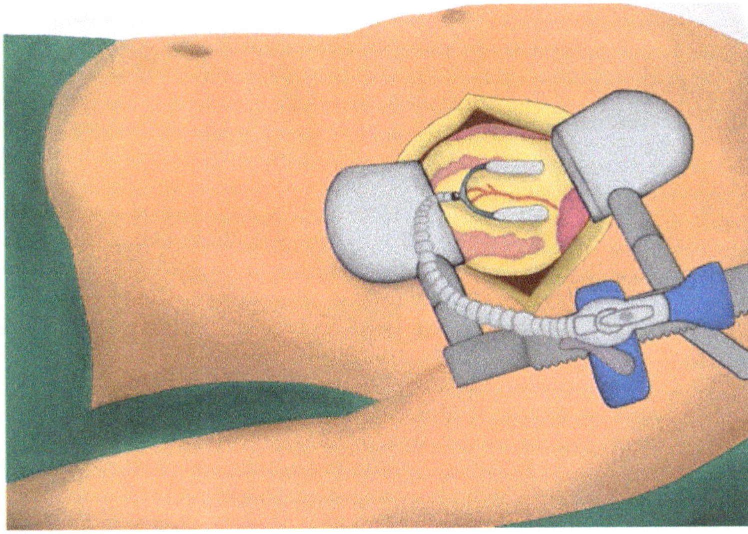

Figure 2. Left thoracotomy for MIDCABG with a heart stabilising device.

7.1.4. Evidence

Patel et al. published the best evidence on this topic by comparing MIDCABG and PCIs for patients with isolated LAD disease in 2014 [44]. They looked at 13 studies and concluded that both are effective treatments. The PCI has higher rates of need for reintervention for symptom recurrence. Despite having a higher upfront cost, MIDCABG is more cost-effective due to the lower rate of reintervention. There was no significant difference in mortality between both groups.

In 2015, Raja et al. [45], on behalf of the Harefield Cardiac Outcomes Research Group, compared propensity score-matched patients undergoing MIDCABG versus full sternotomy revascularisation for isolated LAD disease, with 143 matched sets. In 2018, they compared the short- and long-term outcomes of MIDCABG versus full sternotomy off-pump LIMA to LAD anastomosis for isolated proximal LAD stenosis [46]. They looked at 668 patients, with 508 patients in the MIDCABG group and 160 patients in the full sternotomy off-pump group. The average operative time was significantly shorter in the full sternotomy group, 141 +/− 12 min in the median sternotomy group versus 177 +/− 32 min in the MIDCABG group, $p = 0.003$. There was no significant difference between both groups in terms of the short-term outcomes. The long-term mortality at a median follow-up of 12.95 +/− 0.45 years was 25% in the full sternotomy off-pump group compared to 22.24% in the MIDCABG group, $p = 0.64$.

A study by Repossini et al. in 2019 [47] looked at 1060 patients undergoing MIDCABG, 646 of which had isolated proximal LAD disease and the rest had multivessel disease managed either with HCR or MIDCABG and optimal medical therapy. The reported survival was 92.1 +/− 4.6% at 5 years and 85.3 +/− 6.3% at 15 years, with an overall perioperative mortality of 0.8%.

Manuel et al. [48] recently published their 20-year outcomes of MIDCABG surgery in patients undergoing LIMA to LAD anastomosis. Their cohort consisted of 271 patients—the overall survival was 91.9%, 84.7%, 71.3%, and 56.5% at 5, 10, 15, and 20 years, respectively, with patients with isolated LAD disease doing significantly better than patients with multivessel disease ($p = 0.0035$). There were no patients who required reintervention on the LAD post-operatively.

Ultimately, there are no robust RCTs comparing MIDCABG and PCIs or MIDCABG and conventional CABG via a median sternotomy, and this presents a gap in the literature.

7.2. TECABG/RACABG

7.2.1. Description

TECABG is currently the least invasive form of surgical coronary artery revascularisation. It is performed via a few port sites, occasionally using a remotely controlled robotic system. Robotic-assisted TECABG can be further divided into three surgical techniques: TECABG without CPB, TECABG with CPB, and robotic-assisted LIMA harvest followed by off-pump LIMA to LAD manual anastomosis. Other options also include a video-assisted LIMA harvest, followed by manual LIMA to LAD anastomosis via a small anterior mini-thoracotomy.

7.2.2. Positioning and Monitoring

The position of the patient depends on the approach. If the procedure is performed without robotic assistance and by using video thoracoscopic assistance, the patient is placed in a left lateral decubitus position, 30–60 degrees from the horizontal line with the arm above their head [49]. If robotic-assisted TECABG is performed, the patient is placed supine with the left side elevated to 30 degrees and the left arm tucked in at the side [50,51].

Defibrillation pads are plated on the patient pre-operatively. Monitoring is similar to MIDCABG.

7.2.3. Operative Steps

TECABG is performed with the help of video-assisted thoracoscopy (VATS) or robot-assisted thoracoscopy (RATS). A controlled pneumothorax is induced using carbon dioxide insufflation. This can help create a visual field without one-lung ventilation. However, sometimes, one-lung ventilation may be required, in which case either a double-lumen endotracheal tube or a bronchial blocker can be used. The LIMA and/or RIMA can both be harvested from the left chest using VATS or RATS instruments via ports in the second, third, and fourth intercostal spaces, approximately 2 cm above and below the anterior axillary line, triangulating towards the mediastinum (Figure 3). However, the port placement can be changed depending on the surgeon, patient body habitus, and position of the target vessels. The patient is then heparinised, and the distal ends of the mammary arteries are transected. The pericardium is opened longitudinally, anterior to the left phrenic nerve, and all target vessels are identified and correlated with angiographic findings. Once the target vessels are identified and located, a 3–4 cm port is created directly above the heart close to the midline in the selected intercostal space. CPB can be instituted peripherally via the femoral vessels. A pledgeted purse-string suture for antegrade cardioplegia is inserted in the ascending aorta. After decompression of the right atrium on CPB, an endoscopic transthoracic clamp is inserted in the second right intercostal space in the anterior axillary line and placed across the ascending aorta. Cardioplegia is then delivered in an antegrade fashion via an endoscopically placed vent needle in the proximal ascending aorta. It should be noted in cases of robotic-assisted TECABG, aortic occlusion in on-pump procedures can also be achieved using an endovascular occluding balloon placed and inflated in the ascending aorta under transoesophageal ultrasound guidance. If the procedure is being carried out off-pump, one of the ports is used to insert tissue-stabilising devices. In procedures where only the LIMA harvest is performed using the robotic system, once the LIMA is harvested, the robot is undocked, and the remainder of the procedure is performed, as per MIDCABG. Pericardial stay sutures, epicardial stay sutures, or gentle traction of the emptied heart through a small subxiphoid incision can help visualise the target vessels to facilitate anastomosis. In cases where the remainder of the procedure is performed using the MIDCABG technique, the heart is positioned close to the utility port in the fourth intercostal space close to the midline, and the anastomosis is performed manually. If the robotic system is being used for the distal anastomoses as well, the pericardium is opened, and the robotic arms are used to manipulate the heart and perform the anastomosis, which is described in detail by Bonatti et al. [50] and Lee et al. in 2012 [52]. Y-grafts to the LIMA are generally used for the non-LAD vessels to avoid aortic manipulation. Alternatively, saphenous vein grafts can be sutured to the axillary artery prior to performing the distal anastomosis—they are endoscopically transferred into the left pleural space through an opening next to the LIMA harvest site. After all anastomoses are completed, haemostasis is performed, and the heparin is reversed with protamine. The pericardium is closed using interrupted sutures apart from channels for the LIMA and/or RIMA. Drains are placed in each intra-thoracic cavity. Ports are closed in a standard fashion, in layers [53].

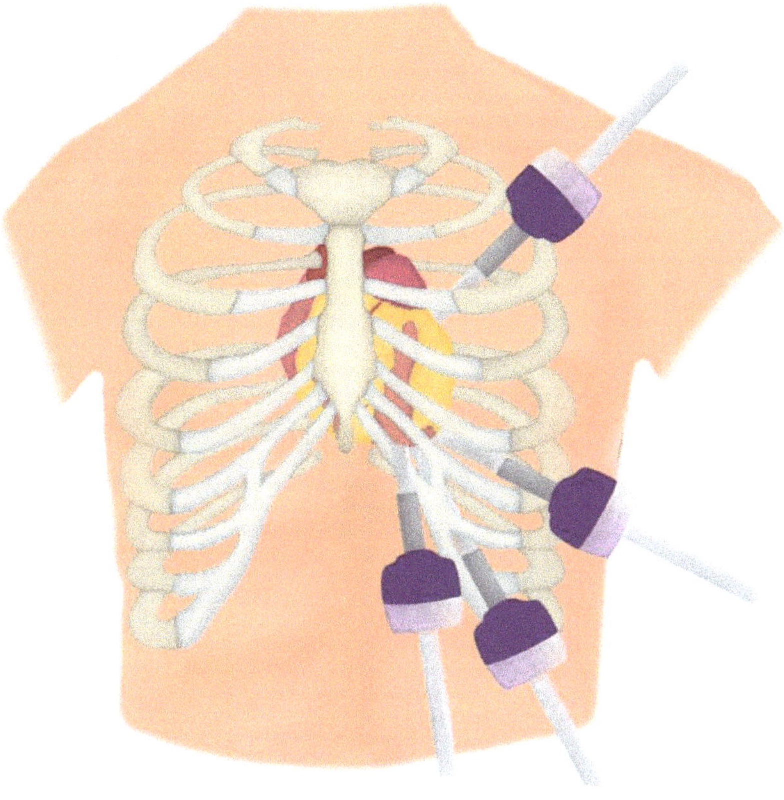

Figure 3. Example of port positions for TECABG—the ports are placed in such a way as to triangulate to the mediastinum, bearing in mind the patient's body habitus and target vessels.

7.2.4. Evidence

There has been no RCT comparing the different types of TECABG and comparing TECABG to conventional CABG.

A systematic review by Cao et al. [54] included 44 studies and a total of 8034 patients and revealed a pooled perioperative mortality rate of 1.7% and 1.0% after off-pump TECAB and robotic-assisted MIDCABG groups, bearing in mind that in the majority of studies, the number of anastomoses was relatively few and patients were relatively young, with a mean age of 60 and good pre-operative left ventricular function, with a mean ejection fraction of more than 55%. Unfortunately, long-term survival was not available due to limited follow-up rates in the included studies.

Although there have been no RCTs comparing outcomes of conventional CABG and TECABG, a study by Kofler et al. 2017 [55] compared 134 propensity score-matched pairs of conventional CABG and robotic TECABG. The primary endpoints were long-term survival and freedom from major adverse cardiac and cerebral events (MACCEs). There was no significant difference in the primary endpoints between both groups at 1, 5, and 10 years.

The survival at 1, 5, and 10 years was 99.3%, 96.9%, and 81.3%, respectively, in the robotic group versus 96.3%, 92.2%, and 82.6% in the conventional group, $p = 0.960$. Freedom from MACCE in the robotic group at 1, 5, and 10 years was 97.6%, 96.8%, and 96.8%, respectively, versus 100%, 97.7%, and 92.8% in the conventional group, $p = 0.790$. Of note, robotic TECABG had significantly longer CPB times (robotic 112 +/− 100 min versus conventional 67 +/− 48 min, $p < 0.001$) and cross-clamp times (robotic 68 +/− 54 min versus 38 +/− 27 min in the conventional group, $p < 0.001$.)

A meta-analysis by Leonard et al. in 2018 looking at the outcomes of TECABG including 17 studies and 3721 patients demonstrated that TECABG has acceptably low operative risk [56], but there was a severe dearth of data to confidently recommend TECABG. The pooled operative mortality for 3676 patients was 0.8% with a 95% CI of 0.6–1.2%. The pooled perioperative myocardial infarction event rate for 2556 patients was 2.28% with a 95% CI of 1.7–3%. The overall pooled graft patency rate was 94.8%. The pooled event rate for perioperative stroke was 1.5% with a 95% CI of 1.1–1% with 3353 patients being included.

Gobolos et al. [57] published a systematic review of the clinical outcomes of TECABG over the last 20 years in 2019. The pooled results included 2397 cases and reported a perioperative mortality of 0.8%, with conversion rates of 11.5% and an average surgical time of 291 +/− 57 min. Comparing beating heart TECABG (BH-TECABG) and arrested heart TECABG (AH-TECABG) revealed perioperative mortality of nearly 1% for BH-TECABG and 0.6% for AH-TECABG.

Similarly, a meta-analysis in 2020 by Hammal et al. looking specifically at robotic TECABG and 13 studies and reported that although robotic coronary artery surgery was feasible and certainly an appealing alternative to conventional surgery [58], the level of evidence was too low to make any significant conclusions regarding the benefit of robotic TECABG over conventional CABG in terms of short- and long-term outcomes including perioperative mortality, long-term survival, perioperative stroke, perioperative or late MI, and the rate of revascularisation. The data were too heterogenous to compare pooled event rates between robotic TECABG and conventional CABG.

7.3. HCR

7.3.1. Definition

CABG remains the guideline-recommended management option for many patients with multivessel coronary artery disease and has superior long-term survival rates [59]. It has been posited that the superiority of CABG lies with the LIMA to LAD anastomosis [60]. For non-LAD lesions, the PCI potentially confers similar long-term results as saphenous vein grafts. This principle forms the basis of hybrid minimal-access surgery, where LIMA to LAD anastomosis is performed by minimal-access surgery, and the other lesions are managed percutaneously [61].

Hybrid coronary artery revascularisation combines the prognostic benefit of LIMA to LAD anastomosis through minimal-access surgery with the advantages of less pain, decreased length of hospital stays, and the ability to continue dual antiplatelet agents that the PCI confers [62,63]. While it is difficult to specify a target patient population owing to the lack of RCT evidence, the ideal patient would be a high-risk surgical patient with complex or non-stentable LAD lesions who would reap the benefits of LIMA to LAD anastomosis with concurrent stentable non-LAD lesions.

There are three options for HCR: simultaneous revascularisation in a hybrid theatre, surgery followed by PCIs, or PCIs followed by surgery [64,65]. The latter option could follow such an example, where the culprit artery causing an infarct is a non-LAD artery that can be stented, perhaps acutely, with concurrent LAD lesions requiring surgery performed soon thereafter. Whether the surgery is performed via MIDCABG or TECABG is up to the heart team and the institution's experience.

7.3.2. Evidence

The POL-MIDES (HYBRID) trial in 2014 published by Gasior et al. randomided 200 patients with multivessel disease to undergo either HCR ($n = 98$) or CABG ($n = 100$). The primary endpoint was evaluating the feasibility of HCR, which was defined as the percentage of patients who had a completely hybrid approach with LIMA to LAD followed by PCIs with drug-eluting stents. A total of 93.9% of the patients randomised in the HCR group had a complete hybrid procedure, with 6.1% converting to a standard CABG. The secondary endpoints were post-procedure and angiographic measurements of the graft patency and restenosis rates at 12 months, among others. The mortality from CABG was 2.9% compared to 2% in the HCR group, $p = 0.1$. HCR had a higher HYBRID patency score (free of stenosis/occlusions grafted or ratio of stented arteries to the total number of grafted and stented arteries) at 90% compared to 81% in the CABG group, $p = 0.01$ [26].

In 2019, Ganyukov et al., in the Hybrid coronary REvascularisation Versus Stenting or Surgery (HREVS) prospective randomised safety and efficacy study compared conventional CABG ($n = 50$), HCR ($n = 52$), or multivessel PCIs ($n = 53$), with residual ischaemia as their primary endpoint. They concluded that the percentage of ischaemic myocardium in CABG, HCR, and PCIs was 6.7% (95% CI 4.6–8.8%), 6.4% (95% CI 4.3–8.5%), and 7.9% (95% CI 5.9–9.8%), respectively, $p = 0.45$. The rates of MACCE, one of their secondary endpoints, in CABG, HCR, and PCIs were 12%, 13.4%, and 13.2%, respectively, $p = 0.83$. The main limitation quoted was that the study was severely underpowered and, therefore, not conclusive [66].

In 2020, Esteves et al. published their results of a pilot RCT, the myocardial hybrid revascularization versus coronary artery bypass GraftING (MERGING study) for complex triple-vessel disease comparing HCR to conventional CABG, with 40 patients in the hybrid arm and 20 patients in the conventional CABG arm. They concluded that HCR, while feasible, was associated with higher rates of MACCE defined as all-cause death, stroke, MI, and unplanned revascularisation during the first 2 years as compared to conventional surgery, with a 19.3% MACCE rate at 2 years in the HCR group versus a 5.9% MACCE rate in the conventional group [67].

Guan et al. in 2019 [29] published a meta-analysis comparing other modalities of minimal-access CABG with HCR, which summarised eight observational studies and concluded that HCR was non-inferior to other modalities of minimal-access CABG, in terms of in-hospital mortality, rates of MACCE, shock, perioperative MI, long-term survival, cost, and surgical complications. On the other hand, Nagraj et al. in 2022 concluded in their meta-analysis of twelve observational studies and two RCTs comparing HCR to conventional CABG via a median sternotomy in multivessel coronary artery disease that although feasible, HCR did not have any clear benefits over conventional surgery [68].

Dixon et al. in 2022 [69] published a systematic review and meta-analysis comparing HCR and CABG for multivessel coronary artery disease. Their analysis included 16 studies and concluded that HCR had comparable outcomes to CABG in terms of mid-term survival and rates of MACCE, but patients had a shorter ITU stay and decreased need for blood transfusion. This did not translate into better short-term outcomes of HCR compared to CABG, with a higher incidence of short-term mortality in the HCR group (0.73% versus 0.64% in the CABG group). However, it should be mentioned that the results reported in the HCR group had a much wider confidence interval, indicating a lack of statistical power. Therefore, they were unable to definitely conclude any advantage of HCR over CABG or vice versa. Table 2 summarises some of the major studies regarding minimal access surgical coronary artery revascularisation.

Table 2. Summary of major studies (>150 patients) looking at the outcomes of minimal-access coronary revascularisation ((-) means that the data were not reported by the authors).

Authors	Surgical Technique	Patients	Retrospective vs. Prospective	Survival	Follow-Up/Months	Sternotomy Conversion	Peri-Op Stroke	LOS	Number of Grafts	Complete Revascularisation	LIMA–LAD Patency	Repeat Revascularisation
McGinn et al. (2009) [35]	MIDCABG	450	Retrospective	98.7%	1	3.8%	0.4%	5.9 +/− 3.4	2.1 +/− 0.7	95%	-	2.7%
Lapierre et al. (2011) [70]	MIDCABG	150	Retrospective	100.0%	3	6.7%	0.0%	5.0	1.8 +/− 0.7	100%	-	3.3%
Zianku et al. (2015) [71]	MIDCABG	151	Retrospective	99.3%	40.3	2.7%	0.0%	4.5	2.9 +/− 0.5	100%	100.0%	-
Rodriguez et al. (2017) [72]	MIDCABG	306	Retrospective	100.0%	33.6	3.3%	0.0%	5.8 +/− 5.5	1.8 +/− 0.7	93%	-	6.9%
Nambiar et al. (2019) [73]	MIDCABG	940	Retrospective	99.1%	2.9	0.6%	0.2%	3.1 +/− 1.2	3.2	97.90%	99.80%	1.1%
Bonaros et al. (2013) [74]	TECABG	500	Retrospective	99.0%	120	10.0%	9.0%	6.0	-	-	90–95%	-
Weldinger et al. (2014) [75]	TECABG	384	Retrospective	99.2%	60	14.0%	1.8%	7.0	-	-	-	-
Kitahara et al. (2018) [76]	TECABG	263	Retrospective	98.5%	1	3.0%	0.0%	3.5 +/− 2.9	-	-	-	-
Repossini et al. (2013) [77]	HCR with MIDCABG	166	Retrospective	95.8%	54	2.4%	N/A	6.5	-	Functionally complete 100%, anatomically incomplete 16.9%	100% before PCI	7.2%
Halkos et al. (2014) [78]	HCR with RA-MIDCABG	300	Retrospective	98.7%	1	2.0%	1.0%	5.0	-	-	97.60%	4.3%
Puskas et al. (2016) [79]	HCR (variable)	200	Prospective	98.5%	1.5 years	0.5%	0.0%	-	-	75.20%	-	7.0%

8. Nomenclatures

The large variation in the nomenclature used to describe minimal-access surgical techniques for coronary artery revascularization renders the interpretation of the literature challenging and makes comparisons of the different techniques challenging. Just to name a few, the terms MIDCABG, MICS CABG, TECABG, AH-TECABG [80], PA CABG [81], and RACABG have all been used to describe various minimal-access cardiac surgery. Some of these terms are used interchangeably by some authors but considered distinct by others. For example, some papers claim that MIDCABG and MICS CABG are completely different modalities, while others use the terms interchangeably. Similarly, some papers consider TECABG and RACABG to be distinct modalities, while some authors describe, in detail, how they use either VATS or RATS to perform TECABG. We would posit that the standardization of terms is an imperative step to allow robust comparison of minimal-access techniques, be it as compared to each other or conventional CABG.

9. Future Perspectives

Minimal-access techniques are gaining popularity in all areas of surgery. The number of cardiac surgical centres with access to minimal-access techniques and surgical robots is continuously increasing. Mitral valve surgery is a particularly hot area for minimal-access surgery—and the publication of the results of the UK Mini Mitral Trial is eagerly awaited. For coronary revascularization, it is important that these new techniques are cautiously adopted and experience is accumulated. For this, large RCTs are required to develop the evidence base to support the use of these techniques and demonstrate conclusively that they are beneficial to patient outcomes. Demonstrating this through trials will be essential to gaining wider adoption of these techniques and for some, the ability to justify the expense of the technology to hospital management.

Thankfully, there are trials ongoing. For example, the Minimally Invasive Coronary Surgery Compared to STernotomy Coronary Artery Bypass Grafting RCT (MIST trial) is an upcoming prospective RCT. It compares the outcomes of minimal-access coronary revascularization to conventional CABG [82]. The primary outcome is the quality of life using the physical function score of the Short Form Health Survey (SF-36) four weeks after surgery. Secondary outcomes include MACCE and target vessel revascularisation at 1 year after surgery, the number of bypass grafts, the percentage of arterial graft use, the use of transfusion intra-operatively and post-operatively, the rates of re-exploration for bleeding, post-operative pain, duration of intubation, length of stay in the intensive care unit, length of hospital stay, the rates of post-operative atrial fibrillation and wound infection, and post-operative angina and quality of life in terms of mental health. It is currently still in the enrolment phase and is projected to be completed primarily in March 2024.

10. Conclusions

Minimal-access surgery is becoming increasingly popular and may become the future. It is increasingly demanded by referring cardiologists and also patients who perceive the surgery to be superior. Minimal-access coronary artery revascularization represents a very appealing management approach to coronary artery disease. It incorporates the benefits of surgical revascularization with some of the advantages of off-pump surgery and PCIs with less pain, shorter hospital stays, earlier mobilization, and earlier return to work for patients. However, the challenge is to ensure that the benefits of surgical revascularization with complete revascularization and patency of grafts remain uncompromised by using a minimal-access approach. Given the paucity of RCTs regarding methods of minimal-access coronary artery revascularization, it is challenging to make any robust recommendations. Part of this comes from the large variation in the nomenclature of the methods of minimal-access coronary artery revascularization and the very slow uptake of minimal-access methods across different surgical units.

Author Contributions: Conceptualization, J.A.; methodology, R.P.; writing—original draft preparation, R.P. and T.W.; writing—review and editing, R.P., T.W. and J.A.; supervision, J.A. All authors have read and agreed to the published version of the manuscript.

Funding: This review received no external funding.

Institutional Review Board Statement: Not applicable.

Informed Consent Statement: Not applicable.

Data Availability Statement: Not applicable.

Conflicts of Interest: The authors declare no conflict of interest.

Abbreviations

AH-TECABG	Totally Endoscopic Arrested Heart Coronary Artery Bypass Grafting
CABG	Coronary Artery Bypass Grafting
CPB	Cardiopulmonary bypass
HCR	Hybrid Coronary Revascularisation
LAD	Left Anterior Descending Artery
LIMA	Left Internal Mammary Artery
MICS CABG	Minimally Invasive Coronary Artery Bypass Grafting
MIDCABG	Minimally invasive Coronary Artery Bypass Grafting
PA CABG	Port-Access Coronary Artery Bypass Grafting
RACABG	Robotic-Assisted Coronary Artery Bypass Grafting
RATS	Robot-Assisted Thoracoscopic Surgery
RCT	Randomised Control Trial
RIMA	right Internal Mammary Artery
TECABG	Totally Endoscopic Coronary Artery Bypass Grafting
VATS	Video-Assisted Thoracoscopic Surgery

References

1. Carrel, A., VIII. On the Experimental Surgery of the Thoracic Aorta and Heart. *Ann. Surg.* **1910**, *52*, 83–95. [CrossRef] [PubMed]
2. Melly, L.; Torregrossa, G.; Lee, T.; Jansens, J.-L.; Puskas, J.D. Fifty years of coronary artery bypass grafting. *J. Thorac. Dis.* **2018**, *10*, 1960–1967. [PubMed]
3. Diodato, M.; Chedrawy, E.G. Coronary artery bypass graft surgery: The past, present, and future of myocardial revascularisation. *Surg. Res. Pract.* **2014**, *2014*, 726158. [PubMed]
4. Vineberg, A.; Miller, G. Internal mammary coronary anastomosis in the surgical treatment of coronary artery insufficiency. *Can. Med. Assoc. J.* **1951**, *64*, 204–210.
5. Thomas, J.L. The Vineberg legacy: Internal mammary artery implantation from inception to obsolescence. *Tex. Heart Inst. J.* **1999**, *26*, 107–113.
6. Rozsival, V. Outcome of Vineberg's operation after 31 years. *Heart* **2006**, *92*, 1070. [CrossRef]
7. Sabiston, D.C., Jr. The William F. Rienhoff, Jr. lecture. The coronary circulation. *Johns Hopkins Med. J.* **1974**, *134*, 314–329.
8. Goetz, R.H.; Rohman, M.; Haller, J.D.; Dee, R.; Rosenak, S.S. Internal mammary-coronary artery anastomosis. A nonsuture method employing tantalum rings. *J. Thorac. Cardiovasc. Surg.* **1961**, *41*, 378–386.
9. Bailey, C.P.; May, A.; Lemmon, W.M. Survival after coronary endarterectomy in man. *J. Am. Med. Assoc.* **1957**, *164*, 641–646. [CrossRef]
10. Sones, F.M., Jr.; Shirey, E.K. Cine coronary arteriography. *Mod. Concepts Cardiovasc. Dis.* **1962**, *31*, 735–738.
11. Garrett, H.E.; Dennis, E.W.; DeBakey, M.E. Aortocoronary bypass with saphenous vein graft. Seven-year follow-up. *JAMA* **1973**, *223*, 792–794. [CrossRef] [PubMed]
12. Kolessov, V.I. Mammary artery-coronary artery anastomosis as method of treatment for angina pectoris. *J. Thorac. Cardiovasc. Surg.* **1967**, *54*, 535–544. [PubMed]
13. Green, G.E.; Stertzer, S.H.; Reppert, E.H. Coronary arterial bypass grafts. *Ann. Thorac. Surg.* **1968**, *5*, 443–450. [CrossRef] [PubMed]
14. Favaloro, R.G. Saphenous vein autograft replacement of severe segmental coronary artery occlusion: Operative technique. *Ann. Thorac. Surg.* **1968**, *5*, 334–339. [CrossRef]
15. Marti, M.C.; Bouchardy, B.; Cox, J.N. Aorto-coronary by-pass with autogenous saphenous vein grafts: Histopathological aspects. *Virchows Arch. A Pathol. Pathol. Anat.* **1971**, *352*, 255–266. [CrossRef]
16. Cuminetti, G.; Gelsomino, S.; Curello, S.; Lorusso, R.; Maessen, J.G.; Hoorntje, J.C.A. Contemporary use of arterial and venous conduits in coronary artery bypass grafting: Anatomical, functional and clinical aspects. *Neth. Heart J.* **2017**, *25*, 4–13. [CrossRef]

17. Carpentier, A.; Guermonprez, J.L.; Deloche, A.; Frechette, C.; DuBost, C. The aorta-to-coronary radial artery bypass graft. A technique avoiding pathological changes in grafts. *Ann. Thorac. Surg.* **1973**, *16*, 111–121. [CrossRef]
18. Acar, C.; Jebara, V.A.; Portoghese, M.; Beyssen, B.; Pagny, J.Y.; Grare, P.; Chachques, J.C.; Fabiani, J.N.; Deloche, A.; Guermonprez, J.L. Revival of the radial artery for coronary artery bypass grafting. *Ann. Thorac. Surg.* **1992**, *54*, 652–659, discussion 659–660. [CrossRef]
19. Acar, C.; Ramsheyi, A.; Pagny, J.Y.; Jebara, V.; Barrier, P.; Fabiani, J.N.; Deloche, A.; Guermonprez, J.L.; Carpentier, A. The radial artery for coronary artery bypass grafting: Clinical and angiographic results at five years. *J. Thorac. Cardiovasc. Surg.* **1998**, *116*, 981–989. [CrossRef]
20. Loop, F.D.; Lytle, B.W.; Cosgrove, D.M.; Stewart, R.W.; Goormastic, M.; Williams, G.W.; Golding, L.A.; Gill, C.C.; Taylor, P.C.; Sheldon, W.C.; et al. Influence of the internal-mammary-artery graft on 10-year survival and other cardiac events. *N. Engl. J. Med.* **1986**, *314*, 1–6. [CrossRef]
21. Gruntzig, A. Transluminal dilatation of coronary-artery stenosis. *Lancet* **1978**, *1*, 263. [CrossRef]
22. Calafiore, A.M.; Giammarco, G.D.; Teodori, G.; Bosco, G.; D'Annunzio, E.; Barsotti, A.; Maddestra, N.; Paloscia, L.; Vitolla, G.; Sciarra, A.; et al. Left anterior descending coronary artery grafting via left anterior small thoracotomy without cardiopulmonary bypass. *Ann. Thorac. Surg.* **1996**, *61*, 1658–1663. discussion 1664–1665.
23. Fann, J.I.; Burdon, T.A.; Pompili, M.F. Minimally invasive cardiac surgery using the HEARTPORT technique. *Asia Pac. Heart J.* **1999**, *8*, 19–26. [CrossRef]
24. Loulmet, D.; Carpentier, A.; d'Attellis, N.; Berrebi, A.; Cardon, C.; Ponzio, O.; Aupecle, B.; Relland, J.Y. Endoscopic coronary artery bypass grafting with the aid of robotic assisted instruments. *J. Thorac. Cardiovasc. Surg.* **1999**, *118*, 4–10. [CrossRef] [PubMed]
25. Neumann, F.-J.; Sousa-Uva, M.; Ahlsson, A.; Alfonso, F.; Banning, A.P.; Benedetto, U.; Byrne, R.A.; Colet, J.; Falk, V.; Head, S.J.; et al. 2018 ESC/EACTS Guidelines on myocardial revascularization. *Eur. Heart J.* **2018**, *40*, 87–165.
26. Gasior, M.; Zembala, M.O.; Tajstra, M.; Filipiak, K.; Gierlotka, M.; Hrapkowicz, T.; Hawranek, M.; Polonski, L.; Zembala, M.; POL-MIDES (HYBRID) Investigators. Hybrid revascularization for multivessel coronary artery disease. *JACC Cardiovasc. Interv.* **2014**, *7*, 1277–1283. [PubMed]
27. Tajstra, M.; Hrapkowicz, T.; Hawranek, M.; Filipiak, K.; Gierlotka, M.; Zembala, M.; Gasior, M.; Zembala, M.O. Hybrid coronary revascularization in selected patients with Multivessel disease. *JACC Cardiovasc. Interv.* **2018**, *11*, 847–852. [PubMed]
28. Lawton, J.S.; Tamis-Holland, J.E.; Bangalore, S.; Bates, E.R.; Beckie, T.M.; Bischoff, J.M.; Bittl, J.A.; Gohen, M.G.; DiMaio, J.M.; Don, C.W.; et al. 2021 ACC/AHA/SCAI guideline for Coronary artery revascularization: A report of the american college of cardiology/american heart association joint committee on clinical practice guidelines. *Circulation* **2022**, *145*, e4–e17. [PubMed]
29. Guan, Z.; Zhang, Z.; Gu, K.; Wang, H.; Lin, J.; Zhou, W.; Wan, F. Minimally invasive CABG or hybrid coronary revascularization for Multivessel Coronary Diseases: Which is best? A systematic review and metaanalysis. *Heart Surg. Forum* **2019**, *22*, E493–E502.
30. Misfeld, M.; Brereton, R.J.; Sweetman, E.A.; Doig, G.S. Neurologic complications after off-pump coronary artery bypass grafting with and without aortic manipulation: Meta-analysis of 11,398 cases from 8 studies. *J. Thorac. Cardiovasc. Surg.* **2011**, *142*, e11–e17.
31. Czerny, M.; Baumer, H.; Kilo, J.; Lassnigg, A.; Hamwi, A.; Vukovich, T.; Wolner, E.; Grimm, M. Inflammatory response and myocardial injury following coronary artery bypass grafting with or without cardiopulmonary bypass. *Eur. J. Cardiothorac. Surg.* **2000**, *17*, 737–742. [PubMed]
32. Shroyer, A.L.; Hattler, B.; Wagner, T.H.; Collins, J.F.; Baltz, J.H.; Quin, J.A.; Hossein Almassi, G.; Kozora, E.; Bakaeen, F.; Cleveland, J.C., Jr.; et al. Five-year outcomes after on-pump and off-pump coronary-artery bypass. *N. Engl. J. Med.* **2017**, *377*, 623–632. [PubMed]
33. Diegeler, A.; Walther, T.; Metz, S.; Falk, V.; Krakor, R.; Autschbach, R.; Mohr, F.W. Comparison of MIDCAB versus conventional CABG surgery regarding pain and quality of life. *Heart Surg. Forum* **1999**, *2*, 290–295. [PubMed]
34. Garg, S.; Raja, S.G. Minimally invasive direct coronary artery bypass (MIDCAB) grafting. *AME Med. J.* **2020**, *5*, 19.
35. McGinn, J.T.; Usman, S.; Lapierre, H.; Pothula, V.R.; Mesana, T.G.; Ruel, M. Minimally invasive coronary artery bypass grafting. *Circulation* **2009**, *120* (Suppl. 1), S78–S84. [PubMed]
36. Subramanian, V.A. Midcab approach for Single Vessel Coronary Artery Bypass Graft. *Oper. Tech. Card. Thorac. Surg.* **1998**, *3*, 2–15. [CrossRef]
37. Ruel, M. Nonsternotomy multivessel coronary artery bypass grafting: A key development in cardiac surgery. *J. Thorac. Cardiovasc. Surg. Tech.* **2021**, *10*, 162–167.
38. Bonatti, J.; Schachner, T.; Bonaros, N.; Oehlinger, A.; Ruetzler, E.; Friedrich, G.; Feuchner, G.; Laufer, G. How to improve performance of robotic totally endoscopic coronary artery bypass grafting. *Am. J. Surg.* **2008**, *195*, 711–716.
39. Ruel, M.; Shariff, M.A.; Lapierre, H.; Goyal, N.; Dennie, C.; Sadel, S.M.; Sohmer, B.; McGinn, J.T., Jr. Results of the minimally invasive coronary artery bypass grafting angiographic patency study. *J. Thorac. Cardiovasc. Surg.* **2014**, *147*, 203–209.
40. Bonatti, J.; Schachner, T.; Bernecker, O.; Chevtchik, O.; Bonaros, N.; Ott, H.; Friedrich, G.; Weidiner, F.; Laufer, G. Robotic totally endoscopic coronary artery bypass: Program development and learning curve issues. *J. Thorac. Cardiovasc. Surg.* **2004**, *127*, 504–510.
41. Van Praet, K.M.; Kofler, M.; Nazari Shafti, T.Z.; El Al, A.A.; van Kampen, A.; Amabile, A.; Torregrossa, G.; Kempfert, J.; Falk, V.; Balkhy, H.H.; et al. Minimally invasive coronary revascularisation surgery: A focused review of the available literature. *Interv. Cardiol. Rev.* **2021**, *16*, e08.

42. Ruel, M. Commentary: Sternotomy for every cardiac surgery patient ain't the future, so let's get going. *J. Thorac. Cardiovasc. Surg.* **2023**, *165*, 129–131. [PubMed]
43. Greenspu, H.G.; Adourian, U.A.; Fonger, J.D.; Fan, J.S. Minimally invasive direct coronary artery bypass (MIDCAB): Surgical techniques and anesthetic considerations. *J. Cardiothorac. Vasc. Anes.* **1996**, *10*, 507–509.
44. Patel, A.J.; Yates, M.T.; Soppa, G.K. What is the optimal revascularization technique for isolated disease of the left anterior descending artery: Minimally invasive direct coronary artery bypass or percutaneous coronary intervention? *Interact. Cardiovasc. Thorac. Surg.* **2014**, *19*, 144–148. [CrossRef]
45. Raja, S.G.; Benedetto, U.; Alkizwini, E.; Gupta, S.; Amrani, M.; Harefield Cardiac Outcomes Research Group. Propensity Score Adjusted Comparison of MIDCAB Versus Full Sternotomy Left Anterior Descending Artery Revascularization. *Innovations* **2015**, *10*, 174–178. [CrossRef]
46. Raja, S.G.; Garg, S.; Rochon, M.; Daley, S.; De Robertis, F.; Bahrami, T. Short-term clinical outcomes and long-term survival of minimally invasive direct coronary artery bypass grafting. *Ann. Cardiothorac. Surg.* **2018**, *7*, 621–627. [CrossRef] [PubMed]
47. Repossini, A.; Di Bacco, L.; Nicoli, F.; Passaretti, B.; Stara, A.; Jonida, B.; Muneretto, C. Minimally invasive coronary artery bypass: Twenty-year experience. *J. Thorac. Cardiovasc. Surg.* **2019**, *158*, 127–138.e1. [CrossRef]
48. Manuel, L.; Fong, L.S.; Betts, K.; Bassin, L.; Wolfenden, H. LIMA to LAD grafting returns patient survival to age-matched population: 20-year outcomes of MIDCAB surgery. *Interact. Cardiovasc. Thorac. Surg.* **2022**, *35*, ivac243. [CrossRef]
49. Benetti, F.J.; Ballester, C.; Sani, G.; Doonstra, P.; Grandjean, J. Video assisted coronary bypass surgery. *J. Card. Surg.* **1995**, *10*, 620–625. [CrossRef]
50. Bonatti, J.; Wehman, B.; de Biasi, A.R.; Jeudy, J.; Griffith, B.; Lehr, E.J. Totally endoscopic quadruple coronary artery bypass grafting is feasible using robotic technology. *Ann. Thorac. Surg.* **2012**, *93*, e111–e112. [CrossRef]
51. Balkhy, H.H. Robotic totally endoscopic coronary artery bypass grafting: It's now or never! *JTCVS Tech.* **2021**, *10*, 153–157. [CrossRef]
52. Lee, J.D.; Srivastava, M.; Bonatti, J. History and current status of robotic totally endoscopic coronary artery bypass. *Circ. J.* **2012**, *76*, 2058–2065. [CrossRef]
53. Yilmaz, A.; Robic, B.; Starinieri, P.; Polus, F.; Stinkens, R.; Stessel, B. A new viewpoint on endoscopic CABG: Technique description and clinical experience. *J. Cardiol.* **2020**, *75*, 614–620. [PubMed]
54. Cao, C.; Indraratna, P.; Doyle, M.; Tian, D.H.; Liou, K.; Munkholm-Larsen, S.; Uys, C.; Virk, S. A systematic review on robotic coronary artery bypass graft surgery. *Ann. Cardiothorac. Surg.* **2016**, *5*, 530–543. [CrossRef] [PubMed]
55. Kofler, M.; Stastny, L.; Reinstadler, S.; Dumfarth, J.; Kilo, J.; Friedrich, G.; Schachner, T.; Grimm, M.; Bonatti, J.; Bonaros, N. Robotic Versus Conventional Coronary Artery Bypass Grafting. Direct Comparison of Long-Term Clinical Outcome. *Innovations* **2017**, *12*, 239–246. [PubMed]
56. Leonard, J.R.; Rahouma, M.; Abouarab, A.A.; Schwann, A.N.; Scuderi, G.; Lau, C.; Guy, T.S.; Demetres, M.; Puskas, J.D.; Taggart, D.P.; et al. Totally endoscopic coronary artery bypass surgery: A meta-analysis of the current evidence. *Int. J. Cardiol.* **2018**, *261*, 42–46.
57. Göbölös, L.; Ramahi, J.; Obeso, A.; Bartel, T.; Hogan, M.; Traina, M.; Edris, A.; Hasasn, F.; El Banna, M.; Tuzcu, E.M.; et al. Robotic Totally Endoscopic Coronary Artery Bypass Grafting: Systematic Review of Clinical Outcomes from the Past two Decades. *Innovations* **2019**, *14*, 5–16. [CrossRef]
58. Hammal, F.; Nagase, F.; Menon, D.; Ali, I.; Nagendran, J.; Stafinski, T. Robot-assisted coronary artery bypass surgery: A systematic review and meta-analysis of comparative studies. *Can. J. Surg.* **2020**, *63*, E491.
59. Holm, N.R.; Mäkikallio, T.; Lindsay, M.M.; Spence, M.S.; Erglis, A.; Menown, I.B.; Trovik, T.; Kellerth, T.; Kalinaukas, G.; Mogensen, L.J.H.; et al. Percutaneous coronary angioplasty versus coronary artery bypass grafting in the treatment of unprotected left main stenosis: Updated 5-year outcomes from the randomised, non-inferiority Noble trial. *Lancet* **2020**, *395*, 191–199.
60. Kappetein, A.P.; Head, S.J. CABG, stents, or hybrid procedures for left main disease? *EuroIntervention* **2015**, *11* (Suppl. V), V111–V114.
61. Katz, M.R.; Van Praet, F.; de Canniere, D.; Murphy, D.; Siwek, L.; Seshadri-Kreaden, U.; Friedricj, G.; Bonatti, J. Integrated coronary revascularization: Percutaneous coronary intervention plus robotic totally endoscopic coronary artery bypass. *Circulation* **2006**, *114*, I473–I476. [CrossRef]
62. Deppe, A.-C.; Liakopoulos, O.J.; Kuhn, E.W.; Slottosch, I.; Scherner, M.; Choi, Y.-H.; Rahmanian, P.B.; Wahlers, T. Minimally invasive direct coronary bypass grafting versus percutaneous coronary intervention for single-vessel disease: A meta-analysis of 2885 patients. *Eur. J. Cardiothorac. Surg.* **2014**, *47*, 397–406. [PubMed]
63. Kiaii, B.; Teefy, P. Hybrid coronary artery revascularization: A review and current evidence. *Innov. Technol. Tech. Cardiothorac. Vasc. Surg.* **2019**, *14*, 394–404.
64. Saha, T.; Naqvi, S.Y.; Goldberg, S. Hybrid revascularization: A Review. *Cardiology* **2018**, *140*, 35–44. [PubMed]
65. Harskamp, R.E.; Zheng, Z.; Alexander, J.H.; Williams, J.B.; Xian, Y.; Halkos, M.E.; Brennan, J.M.; de Winter, R.J.; Smith, P.K.; Lopes, R.D. Status quo of hybrid coronary revascularization for multi-vessel coronary artery disease. *Ann. Thorac. Surg.* **2013**, *96*, 2268–2277.
66. Ganyukov, V.; Kochergin, N.; Shilov, A.; Tarasov, R.; Skupien, J.; Szot, W.; Kokov, A.; Popov, V.; Kozyrin, K.; Barbarash, O.; et al. Randomized clinical trial of surgical vs. Percutaneous vs. hybrid revascularization in multivessel coronary artery disease:

Residual myocardial ischemia and clinical outcomes at one year—Hybrid coronary revascularization versus stenting or surgery (HREVS). *J. Interv. Cardiol.* **2020**, *2020*, 5458064. [PubMed]
67. Esteves, V.; Oliveira, M.A.; Feitosa, F.S.; Mariani, J.; Campos, C.M.; Hajjar, L.A.; Lisboa, L.A.; Jatene, F.B.; Filho, R.K.; Lemos Neto, P.A. Late clinical outcomes of myocardial hybrid revascularization versus coronary artery bypass grafting for complex triple-vessel disease: Long-term follow-up of the randomized merging clinical trial. *Catheter. Cardiovasc. Interv.* **2020**, *97*, 259–264. [PubMed]
68. Nagraj, S.; Tzoumas, A.; Kakargias, F.; Giannopoulos, S.; Ntoumaziou, A.; Kokkinidis, D.G.; Villela, M.A.; Latib, A. Hybrid coronary revascularization (HCR) versus coronary artery bypass grafting (CABG) in multivessel coronary artery disease (MVCAD): A meta-analysis of 14 studies comprising 4226 patients. *Catheter. Cardiovasc. Interv.* **2022**, *100*, 1182–1194. [PubMed]
69. Dixon, L.K.; Akberali, U.; Di Tommaso, E.; George, S.J.; Johnson, T.W.; Bruno, V.D. Hybrid coronary revascularization versus coronary artery bypass grafting for Multivessel coronary artery disease: A systematic review and meta-analysis. *Int. J. Cardiol.* **2022**, *359*, 20–27. [CrossRef] [PubMed]
70. Lapierre, H.; Chan, V.; Sohmer, B. Minimally invasive coronary artery bypass grafting via a small thoracotomy versus off-pump: A case-matched study. *Eur. J. Cardiothorac. Surg.* **2011**, *40*, 804–810.
71. Ziankou, A.; Ostrovsky, Y. Early and midterm results of notouch aorta multivessel small thoracotomy coronary artery bypass grafting: A propensity score-matched study. *Innovations* **2015**, *10*, 258–267. [PubMed]
72. Rodriguez, M.L.; Lapierre, H.R.; Sohmer, B.F.; Ruel, M.A. Repeat revascularization after minimally invasive coronary artery bypass grafting: Is it a problem? *Innovations* **2017**, *12*, 269–274. [PubMed]
73. Nambiar, P.; Kumar, S.; Mittal, C.M.; Sarkar, I.C. Outcomes of bilateral internal thoracic arteries in minimally invasive coronary artery bypass grafting with analogy to the SYNTAX trial. *Innovations* **2019**, *14*, 227–235.
74. Bonaros, N.; Schachner, T.; Lehr, E.; Kofler, M.; Wiedemann, D.; Hong, P.; Wehman, B.; Zimrin, D.; Vesely, M.K.; Friedrich, G.; et al. Five hundred cases of robotic totally endoscopic coronary artery bypass grafting: Predictors of success and safety. *Ann. Thorac. Surg.* **2013**, *95*, 803–812. [PubMed]
75. Weidinger, F.; Schachner, T.; Bonaros, N.; Hofauer, B.; Lehr, E.J.; Vesely, M.; Zimrin, D.; Bonatti, J. Predictors and consequences of postoperative atrial fibrillation following robotic totally endoscopic coronary bypass surgery. *Eur. J. Cardiothorac. Surg.* **2014**, *45*, 318–322. [PubMed]
76. Kitahara, H.; McCrorey, M.; Patel, B.; Nisivaco, S.; Balkhy, H.H. Does robotic beating heart connector totally endoscopic coronary artery bypass bridge the gender gap in coronary bypass surgery? *Innovations* **2018**, *13*, 35–39. [PubMed]
77. Repossini, A.; Tespili, M.; Saino, A.; Kotelnikov, I.; Moggi, A.; Di Bacco, L.; Muneretto, C. Hybrid revascularization in multivessel coronary artery disease. *Eur. J. Cardiothorac. Surg.* **2013**, *44*, 288–294.
78. Halkos, M.E.; Walker, P.F.; Vassiliades, T.A.; Douglas, J.S.; Devireddy, C.; Guyton, R.A.; Finn, A.V.; Tanveer Rab, S.; Puskas, J.D.; Liberman, H.A. Clinical and angiographic results after hybrid coronary revascularization. *Ann. Thorac. Surg.* **2014**, *97*, 484–490.
79. Puskas, J.D.; Halkos, M.E.; DeRose, J.J.; Bagiella, E.; Miller, M.A.; Overbey, J.; Bonatti, J.; Srinivas, V.S.; Vesely, M.; Sutter, F.; et al. Hybrid coronary revascularization for the treatment of multivessel coronary artery disease: A multicenter observational study. *J. Am. Coll. Cardiol.* **2016**, *68*, 356–365.
80. Bonatti, J.; Schachner, T.; Bonaros, N.; Öhlinger, A.; Danzmayr, M.; Jonetzko, P.; Friedrich, G.; Kolbitsch, C.; Mair, P.; Laufer, G. Technical challenges in totally endoscopic robotic coronary artery bypass grafting. *J. Thorac. Cardiovasc. Surg.* **2006**, *131*, 146–153.
81. Groh, M.A.; Sutherland, S.E.; Burton, H.G.; Johnson, A.M.; Ely, S.W. Port-access coronary artery bypass grafting: Technique and comparative results. *Ann. Thorac. Surg.* **1999**, *68*, 1506–1508. [PubMed]
82. Guo, M.H.; Wells, G.A.; Glineur, D.; Fortier, J.; Davierwala, P.M.; Kikuchi, K.; Lemma, M.G.; Mishra, Y.K.; McGinn, J.; Ramchandani, M.; et al. Minimally invasive coronary surgery compared to sternotomy coronary artery bypass grafting: The MIST trial. *Contemp. Clin. Trials* **2019**, *78*, 140–145. [PubMed]

Journal of
Cardiovascular
Development and Disease

MDPI

Review

Minimal Access Aortic Valve Surgery

Bilal H. Kirmani [1,*] and Enoch Akowuah [2,3]

1 Department of Cardiothoracic Surgery, Liverpool Heart and Chest Hospital, Liverpool L14 3PE, UK
2 Cardiac Surgery, Faculty of Medical Sciences, Newcastle University, Newcastle upon Tyne NE2 4HH, UK; enoch.akowuah@nhs.net
3 Academic Cardiovascular Unit, South Tees NHS Foundation Trust, Middlesbrough TS4 3BW, UK
* Correspondence: bil.kirmani@lhch.nhs.uk

Abstract: Minimally invasive approaches to the aortic valve have been described since 1993, with great hopes that they would become universal and facilitate day-case cardiac surgery. The literature has shown that these procedures can be undertaken with equivalent mortality rates, similar operative times, comparable costs, and some benefits regarding hospital length of stay. The competing efforts of transcatheter aortic valve implantation for these same outcomes have provided an excellent range of treatment options for patients from cardiology teams. We describe the current state of the art, including technical considerations, caveats, and complications of minimal access aortic surgery and predict future directions in this space.

Keywords: minimally invasive; aortic valve; surgery

1. Introduction

Aortic valve disease is common, affecting 1 in 100 adults in the United States and some six million or so individuals worldwide [1–3]. A heterogeneous spectrum of conditions with different aetiologies and pathophysiologies can lead to valve stenosis, regurgitation, and endocarditis. The natural history of these conditions is progressive, with symptom progression from angina, breathlessness, or syncope eventually culminating in heart failure and death. In the western world, senile degenerative stenosis predominates, whilst elsewhere, rheumatic disease is more prevalent. The onset of symptoms is thought to mark an inflection point at which compensatory mechanisms are exhausted, and prognosis worsens quickly. Most patients with severe aortic stenosis will develop symptoms within five years, and event-free survival may be as low as 21% at two years [4,5]. Even with moderate aortic stenosis, progression leads to poor prognostic disease in 38% of patients within five years [6]. No medical treatments influence the natural history of aortic stenosis [7].

Treatment for aortic valve conditions, therefore, invariably consists of replacement of the diseased valve in 99% of cases [8]. While repair procedures have gained traction in some cases, replacement of the valve has remained the principal strategy since its inception in 1958. Outcomes have been excellent, with mortality from isolated, uncomplicated, and conventional aortic valve replacement consistently less than 1% [9].

Despite excellent outcomes for surgery, a 33% rate of surgical turn-down for patients over the age of 75 y in the Euro Heart Survey prompted a search for less invasive means of treatment for aortic valve disease [10]. The first percutaneous transcatheter aortic valve implantation (TAVI) in humans was performed in 2002 [11]. Over the last two decades, the technology has matured and increased in efficacy and scope, leading to increasingly liberal recommendations for its use in the guidelines [12]. Conversely, the 2017 European Society of Cardiology/European Association of Cardio-Thoracic Surgery guidelines did not reference minimal access approaches for valve surgery at all, and when updated in 2021, these approaches were still not discussed [13]. Transcatheter techniques, with a compellingly short recovery time even in highly comorbid patients, have been a driver reducing the invasiveness of conventional surgical approaches. Complications associated with TAVI, such as cerebrovascular embolic events, vascular complications, conduction disorders, and prosthetic valve dysfunction, are gradually being addressed, and they provide a good rationale to consider the known excellent pedigree of surgical valve replacement as a first-line treatment for the majority of patients requiring interventions.

Having both approaches available in the armamentarium of cardiology teams serves the needs of patients well. Nevertheless, there remains an appetite to marry the reduced invasiveness of TAVI with the meticulous decalcification and directly visualized seating of uncrimped valves. At the turn of the millennium, Chitwood predicted that 21st century cardiac surgery procedures would be performed minimally invasively as day-cases, with patients returning to normal activity within one or two weeks [14]. Nearly 25 years later, this belief has proven true for percutaneous interventions, but it remains an elusive goal in surgery.

Numerous systematic reviews, referenced through this paper, have previously documented defined outcomes for minimally invasive aortic valve surgery against the current standard of care. We do not replicate this format here but synthesize our experience and opinion as both practitioners and as authors of a Cochrane review on the subject. We have not systematically searched the literature but rather seek to fill the gaps with other existing systematic reviews. In this state-of-the-art review, we describe advances in surgical techniques that have improved the quality and outcomes of minimal access aortic valve surgery, and we present a vision for future direction.

2. Minimal Access Options

While the terms *minimal invasiveness* and *minimal access* are often used interchangeably, these overlapping philosophies can be disparate. In particular, the relative technical challenges of performing surgery through reduced access incisions can increase cardiopulmonary bypass and ischaemic surgical time, paradoxically increasing the invasiveness of the procedure. The invasiveness of cardiac surgery, some have posited, is as much contributed to by the deleterious effects of cardiopulmonary bypass as it is by the trauma of sternotomy, which is generally well tolerated [15,16]. Efforts to mitigate for both to make incremental gains have included a plethora of techniques and approaches, each with various advantages, disadvantages, and prerequisites. The most common are summarized here, and it is worth noting that there is a paucity of evidence to support preferring one approach over others [17].

2.1. Approach

2.1.1. Hemi-Sternotomy

The hemi-sternotomy (also known as partial sternotomy or limited sternotomy) approach that is now the most common approach to minimally invasive aortic valve surgery was developed after initial work using mini-thoracotomy [18,19]. The rationale for this approach was to avoid the subcostal neurovascular bundles that can cause post-thoracotomy pain if retracted, as well as to improve access to the great vessels for central cannulation.

The skin incision (Figure 1) is made over the upper midline to access the aorta, with a J-shaped, L-shaped, or chevron sternotomy into the right, left, or bilateral intercostal spaces (Figure 2). The length of the sternotomy can vary and may be into third or fourth intercostal space. Accordingly, the length of the incision can also vary, with 5 cm being a typical lower limit. This modifiable access can be utilized to undertake not only aortic valve replacement but also surgery of the aortic root, ascending aorta, and hemi-arch [20].

The upper hemi-sternotomy approach can provide sufficient access to perform complete central cannulation with conventional instruments and cannulae, if desired, although modifications and training to facilitate surgery have been well described [21,22]. A 2017 Cochrane review of randomized, controlled trials comparing full sternotomy to hemi-sternotomy found that, across 10 included studies, the evidence was of low certainty due to biases and small sample sizes [23]. For most major outcomes, including peri-operative mortality, pain, or quality of life, there was no significant difference. Blood loss was slightly lower with hemi-sternotomy compared to full sternotomy (mean difference 153 mL lower compared to 400 mL), and index admission costs were also higher (a mean difference of £1190 (~$1470) more for hemi-sternotomy). Following the publication of the Cochrane review, the publication of two well-designed trials performed in the UK, MAVRIC and Mini-Stern, prompted a revised review of the literature.

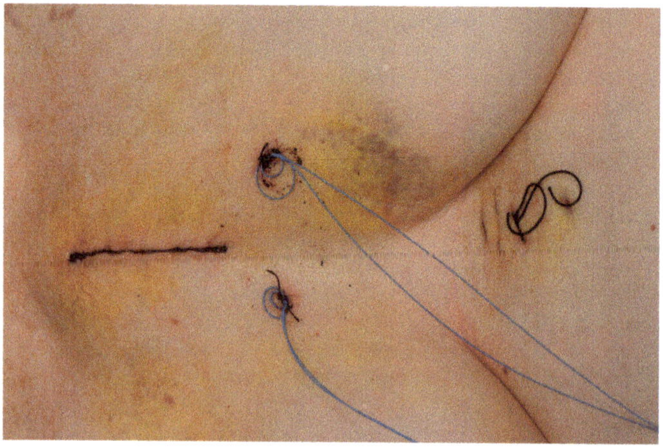

Figure 1. Hemisternotomy incision.

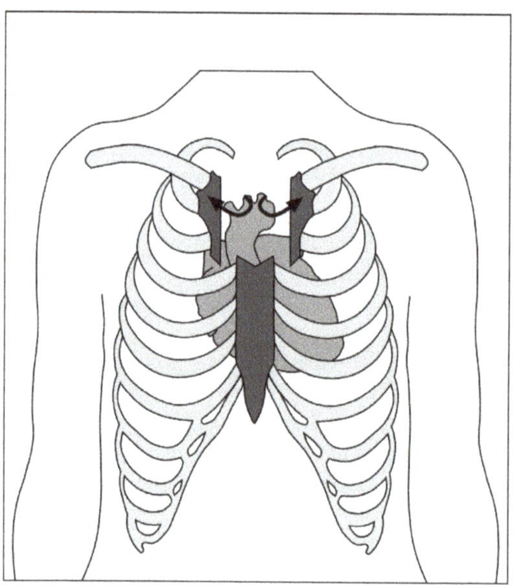

Figure 2. Schematic of chevron-shaped hemi-sternotomy into bilateral second intercostal spaces.

The MAVRIC Trial

The Manubrium-limited Mini-sternotomy versus Conventional Sternotomy for Aortic Valve Replacement (MAVRIC) trial was a single centre, randomized, controlled trial comparing patients undergoing AVR via manubrium-limited mini-sternotomy with an AVR via conventional sternotomy group [24,25].

Patients in the intervention arm received a manubrium-limited mini-sternotomy, performed using a 5- to 7-cm midline skin incision dividing the manubrium from the sternal notch to 1 cm below the manubrium–sternal junction. Cardiopulmonary bypass (CPB) was established with an ascending aortic cannula and percutaneous femoral venous cannulation. Those in the usual care arm received conventional median sternotomy.

The primary outcome was the proportion of patients who received a red cell transfusion postoperatively and within seven days of AVR surgery.

The trial reported that mini-sternotomy was not found to be superior to conventional sternotomy with respect to red cell transfusion requirements within seven days of surgery. The proportion of patients receiving red cell transfusion was 23 of 135 in both groups (odds ratio 1.0 (95% CI: 0.5, 2.0) and risk difference of 0.0 (95% CI: −0.1, 0.1)). However, secondary endpoints showed that there was a statistically significant difference with respect to transfusion volumes of non-red cell blood components. Mini-sternotomy also resulted in a relative reduction in chest drain losses; however, greater blood loss in the conventional group did not translate into red cell transfusions. Patients in the mini-sternotomy group had significantly longer bypass and cross clamp times and worse lung function at fou days post-surgery. Lung function at 12 weeks and adverse event rates were otherwise not different between the groups.

Mini-Stern Trial

Mini-Stern was a multi-centre, open-label, pragmatic, randomized, controlled trial with primary end points of postoperative length of hospital stay and time to fitness for discharge. In total, 222 patients were randomized, and it was found that mini-sternotomy patients had no difference in length of stay (median 7 (interquartile range (IQR 6–10) vs. 7 (IQR 6–10), $p = 0.692$) and no difference in time to fitness for discharge (median 5 (IQR 5–10) vs. median 6 (IQR 5–9), $p = 0.560$). Mini-sternotomy was £1719 more expensive per patient compared to full sternotomy in the first year following surgery. There was no significant difference in EQ-5D-based quality-adjusted life years (QALYs); therefore, at a willingness to pay threshold of £20,000 per QALY, there was only a 3.7% chance that mini-sternotomy was cost-effective.

Current meta-analysis

As of August 2021, there were 15 published randomized, controlled trials of 1395 participants comparing hemisternotomy with full median sternotomy due to be published shortly as an update of the previous Cochrane review. Countries of origin included Austria, the Czech Republic, Spain, Italy, Germany, France, Egypt, Russia, Sweden, Serbia, and the United Kingdom [26–39]. All but one were single-centre studies of elective, isolated aortic valve replacements, typically excluding patients with poor left ventricular function. The European studies were predominantly focused on patients with degenerative heart valve disease and therefore an older population, whereas the study from Egypt included younger patients, presumably with rheumatic heart disease. The surgical strategy was broadly similar between studies, with aortic arterial cannulation and either central or femoral venous cannulation. Venting strategies—often considered a source of concern in minimally invasive aortic valve replacement due to potential compromises in bloodless field, de-airing, or left ventricular decompression—were variable.

The risk ratio for peri-operative mortality was 0.93 (95% confidence interval [CI] 0.45–1.94, in 10 studies, but with low certainty). The mean difference in cardiopulmonary bypass time was 10.7 min longer with ministernotomy (95% CI 3.3–18.0 in 10 studies, but with very low certainty). The mean difference in aortic cross-clamp time was 6.1 min longer with ministernotomy (95% CI 0.8–11.3 across 12 studies but also with very low certainty). Even in this context of uncertainty, these mean differences in extra-corporeal circulation and ischaemic times are likely to have had very little clinical impact. Exclusion of one trial [31] in which rapid deployment valves were used to facilitate expedient surgery in the minimally invasive arm only and not in the full sternotomy arm did not impact the finding of the small increases in bypass and cross-clamp times.

There was a modest reduction in length of stay in patients undergoing mini-sternotomy (mean difference 1.1 days less (95% CI −1.9 to −0.3 days across 11 studies with very low certainty). It is important to note that, for most of these studies, trial protocols were not published *a priori* or at all. Outcome measures, such as hospital length of stay, which might be contingent on different criteria between studies and which was considered at high risk for bias from blinding, were not directly comparable. Similar issues arose with intensive care length of stay, which, in studies at low risk of bias, was marginally shorter with minimally invasive surgery (−0.45 days, 95% CI −0.84 to −0.06).

In-hospital pain assessments were also no different between minimally invasive and full sternotomy approaches (standardized mean difference −0.19 for minimally invasive, 95% CI −0.43 to 0.04 with low certainty). Equally, there was no difference in quality of life measures after discharge from hospital (mean difference 0.03, 95% CI 0.00 to 0.06 across 4 studies with low certainty). Finally, pulmonary function tests—considered a surrogate marker for comfort and capability following disruption of the thoracic skeleton—were also minimally different between the two approaches (mean difference 2.1% higher with mini-sternotomy, 95% CI 0.74 to 3.41).

This new meta-analysis would appear to demonstrate that ministernotomy aortic valve replacement is as safe as full-sternotomy surgery but with few of the anticipated advantages regarding pain, quality of life, or breathing that have been cited as reasons to perform minimally invasive surgery. Length of stay in the hospital and in the intensive care unit was modestly better with minimally invasive surgery but at an increased cost over standard of care.

2.1.2. Right Anterior Mini-Thoracotomy

The right anterior mini-thoracotomy (RAT) approach, using central cannulation, was first described by Rao and Kumar in 1993 [40]. Cosgrove and Sabik first applied the term "minimally invasive" to a 10-cm thoracotomy with excision of two costal cartilages, utilizing a femoral bypass [41]. The current technique accesses the mediastinum through the second intercostal space (Figure 3). The main advantage of this approach is the absolute preservation of sternal integrity and the absence of lateral traction, similar to the parasternal approach described by Cohn [42]. The corollary to these benefits is the need for femoral cannulation because of limited access, necessitating a second incision in the groin and retrograde perfusion, which may offset the cosmetic advantages, quality of life, and satisfaction with minimally invasive surgery [43]. A rate of 1% of non-union of the transected ribs may also cause intractable post-thoracotomy pain.

Initially, meta-analyses found RAT to have shorter hospital stays compared to hemi-sternotomy [44,45], despite higher rates of bleeding, transfusion, and conversion to full sternotomy. A more recent comprehensive network meta-analysis of propensity matched and randomized studies compared full sternotomy, hemi-sternotomy, and right anterior mini-thoracotomy [46]. This study found no differences in surgical time, hospital length of stay, or ventilation time between the two minimally invasive approaches. As with previous meta-analyses, return to the theatre for bleeding was more common with right anterior mini-thoracotomy than with hemi-sternotomy (RR 1.65, 95% CI 1.18–2.30, $p = 0.003$).

The network meta-analysis included 42 studies, including 29 propensity matched studies and 13 randomized, controlled trials. The majority compared median sternotomy to hemisternotomy, with nine comparing RAT to full sternotomy and two comparing RAT to hemisternotomy. Notably, only one randomized study evaluated RAT, so much of the evidence was observational, albeit adjusted with propensity matched techniques. Again, the majority of the included studies were European in origin, and the methodological quality was fraught with uncertainty. That this study identified a significant peri-operative mortality advantage of hemi-sternotomy over median sternotomy (relative risk (RR) 0.60, 95% CI 0.41–0.90) or RAT (RR 0.50, 95% CI 0.27–0.97) should be interpreted with caution. A meta-analysis of randomized trials with didactic scrutiny of methodology and quality found no difference in mortality between hemi-sternotomy and full-sternotomy [23]. There also exists little rationale to explain why hemi-sternotomy should reduce mortality; indeed, all plausible mechanisms for a mortality difference between minimally invasive aortic valve replacement techniques might suggest that minimal access approaches are at *higher* risk than conventional surgery for peri-operative mortality. Therefore, it is our interpretation that, while the network meta-analysis favours hemi-sternotomy as the access of choice for aortic valve surgery (over both full sternotomy and right anterior mini-thoracotomy), the evidence to support this suggestion is scant.

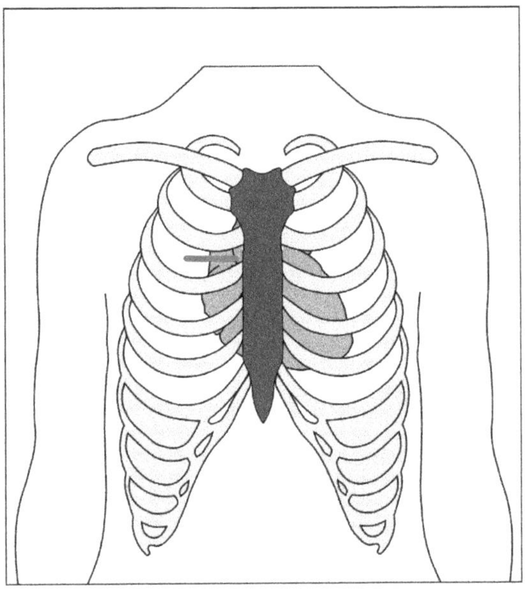

Figure 3. Schematic of right anterior minithoracotomy through second intercostal space.

The authors of a recent consensus statement [47] acknowledged the increased technical challenge of a right anterior mini-thoracotomy approach. Additional equipment, such as thoracosopes, long-handled instruments, and soft tissue retractors, require specific training. Cost comparisons vary across publications. In some, the need for additional equipment and consumables increases the costs of RAT to up to US$4209 higher than full sternotomy, compared to US$290 more for hemisternotomy [48,49]. In others, the costs of RAT have been between US$1891 to US$3887 lower when propensity matched across real-world registry data [50,51].

Right anterolateral mini-thoracotomy (in the third intercostal space) can be used to perform multiple valve replacements, including of the aortic, mitral, and tricuspid valves [52–54]. Table 1 summarises some of the characteristics of the different approaches.

2.1.3. Hybrid Approach (Sternotomy + Transcatheter Aortic Valve Implantation)

While the hybrid approach is not strictly minimal access and ostensibly not minimally invasive, patients not fit for conventional aortic valve replacement who also require coronary artery revascularization may benefit from lower invasiveness using a hybrid approach. Sternotomy may be performed to undertake off-pump coronary artery bypass grafting, with concomitant trans-aortic or trans-femoral TAVI. The procedure avoids the sequelae of cardiopulmonary bypass in patients who may not tolerate it while still allowing for complete revascularization and management of aortic stenosis [55–57].

Table 1. Advantages and disadvantages of aortic valve surgery approaches.

	Full Sternotomy	Hemi-Sternotomy	Right Anterior Minithoracotomy
Access	Unfettered view of whole mediastinum and whole heart	Good access to aortic root, limited to whole heart	Most challenging view
Sternal disruption	Whole sternum	To 2nd–4th intercostal spaces unilaterally or bilaterally	None, although costal cartilages are sometimes divided (may include right mammary artery ligation)
Cannulation	Full central	Variable—from full central to aortic arterial only	Typically requires peripheral cannulation
Instruments	Standard cardiac	Variable—can be standard or long-handled	Typically requires long-handled
Technical difficulty	Baseline	Learning curve easily traversed, including for trainee surgeons	Accepted to be technically challenging
Adjuncts Required	None	Variable—possible with standard equipment. Facilitated by rapid deployment valves, suture placement devices, and knot-tying devices	Facilitated by rapid deployment valves, suture placement devices, and knot-tying devices; Light source advantageous; Single lung ventilation.
Benefits (from most recent meta-analyses) *		Reduced intensive care and hospital length of stay; Reduced ventilation time	Reduced hospital length of stay; Reduced ventilation time; Lower stroke rate; Lower pacemaker rate
Risks *		Increased operative time; Increased costs	Increased operative time; Increased costs (including vs. ministernotomy); Lung herniation

* compared to median sternotomy unless stated otherwise.

2.2. *Cannulation and Cardiopulmonary Bypass*

2.2.1. Central

Hemi-sternotomy to the third or fourth space usually provides sufficient access to the aorta and right atrium to cannulate for arterial inflow and venous drainage centrally. The right superior pulmonary vein may or may not be accessible with this approach. Standard cannulae may be used, although to aid retraction of the pipes out of the field of view, some surgeons prefer angled venous pipes or a flat/low-profile cannula. Vacuum assistance can also help to improve the venous drainage.

2.2.2. Peripheral

Where the incision limits the access to the aorta, there may only be space in the surgical field for the cross-clamp, cardioplegia site, and aortotomy. In this case, peripheral cannulation, typically at the femoral artery, is utilized. Percutaneous methods are possible, but direct surgical access is the more commonly performed approach. Complications arising from groin cannulation may occur in 10.8% of cases, with seromas in up to 5% [48]. Percutaneous cannulation might mitigate some of this risk.

2.2.3. Hypothermia and Systemic Hyperkalaemia

In the context of re-operative minimal access surgery, systemic hypothermia to 20 °C along with systemic hyperkalaemia at 7 mmol/L can support myocardial protection in the presence of patent left internal mammary bypass grafts [58]. This process requires ultrafiltration on cardiopulmonary bypass following cardiac reperfusion. Retrograde flooding of the field from the left coronary ostium in the presence of an unclamped left internal mammary graft can be mitigated using intermittent circulatory arrest to facilitate suture placement or peri-operative percutaneous balloon occlusion of the left internal mammary by cardiology.

2.2.4. Venting (and Imaging)

Reduced access to the left ventricle for inspection or manual decompression mandates the use of a trans-oesophageal echo during minimally invasive aortic valve surgery. Whereas this procedure may be omitted in special circumstances in conventional sternotomy, such as oesophagectomy or oesophageal stricture, the risks are much greater in minimal access surgery, during which the left ventricle cannot be directly assessed.

Dependent on the level of access, left ventricular venting can be achieved in different ways including:

- The right superior pulmonary vein;
- The pulmonary artery;
- Trans-aortically.

Access to the pulmonary veins is typically not possible except in larger partial sternotomy approaches (i.e., fourth intercostal space). The pulmonary artery is usually easily accessible, although the visualization decreases considerably once the cross-clamp is removed, and the efficacy of venting is variable. Access further deteriorates off cardiopulmonary bypass; therefore, it is imperative to achieve haemostasis of the vent site early. The trans-aortic vent approach is usually sufficient to provide a bloodless field for surgery, but it is limited should venting be required during reperfusion since the left ventricle cannot be reached manually.

2.3. *Adjuncts*

2.3.1. Rapid Deployment Valves

Sutureless and rapid deployment valves have been described as obvious companions for minimal access aortic valve replacement to compensate for the increased cardiopulmonary bypass and cross-clamp times that are otherwise seen [31,59]. These procedure typically have excellent haemodynamic profiles, but they have a shorter pedigree and may, with their similarities to transcatheter valves, have a greater propensity towards structural valve deterioration.

2.3.2. Automatic Suture/Knotting Devices

Automatic suture placement or knotting devices reduce invasiveness in minimal access valve surgery by expediting valve implantation and therefore reducing cross-clamp and cardiopulmonary bypass times [60]. The use of the Cor-Knot® device (LSI Solutions, Victor, NY, USA) for valve surgery was noted to also lead to more reproducible valve implantation with lower rates of paravalular leakage [61]. The same manufacturer has also released an automated annular suturing device to expedite this stage of valve implantation, but there are not yet any published series showing that it is effective.

2.3.3. Transvenous Pacing, Cannulation, and Venting

A variety of options exist for percutaneous support of cardiopulmonary bypass from the right jugular. These options include:

- Transvenous pacing can be floated using an inflatable balloon tip into the right ventricle for endocardial pacing if the anterior right ventricle is not accessible;
- Coronary sinus cannulation via the right internal jugular was previously possible using the Proplege device (Edwards LifeSciences, Irvin, CA, USA). but as the strategies for anterograde cardioplegia alone showed good efficacy, it is no longer available;
- Pulmonary artery venting through a percutaneously floated catheter has again lost favour, as trans-aortic and direct pulmonary artery or pulmonary vein venting have been shown to be efficacious and safe.

2.3.4. Thoracoscopes

Direct visualization of the aorta (sufficient to apply a cross-clamp), aortic valve, and aortic annulus is possible through both hemi-sternotomy and right anterior mini-thoracotomy approaches. Thoracoscopes can also be utilized to improve the light and view for areas that might be more difficult to see due to an overhanging thoracic cage. Use of scopes for lighting and/or transmitted video images may, however, limit access for instruments in some cases. This limitation can in part be mitigated using other adjuncts, such as automatic suture placement or knotting devices [47].

2.3.5. Robot Assistance

Robotic aortic valve replacement has been attempted since 2004 [62], with a renewed interest in recent years [63]. In place of either hemi-sternotomy or right anterior mini-thoracotomy, a right *lateral* mini-thoracotomy is utilized as the working port, along with four arms, sparing division of the costal cartilage or sacrifice of the right internal mammary artery. This procedure has the advantage of an intact thoracic skeleton, superior visualization, and virtually unrestricted range of movement in the working space but with a steep learning curve, high capital investment costs, and ongoing consumable expenditures.

2.4. Special Circumstances

2.4.1. Concomitant Procedures

As minimal access incisions have gained favour, indications for procedures amenable to this approach have expanded. The hemi-sternotomy approach has been successfully utilized for aortovascular procedures, including valve sparing root replacement [64].

2.4.2. Re-Do Procedures

Previous sternotomy, even in the presence of patent coronary artery bypass grafts, is not a contraindication for a minimally invasive approach. These procedures can be performed with low-conversion rates of 2.6% [58]. Minimization of the dissection and mobilization of the heart mean that bleeding complications are low. Technical challenges from the presence of patent grafts may require alternative strategies for cardioplegic arrest (including systemic hyperkalaemia, deeper hypothermia, and brief periods of circulatory arrest). However, since transcatheter techniques for aortic valve replacement have improved in safety and reliability, they are often considered the first choice in such anatomical conditions, which can be difficult or hostile for conventional surgery.

3. Minimal Access Pre-Operative Planning/Setup

Additional assessment and preparation are required for minimal access aortic valve surgery. These requirements vary depending on the approach adopted, and not all practitioners employ all these steps. Indeed, some proponents claim that minimal-access aortic valve replacement can be offered to all comers with no patient selection, whereas most would agree that some absolute and relative contraindications exist for each technique. The specific instructions for each technique are beyond the scope of this review.

- A CT scan pre-operatively can allow for assessment of the position of the aorta relative to the incision planned. If peripheral cannulation is intended, CT can also determine whether the femoral vessels are of an adequate calibre and the descending aorta is free of mobile atheroma that may preclude retrograde perfusion.
- Short-acting anaesthetic drugs should be considered to facilitate early extubation and enhanced recovery.
- A sheath in the right internal jugular vein can be introduced at the time of induction of anaesthesia if the usual access limits epicardial pacing wires.
- A bag of saline behind the shoulder blades can elevate and expand the chest, providing an improved approach to the mediastinum.
- External defibrillator pads are required to cardiovert ventricular fibrillation, as internal paddles cannot be applied to the heart.
- Trans-oesophageal echocardiography is mandated for minimally invasive aortic valve surgery, as the direct visualization of the right and left ventricular function is impaired.

- A double lumen tube or bronchial blocker for selective ventilation of the right lung can facilitate the early learning curve [65].
- Carbon dioxide field flooding can aid in de-airing at the end of the case, when cardiac massage is not possible and venting is limited. Passive and limited active de-airing can therefore be supplemented with displacement of air in the cardiac chambers with highly soluble CO_2.

4. Outcomes

It is unlikely that minimally invasive methods of aortic valve surgery would have been permitted to develop if peri-operative mortality was not equivalent to that with conventional full sternotomy. While the excellent current outcomes for isolated aortic valve replacement mean that most series have not had sufficient power to demonstrate a difference, it is apparent that there is no excess mortality.

Some credence has been placed on minimal access surgery to therefore also improve outcomes in other areas and justify the technical challenges and increased costs.

4.1. Pain

For studies that examined post-operative pain scores between minimal-access and full-sternotomy surgery, there has been considerable bias in the reporting [23]. Protocolized analgesic pathways were seldom cited, and blinding was only utilized in one trial. The timing of pain score assessments also varied considerably between studies. The overall assessment following the review was that minimal access aortic valve surgery did not reduce pain compared to sternotomy.

4.2. Respiratory Mechanics

The impact of full median sternotomy on respiratory function following surgery is often cited as a reason to favour minimal access approaches. While there might be small differences in peri-operative lung function parameters between non-sternotomy and full-sternotomy approaches, the main advantage to respiratory mechanics is in the time to return to baseline. For partial sternotomy, this period was one month, whereas for full sternotomy, it was up to three months [66].

4.3. Quality of Life

Five randomized, controlled trials studied quality of life following surgery. Between 6 and 12 weeks following surgery, there was no difference in the quality of life scores between hemi-sternotomy and full-sternotomy [23].

4.4. Complications

While numerous reviews have compared minimal-access and full-sternotomy aortic valve replacement for rates of major complications, such as mortality, stroke, bleeding, etc., some complications are particular to minimal access surgery. Poor visualization or access can increase the chances of iatrogenic injury (especially to great vessels, as well as right ventricular and aortotomy bleeding) and can also increase the likelihood that this injury cannot be controlled. Conversion from minimal-access to full-sternotomy is usually sufficient to resolve the poor exposure and occurs in between 0.8% and 8.0% of cases depending on centre experience, with many reports citing 3–4% conversion rates [67].

5. Discussion

Chitwood's prediction (or aspiration) that cardiac surgery would culminate in routine minimally invasive approaches that would emulate general surgery's day-case model still seem very distant a quarter of century on. Large series initially expounded by forerunners, such as Cohn, Mohr, Roselli, Solinas, Glauber and Lamelas, have inspired considerable growth, but the procedure is far from the standard approach [68]. The benefits of minimal access surgery have not been realized as predicted, and in the intervening decades, transcatheter techniques have improved and expanded their remit to low-risk patients [69]. The cost-effectiveness of percutaneous methods has also improved such that TAVI procedures are now competitive against surgical valves [70].

In the absence of demonstrable superiority, there is therefore more incentive than ever to propagate minimal access approaches to aortic valve replacement. Whereas these procedures can be performed with minimal or no additional equipment, at a similar cost, and with no increase in complications, the new standard should surely be the procedure with the same outcomes, same costs . . . and a smaller incision? Cosmetic superiority, in addition to non-inferiority for all other key metrics, is a convincing argument for minimal access aortic valve surgery, especially when driven by patient preference.

The current state of the art in minimal access aortic valve surgery is advanced. Even in groups such as octogenarians, re-operations, and root/ascending aorta replacements, the results for minimal access aortic surgery can be excellent [71]. The procedure is reproducible and can be undertaken by surgeons in training without compromising patient safety [72]. Peri-operative and one-year mortality rates are no different in a real-world setting, and the length of stay is typically reduced using a minimal-access approach [73].

As transcatheter aortic valve implantation also gathers momentum, gaining approval for increasingly lower-risk patient groups, there is a need to ensure that patients are provided with procedures with good pedigrees. Surgeons seeking to compensate for the increased operative times of minimally invasive aortic valve replacement may turn to sutureless aortic valves, drawing parallels with transcatheter valves. Whereas TAVI valves have higher rates of paravalvular leakage, pacemaker implantation, and vascular complications [74], sutureless valves can offer the advantage of full decalcification and placement under direct vision. Whether these benefits offset the need for thoracic cage disruption, cardiopulmonary bypass, and cross-clamping remains to be seen, particularly in small or calcified roots.

Further research is also still required to elucidate the differences between hemi-sternotomy and right anterior minithoracotomy. The former remains the more accessible minimally invasive approach, with familiar setup, angles, and equipment to those used for training in conventional full sternotomy. Proponents of the right anterior mini-thoracotomy, however, will argue that, if a partial-sternotomy is superior to a full-sternotomy, it stands to reason that no sternotomy should be better still. However, it remains to be compellingly proven that the additional challenges of RAT do not neutralize the benefits provided by maintaining the sternum fully intact. Current syntheses of the existing literature have been disparate in their conclusions.

Future directions for this procedure involve ensuring that it is, indeed, developed as the new standard of care for aortic valve procedures. Once this principle is accepted universally, the process of reducing invasiveness, as well as access, can be developed. Enhanced recovery after surgery (ERAS) has been slow to be adopted in cardiac surgery in general and much less in minimal access cardiac surgery. Protocols are needed for patients with reduced incisions that differ from those used for conventional surgery, which might meaningfully engage and utilize the operative advantages to expedite the patient journey more effectively [75].

6. Conclusions

Minimal access aortic valve surgery is at a watershed moment at which it could plausibly become the new standard of care for aortic valve disease, as laparoscopic procedures have become for general surgery. Unlike the laparotomy versus laparoscopy analogy, however, minimally invasive aortic valve surgery appears to provide few or small benefits over open surgery, so is strongly driven by cosmetic considerations. Economic viability will need to be demonstrated for minimal access to become the default approach, but moreover, a surgical appetite must grow for non-inferior procedures in which the benefits are still being developed and demonstrated.

Author Contributions: All authors contributed to the writing and editing. All authors have read and agreed to the published version of the manuscript.

Funding: This research received no external funding.

Institutional Review Board Statement: Not applicable.

Informed Consent Statement: Not applicable.

Data Availability Statement: Not applicable.

Conflicts of Interest: The authors declare no conflict of interest; E.A. was Chief Investigator for the MAVRIC study (hemi-sternotomy approach).

References

1. Nkomo, V.T.; Gardin, J.M.; Skelton, T.N.; Gottdiener, J.S.; Scott, C.G.; Enriquez-Sarano, M. Faculty Opinions recommendation of Burden of valvular heart diseases: A population-based study. *Lancet* **2006**, *368*, 496161. [CrossRef]
2. Kumar, R.K.; Tandon, R. Rheumatic fever & rheumatic heart disease: The last 50 years. *Indian J. Med. Res.* **2013**, *137*, 643–658.
3. Manjunath, C.; Srinivas, P.; Ravindranath, K.; Dhanalakshmi, C. Incidence and patterns of valvular heart disease in a tertiary care high-volume cardiac center: A single center experience. *Indian Heart J.* **2014**, *66*, 320–326. [CrossRef] [PubMed]
4. Otto, C.M.; Burwash, I.G.; Legget, M.E.; Munt, B.I.; Fujioka, M.; Healy, N.L.; Schwaegler, R.G. Prospective Study of Asymptomatic Valvular Aortic Stenosis Clinical, Echocardiographic, and Exercise Predictors of Outcome. *Circulation* **1997**, *95*, 2262–2270. [CrossRef]
5. Pellikka, P.A.; Sarano, M.E.; Nishimura, R.A.; Malouf, J.F.; Bailey, K.R.; Scott, C.G.; Barnes, M.E.; Tajik, A.J. Outcome of 622 Adults with Asymptomatic, Hemodynamically Significant Aortic Stenosis During Prolonged Follow-Up. *Circulation* **2005**, *111*, 3290–3295. [CrossRef] [PubMed]
6. Gohlke-Bärwolf, C.; Minners, J.; Jander, N.; Gerdts, E.; Wachtell, K.; Ray, S.; Pedersen, T.R. Natural History of Mild and of Moderate Aortic Stenosis—New Insights From a Large Prospective European Study. *Curr. Probl. Cardiol.* **2013**, *38*, 365–409. [CrossRef]
7. Iung, B.; Vahanian, A. Degenerative calcific aortic stenosis: A natural history. *Heart* **2012**, *98*. Available online: http://heart.bmj.com/content/98/Suppl_4/iv7.full.pdf+html (accessed on 6 May 2018). [CrossRef] [PubMed]
8. Iung, B.; Baron, G.; Butchart, E.G.; Delahaye, F.; Gohlke-Bärwolf, C.; Levang, O.W.; Tornos, P.; Vanoverschelde, J.-L.; Vermeer, F.; Boersma, E.; et al. A prospective survey of patients with valvular heart disease in Europe: The Euro Heart Survey on Valvular Heart Disease. *Eur. Heart J.* **2003**, *24*, 1231–1243. [CrossRef]
9. Carabello, B.A. Introduction to Aortic Stenosis. *Circ. Res.* **2013**, *113*, 179–185. [CrossRef] [PubMed]
10. Iung, B.; Cachier, A.; Baron, G.; Messika-Zeitoun, D.; Delahaye, F.; Tornos, P.; Vahanian, A. Decision-making in elderly patients with severe aortic stenosis: Why are so many denied surgery? *Eur. Heart J.* **2005**, *26*, 2714–2720. [CrossRef] [PubMed]
11. Cribier, A.; Eltchaninoff, H.; Bash, A.; Borenstein, N.; Tron, C.; Bauer, F. Percutaneous Transcatheter Implantation of an Aortic Valve Prosthesis for Calcific Aortic Stenosis. *Circulation* **2002**, *106*, 3006–3008. [CrossRef]
12. Bourantas, C.V.; Serruys, P.W. Evolution of Transcatheter Aortic Valve Replacement. *Circ. Res.* **2014**, *114*, 1037–1051. [CrossRef] [PubMed]
13. Baumgartner, H.; Falk, V.; Bax, J.J.; De Bonis, M.; Hamm, C.; Holm, P.J. 2017 ESC/EACTS Guidelines for the management of valvular heart disease. *Eur. Heart J.* **2017**, *38*, 2739–2791. [CrossRef] [PubMed]
14. Elbeery, J.R.; Chitwood, W.R. Minimally invasive cardiac surgery. Heart surgery for the 21st century. *N. C. Med. J.* **1997**, *58*, 374–377.
15. Westaby, S.; Benetti, F.J. Less Invasive Coronary Surgery: Consensus From the Oxford Meeting. *Ann. Thorac. Surg.* **1996**, *62*, 924–931. [CrossRef]
16. Lee, B.Y.; Gleason, T.G.; Sonnad, S.S. Quality of life after aortic valve replacement. *Expert Rev. Pharmacoecon. Outcomes Res.* **2004**, *4*, 265–275. [CrossRef] [PubMed]
17. Mikus, E.; Calvi, S.; Campo, G.; Pavasini, R.; Paris, M.; Raviola, E.; Del Giglio, M. Full Sternotomy, Hemisternotomy, and Mini-thoracotomy for Aortic Valve Surgery: Is There a Difference? *Ann. Thorac. Surg.* **2018**, *106*, 1782–1788. [CrossRef]
18. Liu, J.; Sidiropoulos, A.; Konertz, W. Minimally invasive aortic valve replacement (AVR) compared to standard AVR. *Eur. J. Cardio-Thorac. Surg.* **1999**, *16*, S80–S83. [CrossRef]
19. Autschbach, R.; Walther, T.; Falk, V.; Diegeler, A.; Metz, S.; Mohr, F.W. S-shaped in comparison to L-shaped partial sternotomy for less invasive aortic valve replacement. *Eur. J. Cardiothorac. Surg.* **1998**, *14* (Suppl. 1), S117–S121. [CrossRef]
20. Perrotta, S.; Lentini, S. Ministernotomy approach for surgery of the aortic root and ascending aorta. *Interact. Cardiovasc. Thorac. Surg.* **2009**, *9*, 849–858. [CrossRef]
21. Malaisrie, S.C.; Barnhart, G.R.; Farivar, R.S.; Mehall, J.; Hummel, B.; Rodriguez, E.; Anderson, M.; Lewis, C.; Hargrove, C.; Ailawadi, G.; et al. Current era minimally invasive aortic valve replacement: Techniques and practice. *J. Thorac. Cardiovasc. Surg.* **2014**, *147*, 6–14. [CrossRef] [PubMed]

22. Walther, T.; Falk, V.; Mohr, F.W. Minimally Invasive Surgery for Valve Disease. *Curr. Probl. Cardiol.* **2006**, *31*, 399–437. [CrossRef] [PubMed]
23. Kirmani, B.H.; Jones, S.G.; Malaisrie, S.C.; Chung, D.A.; Williams, R.J. Limited versus full sternotomy for aortic valve replacement. *Cochrane Database Syst. Rev.* **2017**, *4*, CD011793. [CrossRef]
24. Akowuah, E.; Goodwin, A.T.; Owens, W.A.; Hancock, H.C.; Maier, R.; Kasim, A.; Mason, J. Manubrium-limited ministernotomy versus conventional sternotomy for aortic valve replacement (MAVRIC): Study protocol for a randomised controlled trial. *Trials* **2017**, *18*, 46. [CrossRef] [PubMed]
25. Hancock, H.C.; Maier, R.H.; Kasim, A.; Mason, J.; Murphy, G.; Goodwin, A.; Owens, W.A.; Akowuah, E. Mini-sternotomy versus conventional sternotomy for aortic valve replacement: A randomised controlled trial. *BMJ Open* **2021**, *11*, e041398. [CrossRef]
26. Mächler, H.E.; Bergmann, P.; Anelli-Monti, M.; Dacar, D.; Rehak, P.; Knez, I.; Salaymeh, L.; Mahla, E.; Rigler, B. Minimally invasive versus conventional aortic valve operations: A prospective study in 120 patients. *Ann. Thorac. Surg.* **1999**, *67*, 1001–1005. [CrossRef] [PubMed]
27. Gofus, J.; Vobornik, M.; Koblizek, V.; Smolak, P.; Myjavec, A.; Vojacek, J.; Pojar, M. Pulmonary function and quality of life after aortic valve replacement through ministernotomy: A prospective randomized study. *Kardiol. Pol.* **2020**, *78*, 1278–1280. [CrossRef]
28. Aris, A.; Cámara, M.L.; Montiel, J.; Delgado, L.J.; Galán, J.; Litvan, H. Ministernotomy versus median sternotomy for aortic valve replacement: A prospective, randomized study. *Ann. Thorac. Surg.* **1999**, *67*, 1583–1587. [CrossRef]
29. Rodríguez-Caulo, E.A.; Guijarro-Contreras, A.; Otero-Forero, J.; Mataró, M.J.; Sánchez-Espín, G.; Guzón, A.; Porras, C.; Such, M.; Ordóñez, A.; Melero-Tejedor, J.M.; et al. Quality of life, satisfaction and outcomes after ministernotomy versus full sternotomy isolated aortic valve replacement (QUALITY-AVR): Study protocol for a randomised controlled trial. *Trials* **2018**, *19*, 1–8. [CrossRef]
30. Bonacchi, M.; Prifti, E.; Giunti, G.; Frati, G.; Sani, G. Does ministernotomy improve postoperative outcome in aortic valve operation? A prospective randomized study. *Ann. Thorac. Surg.* **2002**, *73*, 460–465. [CrossRef]
31. Borger, M.A.; Moustafine, V.; Conradi, L.; Knosalla, C.; Richter, M.; Merk, D.R.; Doenst, T.; Hammerschmidt, R.; Treede, H.; Dohmen, P.; et al. A Randomized Multicenter Trial of Minimally Invasive Rapid Deployment Versus Conventional Full Sternotomy Aortic Valve Replacement. *Ann. Thorac. Surg.* **2015**, *99*, 17–25. [CrossRef] [PubMed]
32. Dogan, S.; Dzemali, O.; Wimmer-Greinecker, G.; Derra, P.; Doss, M.; Khan, M.F.; Moritz, A. Minimally invasive versus conventional aortic valve replacement: A prospective randomized trial. *J. Heart Valve Dis.* **2003**, *12*, 76–80. [PubMed]
33. Calderon, J.; Richebe, P.; Guibaud, J.P.; Coiffic, A.; Branchard, O.; Asselineau, J.; Janvier, G. Prospective Randomized Study of Early Pulmonary Evaluation of Patients Scheduled for Aortic Valve Surgery Performed by Ministernotomy or Total Median Sternotomy. *J. Cardiothorac. Vasc. Anesth.* **2009**, *23*, 795–801. [CrossRef] [PubMed]
34. Moustafa, M.A.; Abdelsamad, A.A.; Zakaria, G.; Omarah, M.M. Minimal vs Median Sternotomy for Aortic Valve Replacement. *Asian Cardiovasc. Thorac. Ann.* **2007**, *15*, 472–475. [CrossRef]
35. Shneider, Y.u.A.; Tsoi, M.D.; Fomenko, M.S.; Pavlov, A.A.; Shilenko, P.A. Aortic valve replacement via J-shaped partial up-per sternotomy: Randomized trial, mid-term results. *Khirurgiia* **2020**, *7*, 25–30. [CrossRef]
36. Dalen, M.; Oliveira Da Silva, C.; Sartipy, U.; Winter, R.; Franco-Cereceda, A.; Barimani, J.; Svenarud, P. Comparison of right ventricular function after ministernotomy and full sternotomy aortic valve replacement: A randomized study. *Interact. Cardiovasc. Thorac. Surg.* **2018**, *26*, 790–797. [CrossRef]
37. Vukovic, P.M.; Milojevic, P.; Stojanovic, I.; Micovic, S.; Zivkovic, I.; Peric, M.; Milicic, M.; Milacic, P.; Milojevic, M.; Bojic, M. The role of ministernotomy in aortic valve surgery—A prospective randomized study. *J. Card. Surg.* **2019**, *34*, 435–439. [CrossRef]
38. Hancock, H.C.; Maier, R.H.; Kasim, A.S.; Mason, J.M.; Murphy, G.J.; Goodwin, A.T.; Akowuah, E.F. Mini-Sternotomy Versus Conventional Sternotomy for Aortic Valve Replacement. *J. Am. Coll. Cardiol.* **2019**, *73*, 2491–2492. [CrossRef]
39. Nair, S.K.; Sudarshan, C.D.; Thorpe, B.S.; Singh, J.; Pillay, T.; Catarino, P.; Sharples, L.D. Mini-Stern Trial: A randomized trial comparing mini-sternotomy to full median sternotomy for aortic valve replacement. *J. Thorac. Cardiovasc. Surg.* **2018**, *156*, 2124–2132.e31. [CrossRef]
40. Rao, P.N.; Kumar, A.S. Aortic valve replacement through right thoracotomy. *Tex. Heart Inst. J.* **1993**, *20*, 307–308.
41. Cosgrove, D.M., 3rd; Sabik, J.F. Minimally invasive approach for aortic valve operations. *Ann. Thorac. Surg.* **1996**, *62*, 596–597. [CrossRef]
42. Cohn, L.H. Minimally invasive aortic valve surgery: Technical considerations and results with the parasternal approach. *J. Card. Surg.* **1998**, *13*, 302–305. [CrossRef] [PubMed]
43. Detter, C.; Deuse, T.; Boehm, D.H.; Reichenspurner, H.; Reichart, B. Midterm Results and Quality of Life after Minimally Invasive vs. Conventional Aortic Valve Replacement. *Thorac. Cardiovasc. Surg.* **2002**, *50*, 337–341. [CrossRef] [PubMed]
44. Chang, C.; Raza, S.; Altarabsheh, S.E.; Delozier, S.; Sharma, U.M.; Zia, A.; Khan, M.S.; Neudecker, M.; Markowitz, A.H.; Sabik, J.F.; et al. Minimally Invasive Approaches to Surgical Aortic Valve Replacement: A Meta-Analysis. *Ann. Thorac. Surg.* **2018**, *106*, 1881–1889. [CrossRef] [PubMed]
45. Mrcs, M.Y.S.; Hamilton, H.; Rahman, I.; Chien, L.; Rival, P.; Benedetto, U.; Young, C.; Caputo, M.; Angelini, G.D.; Vohra, H.A. Mini-sternotomy vs right anterior thoracotomy for aortic valve replacement. *J. Card. Surg.* **2020**, *35*, 1570–1582. [CrossRef]
46. Ogami, T.; Yokoyama, Y.; Takagi, H.; Serna-Gallegos, D.; Ferdinand, F.D.; Sultan, I.; Kuno, T. Minimally invasive versus conventional aortic valve replacement: The network meta-analysis. *J. Card. Surg.* **2022**, *37*, 4868–4874. [CrossRef]

47. Vohra, H.A.; Salmasi, M.Y.; Mohamed, F.; Shehata, M.; Bahrami, B.; Caputo, M.; Deshpande, R.; Bapat, V.; Bahrami, T.; Birdi, I.; et al. Consensus statement on aortic valve replacement via an anterior right minithoracotomy in the UK healthcare setting. *Open. Heart* **2023**, *10*, e002194. [CrossRef]
48. Balmforth, D.; Harky, A.; Lall, K.; Uppal, R. Is ministernotomy superior to right anterior minithoracotomy in minimally invasive aortic valve replacement? *Interact. Cardiovasc. Thorac. Surg.* **2017**, *25*, 818–821. [CrossRef]
49. Hassan, M.; Miao, Y.; Maraey, A.; Lincoln, J.; Brown, S.; Windsor, J.; Ricci, M. Minimally Invasive Aortic Valve Replacement: Cost-Benefit Analysis of Ministernotomy Versus Minithoracotomy Approach. *J. Heart Valve Dis.* **2015**, *24*, 531–539. [PubMed]
50. Ghanta, R.K.; Lapar, D.J.; Kern, J.A.; Kron, I.L.; Speir, A.M.; Fonner, E.; Quader, M.; Ailawadi, G. Minimally invasive aortic valve replacement provides equivalent outcomes at reduced cost compared with conventional aortic valve replacement: A real-world multi-institutional analysis. *J. Thorac. Cardiovasc. Surg.* **2015**, *149*, 1060–1065. [CrossRef]
51. Rodriguez, E.; Malaisrie, S.C.; Mehall, J.R.; Moore, M.; Salemi, A.; Ailawadi, G.; Economic Workgroup on Valvular Surgery. Right anterior thoracotomy aortic valve replacement is associated with less cost than sternotomy-based approaches: A multi-institution analysis of 'real world' data. *J. Med. Econ.* **2014**, *17*, 846–852. [CrossRef]
52. Gumus, F.; Hasde, A.I.; Bermede, O.; Kilickap, M.; Durdu, M.S. Multiple Valve Implantation Through a Minimally Invasive Approach: Comparison of Standard Median Sternotomy and Right Anterior Thoracotomy. *Heart Lung Circ.* **2020**, *29*, 1418–1423. [CrossRef]
53. Musumeci, F.; Lio, A.; Montalto, A.; Bergonzini, M.; Cammardella, A.G.; Comisso, M.; Nicolò, F.; Ranocchi, F. Minimally invasive treatment of multiple valve disease: A modified approach through a right lateral minithoracotomy. *J. Card. Surg.* **2019**, *35*, 135–139. [CrossRef]
54. Zhao, D.; Wei, L.; Zhu, S.; Zhang, Z.; Liu, H.; Yang, Y.; Wang, Y.; Ji, Q.; Wang, C. Combined Mitral and Aortic Valve Procedure via Right Mini-Thoracotomy versus Full Median Sternotomy. *Int. Heart J.* **2019**, *60*, 336–344. [CrossRef]
55. Manoly, I.; Hasan, R.; Brazier, A.; Farooq, V.; Thompson, T.; Karunaratne, D.; Naylor, H.; Fraser, D. Feasibility of hybrid off pump artery bypass grafting and transaortic transcatheter aortic valve implantation: A case series. *Catheter. Cardiovasc. Interv.* **2016**, *89*, 1273–1279. [CrossRef]
56. Zubarevich, A.; Zhigalov, K.; Szczechowicz, M.; Thielmann, M.; Rabis, M.; Van den Eynde, J.; Wendt, D. Simultaneous trans-aortic transcatheter aortic valve implantation and off-pump coronary artery bypass: An effective hybrid approach. *J. Card. Surg.* **2021**, *36*, 1226–1231. [CrossRef] [PubMed]
57. Mayr, B.; Firschke, C.; Erlebach, M.; Bleiziffer, S.; Krane, M.; Joner, M.; Herold, U.; Nöbauer, C.; Lange, R.; Deutsch, M.-A. Transcatheter aortic valve implantation and off-pump coronary artery bypass surgery: An effective hybrid procedure in selected patients. *Interact. Cardiovasc. Thorac. Surg.* **2018**, *27*, 102–107. [CrossRef]
58. Tabata, M.; Khalpey, Z.; Shekar, P.S.; Cohn, L.H. Reoperative minimal access aortic valve surgery: Minimal mediastinal dissection and minimal injury risk. *J. Thorac. Cardiovasc. Surg.* **2008**, *136*, 1564–1568. [CrossRef]
59. Santarpino, G.; Pfeiffer, S.; Concistrè, G.; Fischlein, T. Perceval S aortic valve implantation in mini-invasive surgery: The simple sutureless solution. *Interact. Cardiovasc. Thorac. Surg.* **2012**, *15*, 357–360. [CrossRef] [PubMed]
60. Morgant, M.-C.; Malapert, G.; Petrosyan, A.; Pujos, C.; Jazayeri, S.; Bouchot, O. Comparison of automated fastener device Cor-Knot versus manually-tied knot in minimally-invasive isolated aortic valve replacement surgery. *J. Cardiovasc. Surg.* **2020**, *61*, 123–128. [CrossRef] [PubMed]
61. Sazzad, F.; Ler, A.; Kuzemczak, M.; Ng, S.; Choong, A.M.; Kofidis, T. Automated Fastener vs Handtied Knots in Heart Valve Surgery: A Systematic Review and Meta-analysis. *Ann. Thorac. Surg.* **2020**, *112*, 970–980. [CrossRef]
62. Folliguet, T.A.; Vanhuyse, F.; Magnano, D.; Laborde, F. Robotic Aortic Valve Replacement: Case Report. *Heart Surg. Forum* **2004**, *7*, E551–E553. [CrossRef] [PubMed]
63. Badhwar, V.; Wei, L.M.; Cook, C.C.; Hayanga, J.W.A.; Daggubati, R.; Sengupta, P.P.; Rankin, J.S. Robotic aortic valve replacement. *J. Thorac. Cardiovasc. Surg.* **2021**, *161*, 1753–1759. [CrossRef] [PubMed]
64. Shrestha, M.; Krueger, H.; Umminger, J.; Koigeldiyev, N.; Beckmann, E.; Haverich, A.; Martens, A. Minimally invasive valve sparing aortic root replacement (David procedure) is safe. *Ann. Cardiothorac. Surg.* **2015**, *4*, 148–153. [CrossRef]
65. Glauber, M.; Miceli, A. Minimally Invasive Aortic Valve Surgery [Internet]. In *Cardiac Surgery: A Complete Guide*; Raja, S.G., Ed.; Springer International Publishing: Cham, Switzerland, 2020; pp. 421–428. [CrossRef]
66. Weissman, C. Pulmonary Complications After Cardiac Surgery. *Semin. Cardiothorac. Vasc. Anesth.* **2004**, *8*, 185–211. [CrossRef]
67. Moscoso Ludueña, M.; Rastan, A.J. Complications and conversions in minimally invasive aortic valve surgery. *Ann. Cardiothorac. Surg.* **2015**, *4*, 94–98.
68. Di Eusanio, M. Minimally invasive aortic valve replacement. *Ann. Cardiothorac. Surg.* **2015**, *4*, 1–2.
69. Mack, M.J.; Leon, M.B.; Thourani, V.H.; Makkar, R.; Kodali, S.K.; Russo, M.; Smith, C.R. Transcatheter Aortic-Valve Replacement with a Balloon-Expandable Valve in Low-Risk Patients. *N. Engl. J. Med.* **2019**, *380*, 1695–1705. [CrossRef]
70. Tam, D.Y.; Azizi, P.M.; Fremes, S.E.; Chikwe, J.; Gaudino, M.; Wijeysundera, H.C. The cost-effectiveness of transcatheter aortic valve replacement in low surgical risk patients with severe aortic stenosis. *Eur. Heart J.-Qual. Care Clin. Outcomes* **2020**, *7*, 556–563. [CrossRef] [PubMed]
71. Tabata, M.; Umakanthan, R.; Cohn, L.H.; Iii, R.M.B.; Shekar, P.S.; Chen, F.Y.; Couper, G.S.; Aranki, S.F. Early and late outcomes of 1000 minimally invasive aortic valve operations. *Eur. J. Cardio-Thorac. Surg.* **2008**, *33*, 537–541. [CrossRef]

72. Soppa, G.; Yates, M.; Viviano, A.; Smelt, J.; Valencia, O.; Van Besouw, J.P.; Jahangiri, M. Trainees can learn minimally invasive aortic valve replacement without compromising safety. *Interact. Cardio Vasc. Thorac. Surg.* **2015**, *20*, 458–462. [CrossRef] [PubMed]
73. Attia, R.Q.; Hickey, G.L.; Grant, S.W.; Bridgewater, B.; Roxburgh, J.C.; Kumar, P.; Young, C.P. Minimally Invasive Versus Conventional Aortic Valve Replacement: A Propensity-Matched Study From the UK National Data. *Innovations* **2016**, *11*, 15–23. [CrossRef] [PubMed]
74. Bilkhu, R.; Borger, M.; Briffa, N.P.; Jahangiri, M. Sutureless aortic valve prostheses. *Heart* **2019**, *105*, s16–s20. [CrossRef]
75. Berretta, P.; De Angelis, V.; Alfonsi, J.; Pierri, M.D.; Malvindi, P.G.; Zahedi, H.M.; Munch, C.; Di Eusanio, M. Enhanced recovery after minimally invasive heart valve surgery: Early and midterm outcomes. *Int. J. Cardiol.* **2022**, *370*, 98–104. [CrossRef] [PubMed]

Journal of
*Cardiovascular
Development and Disease*

MDPI

Review

Minimal Access Tricuspid Valve Surgery

Jean-Alexandre Sauvé *, Yung-Szu Wu, Ravi Ghatanatti and Joseph Zacharias *

Department of Cardiothoracic Surgery, Lancashire Cardiac Centre, Whinney Heys Road, Blackpool FY3 8NR, UK
* Correspondence: jean-alexandre.sauve@nhs.net (J.-A.S.); mr.zacharias@nhs.net (J.Z.)

Abstract: Tricuspid valve diseases are a heterogeneous group of pathologies that typically have poor prognoses when treated medically and are associated with significant morbidity and mortality with traditional surgical techniques. Minimal access tricuspid valve surgery may mitigate some of the surgical risks associated with the standard sternotomy approach by limiting pain, reducing blood loss, lowering the risk of wound infections, and shortening hospital stays. In certain patient populations, this may allow for a prompt intervention that could limit the pathologic effects of these diseases. Herein, we review the literature on minimal access tricuspid valve surgery focusing on perioperative planning, technique, and outcomes of minimal access endoscopic and robotic surgery for isolated tricuspid valve disease.

Keywords: minimal access surgery; tricuspid valve regurgitation; endoscopic and robotic cardiac surgery

1. Introduction

Tricuspid valve disease is a heterogeneous group of pathologies that lead to the impairment of the valve's normal function, which is to ensure the unidirectional flow of blood from the right atrium to the right ventricle. Functional abnormalities (either regurgitation or stenosis) resulting from disease are classified as primary and secondary. Primary causes affect the native tricuspid valve annulus or leaflets and include congenital (Ebstein's), myxomatous degeneration, rheumatic heart disease, infective endocarditis, carcinoid syndrome, iatrogenic valve damage (device leads, endomyocardial biopsies), toxic aetiologies, tumours, and blunt trauma. In Europe, over 90% of tricuspid disease is secondary regurgitation due to pressure and/or volume overload mediated RV dilatation or due to an enlarged atrium/tricuspid annulus due to chronic atrial fibrillation [1]. The prevalence of significant moderate or severe tricuspid regurgitation (TR) increases with age; maybe as high as 0.55% of the general population and has a poor prognosis when left untreated [2,3]. Management of tricuspid valve disease includes medical treatment of the underlying pathology as well as interventional strategies. European guidelines recommend surgery for severe symptomatic primary tricuspid regurgitation, liberally during left-sided surgery in patients with secondary tricuspid regurgitation and significant tricuspid stenosis, as well as in patients with isolated symptomatic secondary disease appropriate for surgery and those with no/mild symptoms but with RV dilatation and severe tricuspid regurgitation [4,5]. A limiting factor of early intervention in isolated tricuspid valve disease is the significant morbidity and mortality associated with a standard sternotomy approach in these older patient populations [6,7]. Additionally, patients presenting late with advanced degrees of RV dilation/dysfunction and/or fixed pulmonary hypertension are unlikely to benefit from the surgery [8]. Minimal access tricuspid valve surgery (MATVS; direct vision, endoscopic and robotic) mitigates some of this risk which could allow for earlier and more appropriate timing of the intervention to promote reverse RV remodeling, avoid organ failure, and improve functional status [9,10].

2. Preoperative Planning

A patient with isolated tricuspid valve disease will initially be assessed using transthoracic echocardiography by his primary physician or cardiologist and once thresholds and guidelines are met will be referred to a surgical or multidisciplinary team to assess the feasibility of an attempt to repair or replace the valve. A new risk score for in-hospital mortality prediction after isolated tricuspid surgery can also be of use to inform the patient and physicians and guide the clinical decision-making process [7]. This score, called the TRI-SCORE, is derived from 466 patients in French centres during a 10-year period and uses a twelve-point scoring system based on eight easy-to-ascertain risk factors to establish a predicted in-hospital mortality rate which ranges from 1% (0 points) to 65% ($\geq$9 points). Once the patient has been informed of the operative plan and has given appropriate consent, further preoperative planning to assess the suitability of the patient for a minimal access approach may proceed.

Patients will typically undergo a routine preoperative workup including a history and physical, a twelve-lead electrocardiogram, a chest X-ray, routine laboratory work, a transthoracic echocardiography, and a coronary angiogram. Due to selective lung ventilation during the procedure, pulmonary function tests are also commonly requested especially when the patient has a long-standing history of smoking or significant pulmonary disease. Depending on the clinician's experience and expertise, an ECG gated contrast thoracoabdominal CT scan with follow-through to the femoral arteries may be requested for evaluation of the thoracic anatomy, cardiac chamber sizes and positioning, ascending aorta size, as well as vascular anatomy [11]. This evaluation is sometimes omitted by certain groups [12]. The use of ultrasound scanning is an alternative in experienced centres with vascular ultrasound expertise.

Commonly, surgeons will also plan their cardiopulmonary bypass strategies at this point with particular attention to cannulation, clamping, and cardioplegia delivery. It is, however, not uncommon for these plans to be modified/adapted to the clinical context at the time of the operation. In MATVS, venous cannulation is almost always peripheral either percutaneous or via cut-down. Arterial cannulation is also commonly peripheral with some groups opting for a central approach [12]. In the case of peripheral cannulation, the common femoral artery was the most common site (either percutaneously or via cut-down) followed by the axillary artery. A femoral artery diameter of 7 mm or more was considered suitable for a cannula starting at 21 Fr [13]. Clamping strategies are either direct using a Chitwood style external clamp or peripheral via an intra-aortic occlusion device (IntraClude device Edwards through an EndoReturn cannula). As per Edwards' recommendation, an ascending aortic diameter of 40 mm or more is unfavourable for IntraClude utilization. Myocardial protection has been shown to be comparable between techniques in certain series [14]. Cardioplegia delivery is often antegrade with direct aortic cannulation or via the central lumen of the IntraClude device. A continuous retrograde delivery strategy has been utilized in some centres (ProPlege, Edwards) [15]. Most of the time, MATVS is performed on an arrested hypothermic heart although, when there is a contraindication to cross-clamping or use of the endovascular device, it may be performed on a beating/fibrillating heart [16].

3. Intraoperative Procedure

3.1. Anesthetic Consideration

General anaesthesia considerations vary widely between centres. MATVS are nearly always elective cases, although some urgent infective endocarditis cases have been reported in the literature [17]. Patients are positioned in the supine position with an inflatable bag or roll placed either transversally at the level of the 4th intercostal space or vertically at the level of the spine. They will typically have the standard anaesthesia monitoring of the respiratory and circulatory system including pulse oximetry, inspired oxygen analyser, capnography, measurement of pulmonary mechanics, non-invasive and invasive blood pressure monitoring (bilateral radial arterial lines often when IntraClude is used to monitor the migration of the balloon), electrocardiogram leads, defibrillation pads, temperature probe(s), peripheral and urinary catheter, quantitative neuromuscular monitoring, and transoesophageal echocardiography (TOE). Cerebral (and/or peripheral) oximetry monitoring and depth of anaesthesia/EEG surveillance are also commonly used. Centres describe a variety of ventilation strategies including intermittent ventilation of a single-lumen endotracheal (ET) tube or lung isolation via either double-lumen ET tubes or single-lumen ET tubes with bronchial blockers [18,19]. Once the patient is under general anaesthesia, central venous lines are placed and, occasionally, Swan-Ganz catheters may be used. Other invasive lines and monitoring may be used depending on the patient's clinical condition and risk factors.

Often, the superior vena cava (SVC) cannula is inserted by the anaesthetist at this stage via the internal jugular vein and properly positioned with the aid of TOE. In redo cases, an arterial embolectomy catheter can be used and inserted through a custom-assembled side arm to occlude SVC before the right atrial opening [13].

3.2. Surgical Technique

Once the patient is positioned, skin disinfected, and draped with sterile sheets, the surgery commences. The skin incision used in isolated MATVS varies between centres but has trended to smaller incisions with the introduction of video assistance. A periareolar skin incision is typically the most cosmetic, delivering patient-satisfying results [20–22]. It can be extended laterally when needed to accommodate for a prosthesis when the valve cannot be repaired or when extensive lysis of adhesions is required. Blunt dissection and muscle splitting of the pectoral muscle allow for entry into the thoracic cavity; sometimes, the muscle is simply divided with diathermy for better haemostasis. Soft tissue retractors are recommended, and a thoracic spreader may be used in certain cases when using direct vision. Additional ports are also installed via 5–10 mm stab incisions; typically, a camera port will be installed in the anterior axillary line at either the 3rd or 4th intercostal space (ICS). A working port at the level of the 4th or 5th ICS (we prefer the 4th ICS; see Figure 1) and an atrial retractor incision may also be made medial to the working port in the 4th ICS. A further 5 mm port is used to introduce a cardiotomy suction device just above the diaphragm in the 6th space in the mid-axillary line. We also use this port to insufflate carbon dioxide. Left atrial retractors may be used, although a novel dedicated right atrial retractor has recently been developed [23]. Cameras used in endoscopic surgery may be 2D or 3D and of varying resolution. Advantages of 3D cameras are enhanced anatomical details and depth perception as well as easier skill acquisition and transfer [24]. Robotic MATVS shares many similarities with the endoscopic techniques. Port configurations are similar: the working port which is typically placed in the third intercostal space (ICS) at the anterior axillary line, the left arm port which is placed in the second ICS (halfway between anterior axillary and midclavicular line), the right arm port in the fifth ICS below the anterior axillary line, and the atrial retractor which is placed in the fourth ICS, 2 cm medial to midclavicular line [25].

As described above, several vascular cannulation strategies are possible and there is great variability between centres. Most commonly, an SVC cannula is inserted by the anaesthetist, and inferior vena cava cannulation (IVC) is performed either percutaneously or via cutdown of the common femoral vein by the surgeon. The IVC cannula is advanced to the junction of the IVC and right atrium. Other strategies of venous cannulation with good outcomes include direct bicaval cannulation using the standard venous cannulas or single multi-stage femoral cannulation [26,27]. An atrial venous shunt may be used once the atriotomy has been performed to provide for adequate drainage of the SVC via the single IVC cannula in certain cases [28]. Snaring of the venae cava can be achieved directly through standard snares or with large bulldog vascular clamps in non-redo operations [13]. In redo cases, arterial embolectomy catheters or vascular occlusion balloons have also been used either through contralateral insertion sites and advancement past the venous cannulas' tips or through a side port of the cannulas themselves (as explained above) [13,29,30]. Others have shown that performing tricuspid surgery without caval occlusion is safe due to the air being captured by the active drainage system [31]. This requires very good communication with the perfusion team to avoid air lock of the venous line in case of excessive vacuum assist.

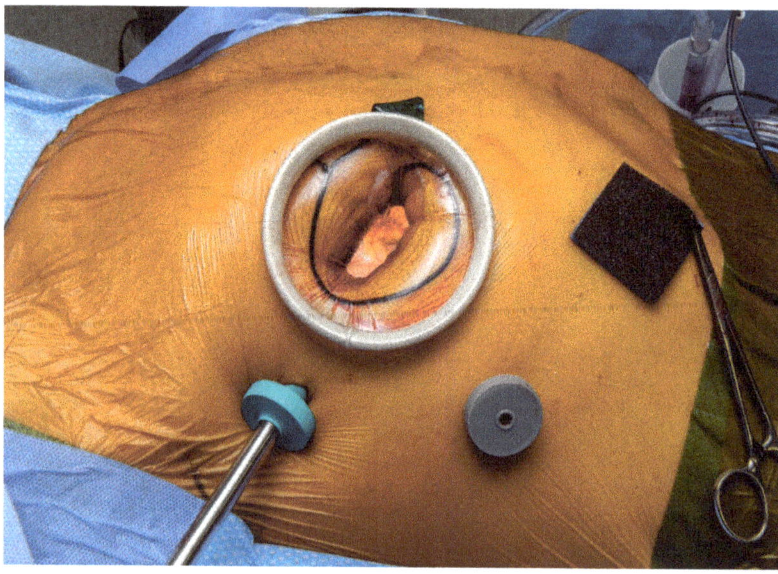

Figure 1. An example of the typical setup for MATVS at the Lancashire cardiac centre. A periareolar skin incision is made with a mini-thoracotomy at the fourth intercostal space with a camera port at the same level (blue trocar). An additional trocar (grey) is placed to facilitate the installation of a cardiotomy succion and/or pericardial stay sutures.

Arterial cannulation in the setting of MATVS is typically femoral but may occasionally be axillary, central, and even, although rarely, via the carotid artery [32]. It may be percutaneous when aortic cross-clamping is done centrally or when no clamping is envisioned. It is more likely by cutdown if the IntraClude device is used given the required larger size of the inflow cannula [33]. Different cardioplegic strategies are possible when arrest is desired with most centres opting for single-dose cardioplegia when available. Other centres avoid cross-clamping by performing beating heart surgery or on a hypothermic fibrillating heart, especially in redo cases (see Figure 2) [16,34].

Techniques for repair and replacement in MATVS are identical to those in open surgery [5]. Knot-tying may be achieved with automatic devices (such as CorKnot, which have several potential intraoperative advantages described elsewhere) or with knot-pushing devices [35]. Given the steep learning curve of MATVS, several learning tools have been suggested. Notably, a 'suture map' has been developed to guide surgeons in the placement of their sutures during annuloplasty repair. A reverse backhand position is suggested for the initial three sutures along the anterior leaflet and the course of the right coronary artery; a reversed forehand position for the next two sutures along the commissure between the anterior and posterior leaflets; a forehand position for the next three sutures along the mid portion of the posterior leaflet to the mid portion of the septal leaflet [36].

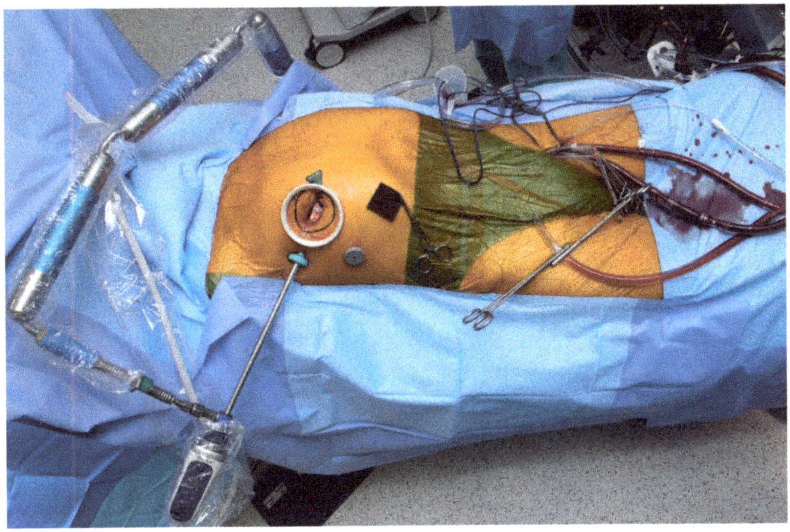

Figure 2. Full cannulation setup. Of note, this case was done on a beating heart with a single venous cannula and no additional shunting or occlusion devices. Furthermore, a 'Y' arterial connection is routinely constructed to facilitate additional arterial cannulation if need be (doubly clamped arterial connection at the bottom of the image). The camera holder is a pneumatically operated arm which can be seen at the top of the image.

The most common method for pacing after an isolated MATVS is to place standard epicardial pacing wires directly on the surface of the right ventricle [13]. In redo cases, where dissection of adhesions is to be avoided, pacing can be achieved through the tricuspid valve using a transvenous pacing catheter inserted preoperatively and repositioned after the repair or replacement [37]. In some cases, the standard epicardial pacing wires may be placed directly into the endocardial surface of the right ventricle and passed through the tricuspid valve and right atriotomy suture line [13]. After weaning from CPB, loose closure of the pericardium with a small drain in the pericardium and another drain in the right pleura is common. In redo cases, a single drain in the right pleura without closing the pericardium may be warranted [13].

4. Postoperative Course

Postoperative care of MATVS is akin to that of sternotomy patients. Fluid replacement in patients with long-term dependence on high-dose diuretic therapy can be challenging. Close attention needs to be given to the right ventricular end-diastolic volumes as overloading the right ventricle in the post-tricuspid valve repair setting can have fatal consequences. Wound monitoring at peripheral cannulation is important, and special attention should be given to the potential development of vascular complications in the initial phase with femoral arterial cannulation (more at risk with percutaneous cannulation) [38,39]. Vascular assessment of peripheral pulses with a doppler and pencil probe may be considered in case of concern. Additionally, given the thoracic approach of MATVS, care must be given to ensure appropriate lung re-expansion after surgery, which can be assessed by chest X-ray. Patients are slightly more at risk of air leaks than their counterparts undergoing open surgery and of pleural effusion/haemothorax, particularly in the initial stages. Some centres advocate for the quick removal of drains, within 24–48 h post-surgery, while others prefer to leave the pericardial drain in place for several days to prevent late pericardial effusion [40,41].

5. Outcomes of MATVS

Minimal access cardiac surgery (MACS) has been shown in multiple case series and propensity-matched analysis to have several advantages when compared to traditional open sternotomy: smaller incisions resulting in less pain, better cosmesis, faster recovery, reduced blood loss, shorter hospital stays, and lowered risk of wound infection [42–44]. When focusing specifically on MATVS, risk/benefit assessments are more difficult to evaluate given that there is a distinct lack of randomized controlled trials comparing the outcomes of MATVS to those undergoing surgery through standard sternotomy when contrasted to minimal access approaches to mitral and aortic valve disease [45]. In 2020, our group summarized our outcomes which included isolated MATVS but also MATVS as a concomitant procedure and in redo settings [10]. Morbidity including cerebrovascular accident (CVA) varied from 0% and 4%, renal complications around 8–13% (which was lower than the 24–35% rate in sternotomy patients), and mortality estimated between 4.1 and 17% in these heterogeneous groups [12,13,40,46–48].

MACS has traditionally been reported to have a higher risk of CVAs as compared to standard sternotomy, which was believed to be due to the use of retrograde cardiopulmonary bypass, leading some centres to shift towards using antegrade cardiopulmonary bypass methods [49]. Recent studies have found, however, that the risk of CVA is similar to the use of retrograde perfusion in selected patients [50]. MATVS in reported series has been shown to have a 0–4% risk of CVA, which is akin to the rates in meta-analyses of open surgery comparing repair vs. replacement (stroke risk 1.5% vs. 0.9%) [51,52].

Patients undergoing isolated tricuspid valve surgery may be at a higher risk of renal complications due to their comorbidities and often delayed referral for surgery. Studies have shown higher rates of renal failure and acute kidney injury (AKI) in patients undergoing redo tricuspid valve surgery, with some studies reporting incidence as high as 30–35% with sternotomy [40,53]. However, studies comparing MATVS to sternotomy have generally reported a lower risk of AKI and a new onset dialysis requirement in the MATVS group. These studies have reported new onset renal replacement therapy ranging from 5.6% to 13% in the MATVS groups as compared to 12.4–15.6% (repair vs. replacement) in the traditional literature [40,51,54]. In high-risk patients undergoing MATVS, the risk of acute renal failure requiring renal replacement therapy is reported to be around 7.8% [46].

One of the causes of the increasing diagnosis of tricuspid valve regurgitation is the increased prevalence of atrial fibrillation (AF) in the general population and the increasing use of device leads [55,56]. Many patients undergoing tricuspid valve surgery, therefore, have underlying rhythm problems and the surgery itself is at risk of causing such issues given the anatomical proximity of the tricuspid valve to the conduction system [36]. Tricuspid valve surgery, therefore, carries a high risk of post-operative arrhythmias and device implantation; with variable rates in the defined MATVS case series.

Tricuspid valve surgery via sternotomy has been shown to have high mortality rates, reaching up to 50% in some cases [2]. On the other hand, MATVS seems to have lower mortality rates when compared to the sternotomy approach. Studies have reported a 30-day mortality rate of 5% for both sternotomy and MATVS in redo settings [40]. In contrast, Färber et al. showed a mortality rate of 8% in primary MATVS and 7% in the redo MATVS group compared to 27% in the redo sternotomy group [47]. Abdelbar et al. showed a 30-day mortality rate of 4.1% in MITS both in primary and redo settings [13]. Additionally, Chen and colleagues have reported a significant reduction in mortality after shifting from median sternotomy to MITS, from 23.3% to 4.6% [48]. While associated with adverse perioperative outcomes, in a series of 79 patients undergoing endoscopic repeat isolated tricuspid valve surgery (RITS) after left-sided valve replacement (LSVR) endoscopic access was acceptable as an alternative to sternotomy [57]. Further retrospective analyses of RITS after LSVR have revealed no difference in early mortality and long-term survival between patients undergoing an endoscopic approach vs. sternotomy, although patients undergoing endoscopic approaches had shorter ICU stays and fewer reoperations [58,59]. MATVS as an isolated procedure in a redo setting was also shown to be a safe procedure with no reported mortality in 47 patients [60].

Potential Additional Benefits of MATVS

As reported previously, MACS has been shown to have several potential benefits when compared to open surgery, and this likely applies to MATVS as well. There are, therefore, likely benefits regarding operative times, blood loss, pain management, and overall cost-benefit advantages. Operative times for MACS have traditionally been longer than for open surgery [61]. As surgical techniques have progressed and technological advances have been made, operative time for MACS cases has consequently diminished. In addition, some studies have reported shorter bypass times for MATVS than median sternotomy, particularly in redo surgery (78 ± 31 min vs. 91 ± 23 min) [40]. Despite this, the use of an endovascular occlusion clamp in some cases can increase bypass times. In any case, operative times for MATVS did not seem to impact mortality. MACS has been shown to have a lower incidence of blood loss compared to standard sternotomy due to its smaller incision and lack of bone division [45]. Studies have also shown that MATVS results in less bleeding during the first 24 h post-surgery, with lower mean total drainage [40]. Re-exploration for bleeding is also lower in redo MATVS as compared to sternotomy [47]. This is reflected in the lower blood transfusion rates after redo MATVS. Additionally, Chen and colleagues reported no blood transfusion at all in their redo MATVS group [48]. As most patients referred for tricuspid valve surgery are likely to have some liver congestion, smaller incisions are more likely to reduce the bleeding risks. There are limited reports specifically on pain scores related to isolated MATVS; however, there is a wealth of evidence detailing to benefits of MACS on pain reduction and faster return to normal activity as compared to standard sternotomy [62–64]. It is believed that the pain reduction is due to preserving sternal integrity, resulting in better thorax stability [65]. While not specific to MATVS, quality-of-life studies have reported that up to 94% of patients reported no or minimal pain after their MACS procedure, and 43% reported having returned to work within three weeks [66]. In more recent years, regional and local anaesthesia techniques have been utilized to reduce post-operative pain even further, with studies reporting a reduction in post-operative narcotics usage and improved pain scores [67,68].

6. Conclusions

In summary, isolated MATVS is a safe and reproducible procedure that can be used to effectively address multiple causes of tricuspid valve disease and notably deal with secondary causes of tricuspid regurgitation, which are becoming more prevalent as the population ages. It offers several potential advantages when compared to open surgery including a lower risk of renal complications, fewer blood transfusions, lesser device implantations, and lower mortality. It also has other benefits such as improved cosmesis, less pain, decreased wound infections, and earlier mobilization. Further studies will now be needed to identify the optimal timing for surgery for isolated functional TR and to truly establish whether an intervention such as surgery can confer survival benefits when compared to medical therapy alone; with current evidence suggesting it may without reaching statistical significance [4,69]. Although current evidence supports the timing range on a variety of factors (including patient characteristics, disease aetiology, and anatomical considerations), and that earlier interventions before significant right ventricular dysfunction, congestive heart failure, and pulmonary hypertension seem to offer better results, additional studies including randomized controlled trials would be of use [5]. Finally, such an approach will eventually need to be compared to transcatheter techniques which are rapidly evolving and for which patient outcome studies are now being conducted [70,71].

Author Contributions: Writing—original draft preparation, J.-A.S.; review and editing, J.-A.S., Y.-S.W. and R.G.; supervision, J.Z. All authors have read and agreed to the published version of the manuscript.

Funding: This research received no external funding.

Conflicts of Interest: The authors declare no conflict of interest.

References

1. Vahanian, A.; Beyersdorf, F.; Praz, F.; Milojevic, M.; Baldus, S.; Bauersachs, J.; Capodanno, D.; Conradi, L.; De Bonis, M.; De Paulis, R.; et al. 2021 ESC/EACTS Guidelines for the management of valvular heart disease: Developed by the Task Force for the management of valvular heart disease of the European Society of Cardiology (ESC) and the European Association for Cardio-Thoracic Surgery (EACTS). *Eur. Heart J.* **2021**, *43*, 561–632. [CrossRef]
2. Topilsky, Y.; Maltais, S.; Medina-Inojosa, J.; Oguz, D.; Michelena, H.; Maalouf, J.; Mahoney, D.W.; Enriquez-Sarano, M. Burden of Tricuspid Regurgitation in Patients Diagnosed in the Community Setting. *JACC Cardiovasc. Imaging* **2019**, *12*, 433–442. [CrossRef]
3. Chorin, E.; Rozenbaum, Z.; Topilsky, Y.; Konigstein, M.; Ziv-Balran, T.; Richert, E.; Keren, G.; Banai, S. Tricuspid regurgitation and long-term clinical outcomes. *Eur. Heart J. -Cardiovasc. Imaging* **2020**, *21*, 157–165. [CrossRef]
4. Axtell, A.L.; Bhambhani, V.; Moonsamy, P.; Het aly, E.W.; Picard, M.H.; Sundt, T.M.; Wasfy, J.H. Surgery Does Not Improve Survival in Patients with Isolated Severe Tricuspid Regurgitation. *J. Am. Coll. Cardiol.* **2019**, *74*, 715–725. [CrossRef]
5. Tagliari, A.P.; Perez-Camargo, D.; Taramasso, M. Tricuspid regurgitation: When is it time for surgery? *Expert Rev. Cardiovasc. Ther.* **2021**, *19*, 47–59. [CrossRef]
6. Kilic, A.; Saha-Chaudhuri, P.; Rankin, J.S.; Contet, J.V. Trends and outcomes of tricuspid valve surgery in North America: An analysis of more than 50,000 patients from the Society of Thoracic Surgeons database. *Ann. Thorac. Surg.* **2013**, *96*, 1546–1552, discussion 1552. [CrossRef]
7. Dreyfus, J.; Audureau, E.; Bohbot, Y.; Coisne, A.; Lavie-Badie, Y.; Bouchery, M.; Flagiello, M.; Bazire, B.; Eggenspieler, F.; Viau, F.; et al. TRI-SCORE: A new risk score for in-hospital mortality prediction after isolated tricuspid valve surgery. *Eur. Heart J.* **2021**, *43*, 654–662. [CrossRef]
8. Hamandi, M.; George, T.J.; Smith, R.L.; Malck, M.J. Current outcomes of tricuspid valve surgery. *Prog. Cardiovasc. Dis.* **2019**, *62*, 463–466. [CrossRef]
9. Dreyfus, G.D.; Corbi, P.J.; Chan, K.M.J.; Bahrami, T. Secondary tricuspid regurgitation or dilatation: Which should be the criteria for surgical repair? *Ann. Thorac. Surg.* **2005**, *79*, 127–132. [CrossRef]
10. Abdelbar, A.; Kenawy, A.; Zacharias, J. Minimally invasive tricuspid valve surgery. *J. Thorac. Dis.* **2020**, *13*, 1982–1992. [CrossRef]
11. Ramchandani, M.; Al Jabbari, O.; Abu Saleh, W.K.; Ramlawi, B. Cannulation Strategies and Pitfalls in Minimally Invasive Cardiac Surgery. *Methodist Debakey Cardiovasc. J.* **2016**, *12*, 10–13. [CrossRef]
12. Lamelas, J. Minimal access tricuspid valve surgery. *Ann. Cardiothorac. Surg.* **2017**, *6*, 283–286. [CrossRef]
13. Abdelbar, A.; Niranjan, G.; Tetnnyson, C.; Saravanan, P.; Knowles, A.; Laskawski, G.; Zacharias, J. Endoscopic Tricuspid Valve Surgery is a Safe and Effective Option. *Innovations* **2020**, *15*, 66–73. [CrossRef] [PubMed]
14. Grazioli, V.; Giroletti, L.; Graniero, A.; Albano, G.; Mazzoni, M.; Panisi, P.G.; Gerometta, P.; Anselmi, A.; Agnino, A. Comparative myocardial protection of endoaortic balloon versus external clamp in minimally invasive mitral valve surgery. *J. Cardiovasc. Med.* **2022**, *24*, 184–190. [CrossRef] [PubMed]
15. Lebon, J.-S.; Couture, P.; Rochon, A.G.; Laliberté, É.; Harvey, J.; Aubé, N.; Cossette, M.; Bouchard, D.; Jeanmart, H.; Pellerin, M. The endovascular coronary sinus catheter in minimally invasive mitral and tricuspid valve surgery: A case series. *J. Cardiothorac. Vasc. Anesth.* **2010**, *24*, 746–751. [CrossRef] [PubMed]
16. Misfeld, M.; Daviet rwala, P.; Banusch, J.; Ender, J.; Mohr, F.-W.; Pfannmüller, B. Minimally invasive, beating heart tricuspid valve surgery in a redo case. *Ann. Cardiothorac. Surg.* **2017**, *6*, 290–293. [CrossRef]
17. Robin, J.; Tronc, F.; Vetdrinne, C.; Chalmpsaur, G. Video-assisted tricuspid valve surgery: A new surgical option in endocarditis on pacemaker. *Eur. J. Cardiothorac. Surg.* **1999**, *16*, 243–245. [CrossRef]
18. White, A.; Patvardhan, C.; Falter, F. Anesthesia for minimally invasive cardiac surgery. *J. Thorac. Dis.* **2021**, *13*, 1886–1898. [CrossRef]
19. Zhang, C.; Yue, J.; Li, M.; Jiang, W.; Pan, Y.; Song, Z.; Shi, C.; Fan, W.; Pan, Z. Bronchial blocker versus double-lumen endobronchial tube in minimally invasive cardiac surgery. *BMC Pulm. Med.* **2019**, *19*, 207. [CrossRef]
20. Poffo, R.; Montanhesi, P.K.; Toschi, A.P.; Pope, R.B.; Mokross, C.A. Periareolar Access for Minimally Invasive Cardiac Surgery: The Brazilian Technique. *Innovations* **2018**, *13*, 65–69. [CrossRef]
21. Van Praet, K.M.; Kofletr, M.; Akansel, S.; Montagner, M.; Meyer, A.; Sündermann, S.H.; Falk, V.; Kempfert, J. Periareolar endoscopic minimally invasive cardiac surgery: Postoperative scar assessment analysis. *Interact. Cardiovasc. Thorac. Surg.* **2022**, *35*, ivac200. [CrossRef] [PubMed]
22. Durdu, M.S.; Baran, C.; Gümüş, F.; Deniz, G.; Çakıcı, M.; Özçınar, E.; Bermede, A.O.; Uçanok, K.; Akar, A.R. Comparison of minimally invasive cardiac surgery incisions: Periareolar approach in female patients. *Anatol. J. Cardiol.* **2018**, *20*, 283–288. [PubMed]
23. Castillo-Sang, M.; Konys, J.; Burkhard, B.; Voetller, R. First Dedicated Minimally Invasive Right Atrial Retractor. *Surg. Technol. Int.* **2022**, *41*, sti41-1584. [CrossRef] [PubMed]
24. Beattie, K.L.; Hill, A.; Horswill, M.S.; Grove, P.M.; Stevenson, A.R.L. Laparoscopic skills training: The effects of viewing mode (2D vs. 3D) on skill acquisition and transfer. *Surg. Endosc.* **2021**, *35*, 4332–4344. [CrossRef] [PubMed]

25. Amabile, A.; LaLonde, M.R.; Mullan, C.W.; Hameed, I.; Degife, E.; Krane, M.; Geirsson, A.; Agrawal, A. Totally endoscopic, robotic-assisted tricuspid valve repair with neochords. *Multimed. Man. Cardiothorac. Surg.* **2022**, *2022*.
26. Kandakure, P.R.; Batra, M.; Garre, S.; Banovath, S.N.; Shalikh, F.; Pani, K. Direct Cannulation in Minimally Invasive Cardiac Surgery with Limited Resources. *Ann. Thorac. Surg.* **2020**, *109*, 512–516. [CrossRef]
27. Peng, R.; Shi, H.; Ba, J.; Wang, C.S. Single Femoral Venous Drainage Versus Both Vena Cava Drainage in Isolated Repeat Tricuspid Valve Surgery. *Int. Heart J.* **2018**, *59*, 518–522. [CrossRef]
28. Wu, S.; Ma, aL.; Li, C.; Ni, Y. Optimizing Venous Drainage for Minimal Access Right Atrial Procedures. *Ann. Thorac. Surg.* **2019**, *108*, e337–e338. [CrossRef]
29. Pfannmuüller, B.; Misfeld, M.; Borger, M.A.; Etz, C.D.; Funkat, A.-K.; Garbade, J.; Mohr, F.W. Isolated reoperative minimally invasive tricuspid valve operations. *Ann. Thorac. Surg.* **2012**, *94*, 2005–2010. [CrossRef]
30. Yamani, N.E.; Lebon, J.-S.; Laliberté, E.; Couture, P.; Desjardins, G.; Coddens, J.; Bouchard, D. Endovascular Vena Cavae Occlusion Technique in Minimally Invasive Tricuspid Valve Surgery in Patients with Previous Cardiac Surgery. *J. Cardiothorac. Vasc. Anesth.* **2021**, *35*, 1334–1340. [CrossRef]
31. Margari, V.; Malvindi, P.G.; De Santis, A.; Kounakis, G.; Visicchio, G.; Ccp, G.M.; Dambruoso, P.; Carbone, C.; Paparella, D. Minimally invasive tricuspid valve surgery without caval occlusion: Short and midterm results. *J. Card. Surg.* **2021**, *36*, 618–623. [CrossRef] [PubMed]
32. Bonaros, N.; Höfetr, aD.; Holfeld, J.; Grimm, M.; Müller, L. Cannulation of the Carotid Artery for Minimally Invasive Mitral or Tricuspid Valve Surgery. *Ann. Thorac. Surg.* **2020**, *110*, e517–e519. [CrossRef] [PubMed]
33. der Merwe, J.V.; Casselman, F.; Van Praet, F. The principles of minimally invasive atrioventricular valve repair surgery utilizing endoaortic balloon occlusion technology: How to start and sustain a safe and effective program. *J. Vis. Surg.* **2019**, *5*, 72. [CrossRef]
34. Lu, S.; eSong, K.; Yao, W.; Xia, L.; Dong, L.; Sun, Y.; Hong, T.; Yalng, S.; Wang, C. Simplified, minimally invasive, beating-heart technique for redo isolated tricuspid valve surgery. *J. Cardiothorac. Surg.* **2020**, *15*, 146. [CrossRef]
35. Jenkin, I.; Prachete, I.; Sokal, P.A.; Harky, A. The role of Cor-Knot in the future of cardiac surgery: A systematic review. *J. Card. Surg.* **2020**, *35*, 2987–2994. [CrossRef] [PubMed]
36. Hamid, U.I.; Aksoy, R.; Nia, P.S. Suture map for endoscopic tricuspid valve repair. *Multimed. Man. Cardiothorac. Surg.* **2022**, *2022*. [CrossRef]
37. Lei, Q.; Wei, X.-C.; Huang, K.-L.; Yu, T.; Zhang, X.-S.; Huang, H.-L.; Guo, H.-M. Intraoperative Implantation of Temporary Endocardial Pacing Catheter During Thoracoscopic Redo Tricuspid Surgery. *Heart Lung Circ.* **2019**, *28*, 1121–1126. [CrossRef]
38. Noori, V.J.; Eldrup-Jørgensen, J. A systematic review of vascular closure devices for femoral artery puncture sites. *J. Vasc. Surg.* **2018**, *68*, 887–899. [CrossRef]
39. Lamelas, J.; Williams, R.F.; Mawad, M.; LaPietra, A. Complications Associated with Femoral Cannulation During Minimally Invasive Cardiac Surgery. *Ann. Thorac. Surg.* **2017**, *103*, 1927–1932. [CrossRef]
40. Maimaiti, A.; Weti, L.; Yang, Y.; Liu, H.; Wang, C. Benefits of a right anterolateral minithoracotomy rather than a median sternotomy in isolated tricuspid redo procedures. *J. Thorac. Dis.* **2017**, *9*, 1281–1288. [CrossRef]
41. Li, M.; Zhang, J.; Gan, T.J.; Qin, G.; Wang, L.; Zhu, M.; Zhang, Z.; Pan, Y.; Ye, Z.; Zhang, F.; et al. Enhanced recovery after surgery pathway for patients undergoing cardiac surgery: A randomized clinical trial. *Eur. J. Cardiothorac. Surg.* **2018**, *54*, 491–497. [CrossRef] [PubMed]
42. Ishikawa, N.; Watanabe, G. Robot-assisted cardiac surgery. *Ann. Thorac. Cardiovasc. Surg.* **2015**, *21*, 322–328. [CrossRef]
43. Iribarne, A.; Easterwood, R.; Chan, E.Y.; Yang, J.; Soni, L.; Russo, M.J.; Smith, C.R.; Algenziano, M. The golden age of minimally invasive cardiothoracic surgery: Current and future perspectives. *Future Cardiol.* **2011**, *7*, 333–346. [CrossRef] [PubMed]
44. Grant, S.W.; Hickey, G.L.; Modi, P.; Hunter, S.; Alkowuah, E.; Zacharias, J. Propensity-matched analysis of minimally invasive approach versus sternotomy for mitral valve surgery. *Heart* **2019**, *105*, 783–789. [CrossRef] [PubMed]
45. Doenst, T.; Diab, M.; Sponholz, C.; Bauetr, M.; Färber, G. The Opportunities and Limitations of Minimally Invasive Cardiac Surgery. *Dtsch. Arztebl. Int.* **2017**, *114*, 777–784. [CrossRef]
46. Ricci, D.; Boffini, M.; Barbero, C.; El Qarra, S.; Marchetto, G.; Rinaldi, M. Minimally invasive tricuspid valve surgery in patients at high risk. *J. Thorac. Cardiovasc. Surg.* **2014**, *147*, 996–1001. [CrossRef]
47. Färber, G.; Tkebuchava, S.; Dawson, R.S.; Kirov, H.; Diab, M.; Schlattmann, P.; Doenst, T. Minimally Invasive, Isolated Tricuspid Valve Redo Surgery: A Safety and Outcome Analysis. *Thorac. Cardiovasc. Surg.* **2018**, *66*, 564–571. [CrossRef]
48. Chen, J.; Hu, K.; Ma, W.; Lv, M.; Shi, Y.; Liu, J.; Wei, L.; Lin, Y.; Hong, T.; Walng, C. Isolated reoperation for tricuspid regurgitation after left-sided valve surgery: Technique evolution. *Eur. J. Cardiothorac. Surg.* **2020**, *57*, 142–150. [CrossRef]
49. Murzi, M.; Cerillo, A.G.; Miceli, A.; Bevilacqua, S.; Kallushi, E.; Farneti, P.; Solinas, M.; Glauber, M. Antegrade and retrograde arterial perfusion strategy in minimally invasive mitral-valve surgery: A propensity score analysis on 1280 patients. *Eur. J. Cardiothorac. Surg.* **2013**, *43*, e167–e172. [CrossRef]
50. Modi, P.; Hassan, A.; Chitwood, W.R., Jr. Minimally invasive mitral valve surgery: A systematic review and meta-analysis. *Eur. J. Cardiothorac. Surg.* **2008**, *34*, 943–952. [CrossRef]
51. Wang, T.K.M.; Griffin, B.P.; Miyasaka, R.; Xu, B.; Popovic, Z.B.; Pettersson, G.B.; Gillinov, A.M.; Desai, M.Y. Isolated surgical tricuspid repair versus replacement: Metaanalysis of 15 069 patients. *Open. Heart* **2020**, *7*, e001227. [CrossRef] [PubMed]
52. Sarris-Michopoulos, P.; Macias, A.E.; Sarris-Michopoulos, C.; Woodhouse, P.; Buitrago, D.; Salerno, T.A.; Magarakis, M. Isolated tricuspid valve surgery—Repair versus replacement: A meta-analysis. *J. Card. Surg.* **2022**, *37*, 329–335. [CrossRef] [PubMed]

53. Moutakiallah, Y.; Aithoussa, M.; Atmani, N.; Seghrouchni, A.; Moujahid, A.; Hatim, A.; Asfalou, I.; Lakhal, Z.; Boulahya, A. Reoperation for isolated rheumatic tricuspid regurgitation. *J. Cardiothorac. Surg.* **2018**, *13*, 104. [CrossRef] [PubMed]
54. Liu, S.; Chen, J.M.; Wang, W.S.; Lu, Y.T.; aMing, Y.; Wei, L.; Wang, C.S. Short-term outcomes of minimally invasive reoperation for tricuspid regurgitation after left-sided valve surgery. *Zhonghua Wai Ke Za Zhi* **2019**, *57*, 898–901.
55. Patlolla, S.H.; Schaff, H.V.; Nishimura, R.A.; Stulak, J.M.; Chambetrlain, A.M.; Pislaru, S.V.; Nkomo, V.T. Incidence and Burden of Tricuspid Regurgitation in Patients with Atrial Fibrillation. *J. Am. Coll. Cardiol.* **2022**, *80*, 2289–2298. [CrossRef]
56. Khoshbin, E.; Abdetlbar, A.; Allen, S.; Hasan, R. The mechanism of endocardial lead-induced tricuspid regurgitation. *BMJ Case Rep.* **2013**, *2013*, bcr2012008191. [CrossRef]
57. Xie, X.J.; Yang, L.; Zhou, K.; Yang, Y.-C.; He, B.-C.; Chen, Z.-R.; Huang, H.-R. Endoscopic repeat isolated tricuspid valve surgery after left-sided valve replacement: Valvuloplasty or replacement. *J. Cardiovasc. Surg.* **2021**, *62*, 515–522. [CrossRef]
58. Yang, L.; Zhou, K.; Yang, Y.; He, B.; Chen, Z.; Tian, C.; Hualng, H. Outcomes of redo-isolated tricuspid valve surgery after left-sided valve surgery. *J. Card. Surg.* **2021**, *36*, 3060–3069. [CrossRef]
59. Dai, X.; Teng, P.; Miao, S.; Zheng, J.; Si, W.; Zheng, Q.; Qin, K.; Ma, L. Minimally Invasive Isolated Tricuspid Valve Repair After Left-Sided Valve Surgery: A Single-Center Experience. *Front. Surg.* **2022**, *9*, 837148. [CrossRef]
60. Wei, S.; Zhang, L.; Cui, H.; Ren, T.; Li, L.; Jiang, S. Minimally Invasive Isolated Tricuspid Valve Redo Surgery Has Better Clinical Outcome: A Single-Center Experience. *Heart Surg. Forum.* **2020**, *23*, E647–E651. [CrossRef]
61. Chaney, M.A.; Durazo-Arvizu, R.A.; Fludetr, E.M.; Sawicki, K.J.; Nikolov, M.P.; Blakeman, B.P.; Bakhos, M. Port-access minimally invasive cardiac surgery increases surgical complexity, increases operating room time, and facilitates early postoperative hospital discharge. *Anesthesiology* **2000**, *92*, 1637–1645. [CrossRef] [PubMed]
62. Glower, D.D.; Landolfo, K.P.; Clements, F.; DeBruijn, N.P.; Stafford-Smith, M.; Smith, P.K.; Duhaylongsod, F. Mitral valve operation via Port Access versus median sternotomy. *Eur. J. Cardiothorac. Surg.* **1998**, *14* (Suppl. S1), S143–S147. [CrossRef] [PubMed]
63. Yamada, T.; Ochiai, R.; Taketda, J.; Shin, H.; Yozu, R. Comparison of early postoperative quality of life in minimally invasive versus conventional valve surgery. *J. Anesth.* **2003**, *17*, 171–176. [CrossRef]
64. Santana, O.; Retyna, J.; Grana, R.; Buendia, M.; Lamas, G.A.; Lamelas, J. Outcomes of minimally invasive valve surgery versus standard sternotomy in obese patients undergoing isolated valve surgery. *Ann. Thorac. Surg.* **2011**, *91*, 406–410. [CrossRef]
65. Mazzeffi, M.; Khelemsky, Y. Poststernotomy pain: A clinical review. *J. Cardiothorac. Vasc. Anesth.* **2011**, *25*, 1163–1178. [CrossRef] [PubMed]
66. Walther, T.; Falk, V.; Metz, S.; Diegeler, A.; Battellini, R.; Autschbach, R.; Mohr, F.W. Pain and quality of life after minimally invasive versus conventional cardiac surgery. *Ann. Thorac. Surg.* **1999**, *67*, 1643–1647. [CrossRef] [PubMed]
67. Sherazee, E.A.; Chetn, S.A.; Li, D.; Frank, P.; Kiaii, B. Pain Management Strategies for Minimally Invasive Cardiothoracic Surgery. *Innovations* **2022**, *17*, 167–176. [CrossRef]
68. Castillo-Sang, M.; Bartone, C.; Palmer, C.; Truong, V.T.; Kelly, B.; Voeller, R.K.; Griffin, J.; Smith, T.; Raidt, H.; Alnswini, G.A. Fifty Percent Reduction in Narcotic Use After Minimally Invasive Cardiac Surgery Using Liposomal Bupivacaine. *Innovations* **2019**, *14*, 512–518. [CrossRef]
69. Lee, J.W.; Song, J.-M.; Park, J.P.; Lee, J.W.; Kang, D.-H.; Song, J.-K. Long-term prognosis of isolated significant tricuspid regurgitation. *Circ. J.* **2010**, *74*, 375–380. [CrossRef] [PubMed]
70. Asmarats, L.; Puri, R.; Latib, A.; Navia, J.L.; Rodés-Cabau, J. Transcatheter Tricuspid Valve Interventions: Landscape, Challenges, and Future Directions. *J. Am. Coll. Cardiol.* **2018**, *71*, 2935–2956. [CrossRef]
71. Lurz, P.; von Bardeleben, R.S.; Weber, M.; Sitges, M.; Sorajja, P.; Hausleiter, J.; Denti, P.; Trochu, J.-N.; Nabauer, M.; Tang, G.H.; et al. Transcatheter Edge-to-Edge Repair for Treatment of Tricuspid Regurgitation. *J. Am. Coll. Cardiol.* **2021**, *77*, 229–239. [CrossRef] [PubMed]

Journal of
Cardiovascular Development and Disease

MDPI

Article

An Individualized, Less-Invasive Surgical Approach Algorithm Improves Outcome in Elderly Patients Undergoing Mitral Valve Surgery

Ulvi Cenk Oezpeker [1,*], Fabian Barbieri [2], Daniel Höfer [1], Can Gollmann-Tepeköylü [1], Johannes Holfeld [1], Florian Sommerauer [1], Julian Wagner [3], Sasa Rajsic [3], Suat Ersahin [4], Nikolaos Bonaros [1,*], Michael Grimm [1] and Müller Ludwig [1]

1 Department of Cardiac Surgery, Medical University of Innsbruck, 6020 Innsbruck, Austria
2 Department of Cardiology, Charité—Universität zu Berlin, Hindenburgdamm 30, 12203 Berlin, Germany
3 Department of Anesthesiology and Intensive Care Medicine, Medical University of Innsbruck, 6020 Innsbruck, Austria
4 Sakarya Eğitim ve Araştırma Hospital, 54100 Adapazarı, Turkey
* Correspondence: cenk.oezpeker@tirol-kliniken.at (U.C.O.); nikolaos.bonaros@tirol-kliniken.at (N.B.); Tel.: +43-505040-22501 (N.B.); Fax: +43-505040-22502 (N.B.)

Abstract: Background: For mitral valve surgery (MVS) in elderly, frail patients with increasing life expectancy, finding the least harmful means of access is a challenge. In the complexity of MVS approach evolution, using three different approaches (mini-thoracotomy (MT), partial upper-sternotomy (PS), full-sternotomy (FS), we developed a personalized, minimized-invasiveness algorithm for MVS. Methods: In this retrospective analysis, 517 elderly patients (≥70 years) were identified who had undergone MVS ± TV repair. MVS was performed via MT (n = 274), FS (n = 128) and PS (n = 115). The appropriate access type was defined according to several clinical patient conditions. Using uni- and multivariate regression models, we analyzed combined operative success (residual MV regurgitation, conversion to MV replacement or larger thoracic incisions); perioperative success (30-days mortality, thoracotomy, ECMO, pacemaker implantation, dialysis, longer ventilation); and reoperation-free long-term survival. An additional EuroSCORE2 adjustment was performed to reduce the bias of clinical conditions between all access types. Results: The EuroSCORE2-adjusted Cox regression analysis showed significantly increased reoperation-free survival in the MT cohort compared to FS (HR 0.640; 95% CI 0.442–0.926; p = 0.018). Mortality was additionally reduced after the implementation of PS (p = 0.023). Combined operative success was comparable between the three access types. The perioperative success was higher in the MT cohort compared to FS (OR 2.19, 95% CI 1.32–3.63; p = 0.002). Conclusion: Less-invasive approaches in elderly patients improve perioperative success and reoperation-free survival in those undergoing MVS procedures.

Keywords: elderly patients; mitral valve surgery; less invasive; surgical trauma reduction; mitral valve repair

1. Introduction

Mitral valve (MV) disease is common in elderly patients and occurs at an increasing frequency with advanced age [1]. However, choosing between conservative, transcatheter and surgical treatment is an individualized process dependent on several factors, which modify morbidity and mortality risk [2–4]. Most critical parameters include age, comorbidities, time point of surgical intervention and possibility of repairing the MV pathology [4–6]. Due to prolonged life expectancy and the accompanying increase in frailty and concomitant heart failure of elderly patients, surgeons need to seek alternative, reproducible and less harmful algorithms to reduce operative trauma and mortality. An increase in minimally invasive heart surgery has been observed in recent decades [7]. Most of the publications about minimally invasive mitral valve surgery (MIMVS) in the elderly focus on low-risk degenerative MV etiologies [6,8,9]. However, despite the increasing adoption of MIMVS, patients with absolute or relative contraindications for MIMVS exist in daily routine cardiac surgery [10,11]. These certain clinical conditions are potentially harmful limitations for safe MVS via the right MT access type, making FS the sole, alternatively preferred, safe and quick access type in 45% of MV surgeries in almost all German centers [7,12]. Moreover, longer operative times and learning curves associated with the use of long-shafted instruments and endoscopic techniques still prevent the broad acceptance of less-invasive procedures [13]. In addition, MV repair rates in complex pathologies are generally based on institutional experience and may additionally limit the number of patients suitable for MIMVS via MT [14]. However, the benefits of MIMVS in elderly patients and data on transcatheter interventions are inconclusive. Some investigations have demonstrated that MIMVS reduces operative trauma, with long-term survival at five and seven years of 55% and 52%, respectively [8,9,15]. Patients who are considered unsuitable for MT undergo operation with conventional FS. Based on more than 20 years of experience in minimally invasive cardiac procedures, including PS and MT for aortic valve replacement and more than 1000 video-assisted or fully endoscopic MV procedures via MT, we adapted partial upper sternotomy as a complementary, less-invasive mode of access for MVS [16]. In the complexity of MVS approach evolution over the decades, we aimed to keep MV repair rates high and chose a tailored approach for MVS, in order to minimize mortality in elderly patients. In this study, we not only focused on MIMVS in elderly patients with low-risk degenerative MV pathologies, but we also tried to include all higher risk heterogenous MV etiologies and patients with contraindications for MT by implementing a personalized and less-invasive algorithm.

2. Methods

2.1. Study Design and Patients

The data for this investigation were obtained from the MVS database of the Department of Cardiac Surgery of the Medical University of Innsbruck, Austria. Survival data were acquired by the national death registry of Austria (Statistik Austria). Patients without an event were censored at the end of the follow up. The follow up was conducted by outpatient visits as well as phone calls to the patients and their attending physicians, who sent us the echocardiographic and ECG findings. Written informed consent for the scientific use of clinical data was obtained from all patients as part of the quality control program of the Medical University of Innsbruck, which was approved by the local ethics committee (13 February 2020; EC Nr.: 1203/2019) and the Austrian Ministry of Health. The investigation complied with the principles outlined in the Declaration of Helsinki.

In this longitudinal retrospective cohort study, in our center, we reviewed the records of 1534 patients who had undergone isolated MVS or combined with TV repair $\pm$ atrial ablation procedures, without coronary artery bypass grafting and aortic valve replacement, between March 2001 and February 2021. Patients with age < 70 years; redo surgery; urgent or salvage surgery with, for example, active endocarditis; and concomitant surgery of the ascending aorta were excluded. Eight patients were excluded due to incomplete data, leaving 517 patients who were finally included in the data analysis. For the analysis, the patients were divided into three groups depending on the surgical approach (MT n = 274; FS n = 128; PS n = 115).

Patient allocation to the adequate approach was dictated by institutional protocols (Table 1, Figure 1). Concomitant cardiac surgery, other than TV repair or atrial ablation procedures; aortic valve regurgitation with a possible risk of aortic valve replacement; severe right-sided pulmonary adhesions; significant mitral annulus calcification with the need for unitary decalcification; severely atherosclerotic aorta descendens or femoral arteries not amenable for peripheral cannulation, and a dilated ascending aorta > 45 mm; systolic pulmonary pressure > 50 mm Hg; and severely impaired left-ventricular function were disregarded as ideal candidates for MT access.

Table 1. Reasons against MT and PS access.

	Era 1 n = 181	Era 2 n = 336	
	FS Instead of MT n = 78	**PS Instead of MT** n = 115	**FS Instead of MT** n = 50
Severe peripheral or aortic atherosclerosis (%, n)	3.3 (6)	20.9 (24)	3.3 (6)
AV regurgitation ≤ moderate (%, n)	3.9 (10)	7.8 (9)	3.9 (10)
Patient in a clinically worse condition (%, n)	11.6 (21)	16.5 (19)	11.6 (21)
Moderate-to-major AC (%, n)	9.9 (18)	34 (34)	9.9 (18)
Pulmonary hypertension ≥ moderate (%, n)	6.6 (12)	18.3 (21)	6.6 (12)
Reduced LVEF ≥ moderate	5.0 (9)	4.3 (5)	5.0 (9)
Right-sided pleural adhesions (%, n)	1.1 (2)	1.7 (2)	1.1 (2)
Surgical training reasons (%, n)	0	0.9 (1)	0

Abbreviations: AC = annulus calcification; AV = aortic valve; FS = full sternotomy; MT = mini-thoracotomy, PS = partial sternotomy.

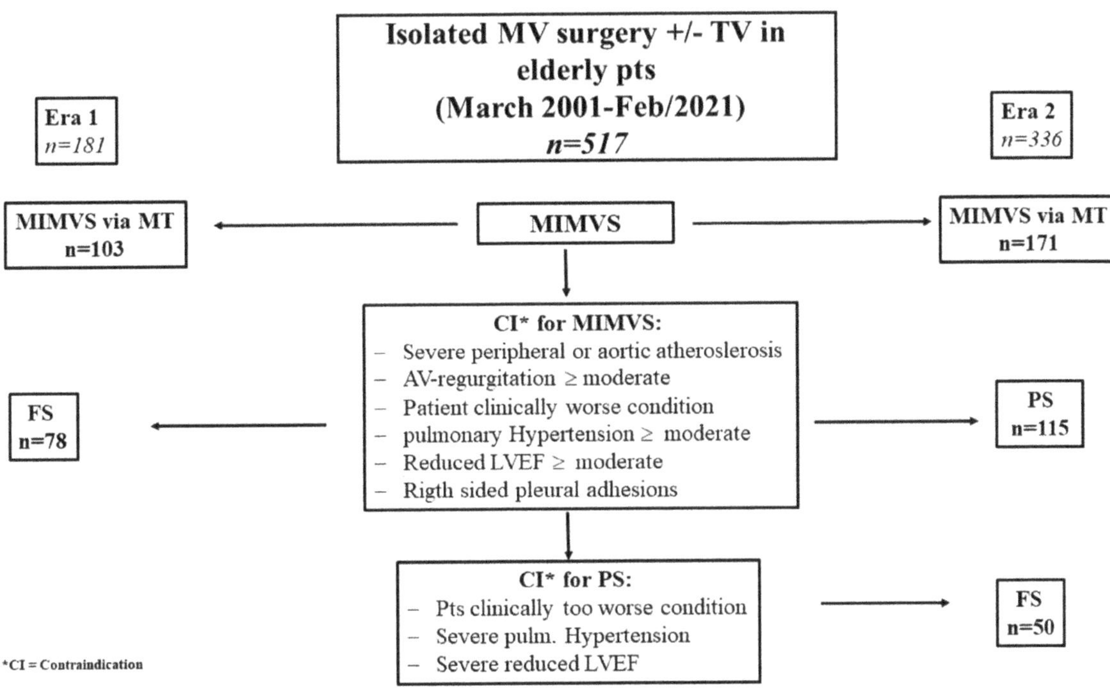

Figure 1. Flowchart for the algorithm of appropriate approach in elderly patients. * CI = contraindication, ± = with or without.

Based on this certain risk profile, MVS was conducted via FS instead of MT up to 2011 (era 1). In 2011, the implementation of PS access started as a complementary, less-invasive access type for patients with clinical contraindications for MT (era 2).

2.2. Surgical Procedures

The institutional operative techniques have been described in detail for all three access types in earlier publications [16,17].

The PS approach with extension of the transseptal incision into the atrial roof was described in detail by Gillinov et al., and Svensson et al. Briefly, we first performed a PS starting at the sternal notch with extension into the fourth intercostal space to the left side. Cannulation for the cardiopulmonary bypass (CPB) was performed via the ascending aorta; the superior vena cava was cannulated directly, while the inferior vena cava (IVC) was cannulated percutaneously or surgically via the femoral vein using Seldinger's technique. Correct positioning was achieved after establishing CPB and the superior and IVC were snared in order to prevent air-lock. After cross-clamping of the ascending aorta cardioplegia was first applied antegrade and, after opening the right atrium, repeated retrograde to the coronary sinus under direct visualization via a catheter. Afterwards the incision of the interatrial septum at the level of the fossa ovalis was performed. This cut was prolonged to the right atrial incision and extended along the roof of the left atrium towards the aorta. With this technique, excellent surgical exposure was achieved.

In the FS access type, the cannulation was similar to the PS approach. The direct cannulation of the IVC was performed. Access to the MV was performed via the dissection of the interatrial groove in every case, independently according to whether a tricuspid valve repair with opening of the right atrium was performed or not.

In the MT cohort, cardiopulmonary bypass was installed via femoro-femoral cannulation with an additional distal leg perfusion to avoid leg perfusion issues. An additional venous cannula was inserted into the right jugular vein in case of TVR or patients with increased body surface area (BSA) for optimal drainage. The MT access was performed through the fourth intercostal space via periareolar or a 3 cm long skin cut lateral to the nipple and a similar incision in the submammary fold was performed depending on a male or female patient. The third intercostal space on the anterior axillary line was used for the scope and the Chitwood clamp. The soft tissue retractor Alexis wound protector was used to avoid rib spreading.

Common mitral-repair techniques, including chordal replacement (single polytetrafluoroethylene (PTFE) chords, secondary chords or pre-fabricated PTFE loops), leaflet resection, sliding plasty or indentation closure, were applied. A semi-rigid annuloplasty ring was used in all procedures. Moreover, a tricuspid valve repair was performed in all patients with severe tricuspid valve regurgitation or annular dilatation above 21 mm/m^2 BSA.

2.3. Definitions

The major outcome parameter was reoperation-free survival defined as freedom from death and reoperation during follow up, due to valve-related complications (native valve-related: new onset of MV-regurgitation > moderate or prosthetic valve-related: paravalvular leakage, valve degeneration, valve thrombosis, endocarditis).

Further major outcome parameters were operative and perioperative success as composite endpoints within the first 30 days. Combined operative success was defined as freedom of death, successful primary MV repair without conversion to replacement or to larger thoracic incisions, and residual mitral regurgitation $\geq$ moderate or prosthetic valve-related paravalvular leakage.

The definition for combined perioperative success was 30-days survival, freedom from perioperative myocardial infarction (Fourth Universal Definition of Myocardial infarction), stroke, extracorporeal membrane oxygenation support, renal failure necessitating dialysis, persistent pacemaker implantation, mechanical ventilation > 24 h and re-operation due to any reason (including bleeding).

The subgroup analyses focused on long-term outcome according to three distinct age classes (70–74, 75–79 and $\geq$80 years of age), the comparison of MV repair versus replacement, and the comparison of reoperation-free survival between degenerative and secondary MV etiologies.

3. Statistical Analysis

Categorical variables are displayed as absolute numbers and percentages, and continuous variables as median and their respective 25th and 75th percentile. The distribution of continuous variables was assessed by an inspection of the histograms and use of the Shapiro-Wilk test. Group-specific differences were analyzed either by an ANOVA or Kruskal-Wallis test for continuous variables, according to their distribution, and by the chi-square test for categorical variables. To estimate the group-specific differences for operative and perioperative success, as well as their components, binary logistic regression models were calculated. The weight of factors limiting long-term survival and reoperation-free survival were calculated by applying Cox regression models. These models were, if indicated, also adjusted for the EuroSCORE2. To determine the potential advantages of the less-invasive methods, FS was used as a reference cohort in all models. A univariate subgroup analysis was calculated by creating Kaplan–Meier curves, and differences were assessed by the log-rank test. The analysis was conducted using IBM SPSS, version 24 (IBM Corporation, Armonk, NY, USA), and graphics were designed using GraphPad PRISM, version 5 (GraphPad Software, Inc., La Jolla, CA, USA). p-values of 0.05 or less were considered statistically significant.

4. Results

4.1. Baseline Characteristics and Intraoperative Parameters

Baseline and intraoperative characteristics are illustrated in Tables 2–4. For most variables, all the given preoperative data show statistically significant highest morbidity in the PS cohort and lowest in the MT cohort. The EuroSCORE2 was found to be highest in the FS group ($p < 0.001$), while the pre-operative NT-proBNP levels were increased in the PS cohort ($p = 0.004$). Patients requiring dialysis before surgery were only present in the PS cohort ($p = 0.030$).

Table 2. Baseline characteristics of the study cohort.

	MVS (Total) $n = 517$	**MT-MVS** $n = 274$	**PS-MVS** $n = 115$	**FS-MVS** $n = 128$	p**-Value**
Age (years) [1]	75 (72–78)	74 (63–77)	76 (72–79)	75 (72–79)	0.006
Gender, females (%, n)	56.5 (292)	52.6 (144)	58.3 (67)	62.5(80)	0.154
Primary MV disease (%, n)	82.6 (427)	79.9 (219)	87.8 (101)	83.6 (107)	0.163
BSA (m^2)	1.80 (1.66–1.94)	1.80 (1.70–2.0)	1.77 (1.62–1.94)	1.74 (1.63–1.87)	<0.001
DM (%, n)	36.2 (187)	52.9 (145)	18.3 (21)	16.4 (21)	<0.001
IDDM (%, n)	4.6 (24)	6.2 (17)	2.6 (3)	3.1 (4)	0.191
Art.hypertension (%, n)	65.8 (340)	52.9 (145)	81.7 (94)	78.9 (101)	<0.001
COPD $\geq$ GOLD 2 (%, n)	18.4 (95)	30.5 (51)	35.4 (58)	30.5 (50)	<0.001
PAOD (%, n)	2.3 (12)	0.7 (2)	6.1 (7)	2.3 (3)	0.006
Dialysis (%, n)	0.4 (2)	0	1.7 (2)	0	0.030
Smoking history (%, n)	9.5 (49)	5.1 (14)	16.5 (19)	12.5 (16)	<0.001
HLP (%, n)	39.1 (202)	28.8 (79)	53.9 (62)	47.7 (61)	<0.001
Prev.CVE (%, n)	4.1 (21)	1.5 (4)	7 (8)	7 (9)	0.006
EuroSCORE2 (%) [1]	3.10 (1.80–4.73)	2.20 (1.31–3.70)	3.70 (2.51–5.20)	4.21 (3.15–6.43)	<0.001
LV-EF (%) [1]	60 (51–64)	60 (52–64)	58 (50–65)	57 (50–63)	0.114
NYHA III (%, n)	56.1 (290)	51.8 (142)	61.7 (71)	60.2 (77)	0.112
NYHA IV (%, n)	5.0 (26)	3.3 (9)	8.7 (10)	5.5 (7)	0.081
i-Afib (%, n)	42.4 (219)	37.2 (102)	43.5 (50)	52.3 (67)	0.016
p-Afib (%, n)	15.3 (79)	9.5 (26)	25.2 (29)	21.1 (27)	<0.001
sPAP > 55 mmHg (%, n)	15.3 (79)	5.1 (14)	32.1 (34)	32 (31)	<0.001
NT-proBNP (ng/l) [1]	1218 (550–2133)	1148 (472–1800)	1410 (705–2979)	1220 (723–2431)	0.004

Abbreviations: BSA = body surface area; COPD = chronic obstructive pulmonary disease; CVE = cerebrovascular event; DM = diabetes mellitus; FS = full sternotomy; HLP = hyperlipidemia; IDDM = insulin-dependent diabetes mellitus; i-Afib = intermittent atrial fibrillation; LV-EF = left-ventricular ejection fraction; MT = mini thoracotomy, MV = mitral valve; MVS = mitral valve surgery; p-Afib = permanent atrial fibrillation; PAOD = peripheral arterial occlusive disease; PS = partial upper sternotomy; sPAP = systolic pulmonary artery pressure; [1] continuous variables are expressed as median and interquartile range.

Regarding etiology, there was no significant difference in the incidence of MV pathology ($p = 0.163$). Overall, the MV repair rate was 74.1% ($n = 383$). The highest rates of MV repair (87.6%, $n = 240$, $p = < 0.001$) and partial additional TV repair (34.3%, $n = 94$, $p = 0.005$) were seen in the MT cohort. In addition, CPB times (198 (158–232) min, $p < 0.001$) and cross-clamp times (106 (84–126) min, $p = 0.004$) were significantly longer in the MT cohort. Comparable frequencies were found for moderate-to-severe annulus calcification in both sternotomy cohorts (32.2% vs. 38.3%), but significantly less in the MT cohort (0.7% $p < 0.001$).

Table 3. Secondary intraoperative outcomes.

Intraoperative Outcomes	MVS (Total) $n = 517$	MT-MVS $n = 274$	PS-MVS $n = 115$	FS-MVS $n = 128$	p-Value
MV repair (%, n)	74.1 (383)	88.97 (242)	62.6 (72)	53.9 (69)	<0.001
Switch MV repair to replacement (intraoperatively) (%, n)	2.7 (14)	1.5 (4)	2.6 (3)	5.5 (7)	0.070
Additional TV repair (%, n)	40.8 (211)	34.3 (94)	46.1 (53)	50 (64)	0.005
Ablation surgical (%, n)	15.3 (79)	17.5 (48)	9.6 (11)	15.6 (20)	0.137
Cardiopulmonary bypass time (min) [1]	168 (137–211)	198 (158–232)	151 (130–176)	144 (113–170)	<0.001
Aortic cross-clamp time (min) [1]	101 (80–123)	106 (84–126)	94 (83–115)	93 (71–118)	0.004
Conversion to FS (%, n)	5.0 (26)	4 (11)	13 (15)	0	<0.001
Second pump run/X-clamp (%, n)	4.3 (22)	3.0 (8)	6.1 (7)	5.5 (7)	0.365
Moderate-to-major annulus calcifications (%, n)	17.0 (88)	0.7 (2)	32.2 (37)	38.3 (49)	<0.001
En bloc decalcifications (%, n)	2.9 (15)	0.7 (2)	3.5 (4)	7.0 (9)	0.002

Abbreviations: FS = full sternotomy; MVS = mitral valve surgery; MT = mini thoracotomy PS = partial upper sternotomy; [1] continuous variables are expressed as median and interquartile range.

Table 4. Secondary postoperative outcomes.

Postoperative Outcomes	MVS (Total) $n = 517$	MT-MVS $n = 274$	PS-MVS $n = 115$	FS-MVS $n = 128$	p-Value
MV regurgitation ≥ 2 after MV-reapair * (%, n)	4.2 (16)	2.9 (7)	1.4 (1)	11.6 (8)	0.040
Mild PVL * (in the MV-replacement group) (%, n)	2.2 (3)	0 (0)	4.7 (2)	1.7 (1)	0.113
30-days mortality (%, n)	2.1 (11)	0.7 (2)	2.6 (3)	4.7 (6)	0.035
1-year mortality (%, n)	4.5 (23)	2.2 (6)	5.2 (6)	8.6 (11)	0.016
Extracorporeal membrane oxygenation, (%, n)	2.5 (13)	3.3 (9)	2.6 (3)	0.8 (1)	0.327
Cardiac low-output syndrome, (%, n)	10.4 (54)	3.3 (9)	14.8 (17)	21.9 (28)	<0.001
Tamponade or excessive bleeding (%, n)	6.2 (32)	5.5 (15)	7.8 (9)	6.3 (8)	0.680
Hemofiltration/-dialysis (%, n)	7.9 (41)	1.1 (3)	20 (23)	11.7 (15)	<0.001
Ventilation >24 hrs (%, n)	15.3 (79)	10.9 (30)	19.1 (22)	21.1 (27)	0.013
Red blood units (total) [1]	1 (1–2)	0 (0–2)	1 (1–3)	1 (1–3)	<0.001
Intensive care unit length (days) [1]	1 (1–2)	1 (1–1)	1 (1–4)	2 (1–9)	<0.001
Hospital stay (days) [1]	8 (7–11)	8 (7–9)	8 (7–12)	10 (8–12)	<0.001
Deep wound infection (%, n)	1.4 (7)	0	1.7 (2)	3.9 (5)	0.006
Cerebrovascular adverse event (%, n)	0.8 (4)	0	0.9 (1)	2.3 (3)	0.044
Pacemaker implantation (%, n)	3.4 (18)	0.4 (1)	8.7 (10)	5.5 (7)	<0.001
Myocardial infarction (%, n)	0.4 (2)	0	0.9 (1)	0.8 (1)	0.648

Abbreviations: FS = full sternotomy; MVS = mitral valve surgery; MT = mini thoracotomy; PS = partial upper sternotomy; PVL = paravalvular leakage; [1] continuous variables are expressed as median and interquartile range; * at 30 days follow up.

4.2. Long-Term Outcome

The total median follow up was 5.6 (IQR 2.7–8.7) years. All-cause mortality was 28.7% ($n = 147$ patients) during this period, while three patients (0.6%) required mitral valve related re-operation. During long-term follow up, 10-year reoperation-free survival was achieved in 65.7% of patients for MT, 64.4 % for PS and 50.2% for FS, while univariate comparison using overall follow up reached statistical significance ($p = 0.016$) (Figure 2). The EuroSCORE2-adjusted Cox regression analysis showed comparable mortality hazard ratios for FS and PS (HR 0.891; 95% CI 0.533–1.490; $p = 0.660$), whereas MT resulted in a significantly lower mortality hazard compared to FS (HR 0.640; 95% CI 0.442–0.926; $p = 0.018$).

4.3. Operative and Perioperative Success

The combined operative success rate was given for all three access types as well as in the EuroSCORE2-adjusted analysis, and it showed no statistically significant difference.

The combined perioperative success rate reached statistical significance with the MT-access and was higher after EuroSCORE2 adjustment (OR 2.19, 95% CI 1.32–3.63; $p = 0.002$) compared to FS. The six-fold higher risk of 30-days mortality was seen in the FS-cohort compared with the MT access type (OR 6.69; 95% CI 1.33–33.61; $p = 0.021$). An advantage of MT compared to FS was also seen in longer ventilation times (OR 2.17; 95% CI 1.23–3.84; $p = 0.007$) and a lower incidence of PM implantations (OR 15.79; 95% CI 1.9–129.8; $p = 0.01$). In addition, more patients required renal replacement therapy in the FS-cohort compared to MT (OR 11.99; 95% CI 3.41–42.23; $p < 0.001$). However, there was no statistical difference between FS and PS (Table 5).

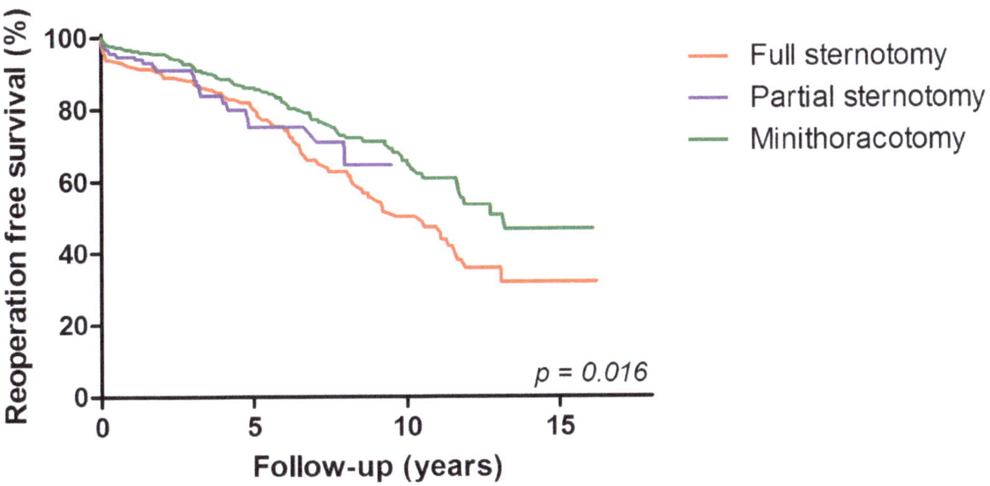

Figure 2. Kaplan-Meier curves: reoperation-free survival, according to the three access types.

In the subgroup analysis, the univariate analyses showed similar reoperation-free long-term survival between primary and secondary MV pathologies ($p = 0.187$). This similarity when comparing the results was also found if the cohorts were broken down into the three access types (FS $p = 0.220$; PS $p = 0.877$; MT $p = 0.253$). In addition, the log-rank test showed a reoperation-free survival benefit of MV repairs (63.6%) over MV replacement (57.8%, $p = 0.030$) (Figure 3).

Moreover, the highest 10-year reoperation-free survival rate was observed for the age group 70–74 years (70.3%), decreasing for 75–79 years (60.2%) and being lowest for patients $\geq$ 80 years (55.8%, $p = 0.012$) (Figure 4). In addition, the long-term mortality was significantly reduced between era 1 and era 2 in this high-risk patient cohort (log rank $p = 0.023$).

Table 5. Operative and perioperative (30-day) success, according to access type *.

	MVS (Total) n = 517	*FS vs. PS n = 243*	*p-Value*	*OR*	*CI*	*FS vs. MT n = 402*	*p-Value*	*OR*	*CI*
Combined operative success—yes (%)	89.0	85.2	0.155	0.60	0.29–1.22	91.0	0.188	1.60	0.80–3.22
EuroSCORE2 adjusted			0.162	0.60	0.29–1.23		0.373	1.39	0.67–2.84
Combined perioperative success—yes (%)	74.1	63.8	0.529	0.85	0.50–1.43	77.6	<0.001	2.60	1.60–4.21
EuroSCORE2 adjusted			0.470	0.82	0.48–1.40		0.002	2.19	1.32–3.63
30-day survival (%)	97.9	96.3	0.398	1.84	0.449–7.52	98.0	0.021	6.69	1.33–33.61
MI (%)	0.6	0.4	0.997	n.a		0.5	0.956	1.07	0.10–11.92
ECMO (%)	2.5	1.6	0.292	0.294	0.030–2.87	2.2	0.168	0.232	0.3–1.85
Renal failure dialysis (%)	7.9	15.6	0.079	0.531	0.26–1.08	4.5	<0.001	11.991	3.41–42.23
>24 h ventilation (%)	15.3	20.1	0.703	1.13	0.60–2.1	14.2	0.007	2.17	1.23–3.84
Reoperation for any reason (%)	7.4	8.6	0.668	1.22	0.49–3.0	4.2	0.256	1.56	0.72–3.38
Reoperation bleeding (%)	6.2	7.0	0.631	0.79	0.29–2.11	5.7	0.755	1.15	0.48–2.8
PM implantation (%)	3.5	7.0	0.329	0.607	0.223–1.652	2.0	0.01	15.79	1.9–129.8
CVE (%)	0.8	1.6	0.386	2.74	0.28–26.68	0	0.99		

*Abbreviations: CI = confidence interval; CVE = cerebrovascular adverse event; ECMO = extracorporeal membrane oxygenation; FS = full sternotomy; MI = myocardial infarction; MVS = mitral valve surgery; OR = odds ratio; PM = pacemaker; * reference access is full sternotomy.*

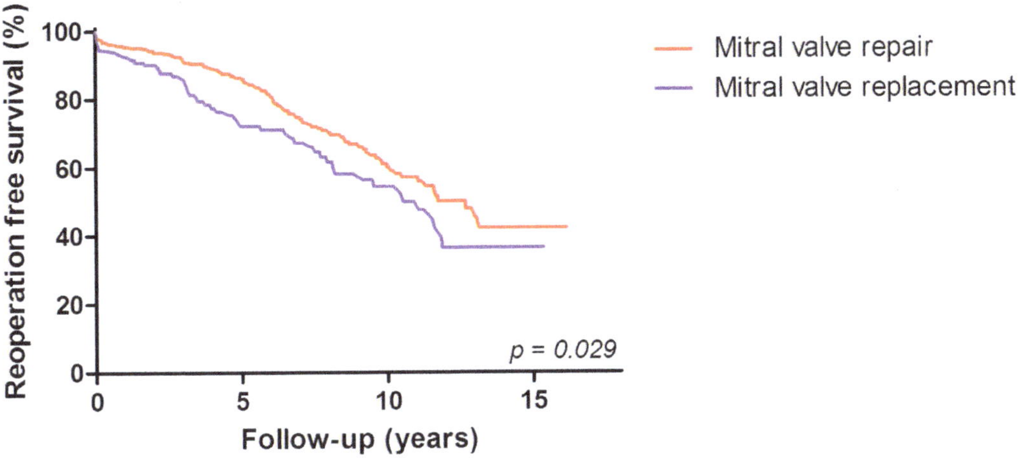

Figure 3. Kaplan–Meier curves: reoperation-free survival benefit of MV repair.

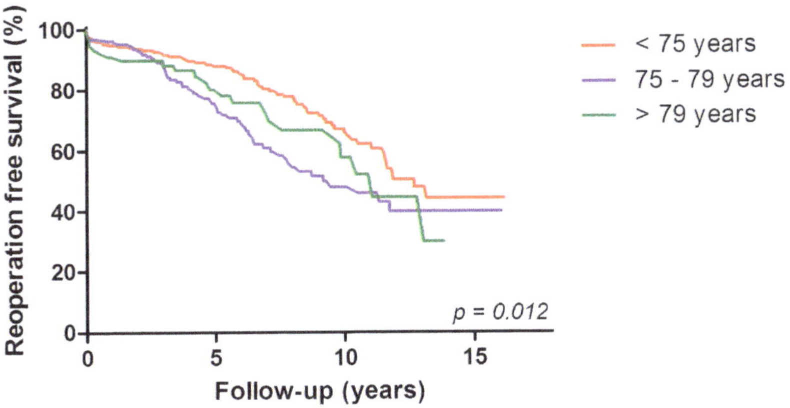

Figure 4. Kaplan-Meier curves: reoperation free survival, according to age groups.

5. Discussion

Safe and reproducible MVS in elderly patients, given their frailty and higher incidence of comorbidities such as heart failure, is a growing challenge due to prolonged life expectancy. Our investigation described the short-term and long-term benefits of an individualized, least-possible invasive surgical algorithm isolated MVS or combined with TVS, in this population. It has to be pointed out that this investigation is not a comparison of three different access types, as MT was the preferred approach in our center. It is an algorithm to reduce the operative trauma in these frail patients to find the least-harmful intervention.

Several studies have described the superiority of MIMVS compared to FS, due to a reduction in operative trauma, especially in elderly patients. However, data on MIMVS either mainly focus on low-risk degenerative MV diseases with high MV repair rates [8,9,15] or, on secondary MV etiologies. As elderly patients who are frail and have accompanying heart failure more often have complex MV pathologies, MV repairs can sometimes be extremely difficult and harmful, pushing many surgeons to opt for straightforward MV replacement or even reject surgery altogether. However, several studies described the superiority of MV repair over replacement, especially regarding survival [18]. Our data are in accordance with these investigations and support the principal strategy to repair the valve whenever possible [17,19], independent of access and complexity. Our data describe an overall figure of 74.1% of MV repair rates, which is higher compared to the study by Seeburger et al. [6], despite including all MV pathologies. In addition, our univariate analyses on reoperation-free long-term survival were similar between primary and secondary MV pathologies; therefore we decided to analyze all MV pathologies together. Our patient cohort included degenerative MV diseases, as well as patients with mitral annular calcifications (17%, n = 88), MV stenosis (8.1% n = 42), inactive endocarditis (3.1%, n = 16) and Barlow disease, which are generally viewed as complex indications for MV repair, especially for less-invasive approaches. Most patients with successful MV repair rates were found in the MT cohort (87%), which reflects the increased survival, safety and reproducibility, even in complex pathologies with this access, despite longer X-clamp and CPB times. It has to be pointed out that the MT cohort contained two patients with peripheral arterial occlusive disease, which is a contraindication for this approach. In these two patients, the right carotid artery was used for arterial cannulation for extracorporeal circulation [20]. However, the data for the two other access types showed similar results, underlining the safety and reproducibility of PS access.

Our data describe the lowest comorbidities, comparable operative but statistically significant highest perioperative success and consecutive 10-year reoperation-free survival rates in the MT cohort, which can be explained by healthier patients and the highest amount of less-operative trauma in this cohort. Overall, the probability of 10-year reoperation-free survival was 71% in our investigation, which is higher than the previous published data, which mainly exclude complex MV pathologies. These data reveal almost equal life expectancy in this cohort compared to the general population of patients, as indicated by Statistik Austria (URL: www.statistik.at), accessed on 1 November 2022. However, selection bias might be the most important factor for outcome. Yet, multivariate analyses with EuroSCORE2 adjustment were applied to reduce this bias, and similar results were obtained. These results are in accordance with the publication of Al Otaibi et al. [21].

Due to limitations for MIMVS, which do exist in daily cardiac surgery [13], FS is the preferred alternative bail-out strategy in almost all centers worldwide. In 47% of the patients in our study cohort, certain clinical or anatomical conditions were considered as contraindications for MT due to the high risk of complications and mortality [10]. We adopted our personalized, least-invasive access strategy with the implementation of PS 2011, resulting in a reduction in the long-term mortality between era 1 and era 2 in this patient cohort. PS was associated with lower postoperative complication rates and survival benefit compared to FS in a previous publication [22], yet this remains unproven in the elderly patient cohort. Nevertheless, the bias of changing surgical and intensive care unit strategies over 20 years may not be excluded by our data, leaving a lack of conclusive evidence for improved outcomes with lower invasiveness.

Despite the high rates of ECMO implantation within the MT access group, the incidence of low cardiac output syndrome was detected most often in the FS and lowest in the MT cohort. This benefit may be explained by the partial integrity of the pericardium in the minimally or less-invasive access types [23,24]. In addition, the regression analyses displayed a lower incidence of prolonged ventilation, which supports the result of several studies, and postoperative new onset of renal replacement therapy in the MT-cohort [25,26]. All these factors together facilitate faster mobilization in elderly patients, which might have an impact on short- and long-term outcomes. Robotic cardiac surgery would probably further reduce operative trauma and improve survival [27].

One of the crucial aspects of our study was that the preoperative data of the PS cohort revealed higher morbidity, but similar perioperative and operative success and long-time survival compared to FS. The reason for the lack of statistical differences between PS over FS can be explained by the low statistical power and the shorter follow-up times in era 2 of these access types.

However, in 5% of the patients, conversion to FS was necessary. In the MT cohort, conversion to FS was necessary due pericardial adhesions n = 4, uncontrollable bleeding *n* = 3, pleural adhesions *n* = 2 and limited surgical exposure *n* = 2. In the PS cohort, the reasons for conversion were pericardial adhesions (*n* = 7), uncontrollable bleeding (*n* = 5, atrioventricular dissection after en bloc decalcification of the mitral annulus) and surgical interventions (*n* = 2, additionally, CABG to the RCX due to cardiac ischemia and ascending aortic replacement due to dissection). Limited exposure was seen in this cohort in one patient; however, the exposure was also very difficult after FS.

Further analysis revealed a lower incidence of PM implantation in the MT cohort and highest in the PS cohort; the cohort might also have an impact on mortality rates. The higher PM implantation rates may be explained by the fact that, for PS access, an extension of the trans-septal incision—which is a subject of controversial discussion [22,28,29]—into the left atrial roof was performed, while for MT and FS, a transatrial or transeptal approach without extension was performed for the exploration of the MV. However, a statistically significant difference was found only between MT and FS.

Limitations

One major limitation of this investigation was the adjudication of patients to one or the other approach with marked preference for MT, potentially creating an allocation bias. With the continuous evolution of surgical techniques and growing experience with MIMVS, the relative contraindications for the MT approach have changed dramatically, leaving only a few indications for PS, and even fewer for FS in recent years. Furthermore, the changing intensive-care therapeutic strategies might have an impact on better outcomes, which cannot be excluded by our investigation.

Further limitations were the retrospective data analysis of a single center experience and the relatively small sample size. Therefore, we may not be able to rule out potential underpowering for the assessment of differences between study groups with regard to the outcome parameters.

In conclusion, the presented results demonstrate that the individualized, least-invasive possible access type with reduced trauma, in combination with the principal intention to repair the MV, reduced mortalities in this high-risk cohort. All minimally invasive or less-invasive access types are safe and reproducible MVS approaches. High rates of MV repair and reduced operative trauma permit short and long-term benefits in elderly patients.

Author Contributions: Conceptualization, methodology, writing—original draft preparation, writing—review and editing, U.C.O.; formal analysis, F.B.; methodology, D.H.; investigation, C.G.-T.; resources, J.H.; visualization, F.S.; resources, J.W.; data curation, S.R., data curation, S.E., writing—review and editing, N.B.; supervision, M.G.; supervision, M.L. All authors have read and agreed to the published version of the manuscript.

Funding: This research received no external funding.

Institutional Review Board Statement: The study was conducted in accordance with the Declaration of Helsinki, and approved by e institutional ethical committee of the Medical University of Innsbruck (Approval 1203/2019) on 13 February 2020.

Informed Consent Statement: Informed consent for the scientific use of clinical data was obtained from all patients as part of the quality control program of the Medical University of Innsbruck.

Data Availability Statement: Data is unavailable due to privacy or ethical restrictions.

Conflicts of Interest: All authors declare that there are no conflict of interest.

References

1. Nkomo, V.T.; Gardin, J.M.; Skelton, T.N.; Gottdiener, J.S.; Scott, C.G.; Enriquez-Sarano, M. Burden of valvular heart diseases: A population-based study. *Lancet* **2006**, *368*, 1005–1011. [CrossRef] [PubMed]
2. O'Brien, S.M.; Shahian, D.M.; Filardo, G.; Ferraris, V.A.; Haan, C.K.; Rich, J.B.; Normand, S.-L.T.; DeLong, E.R.; Shewan, C.M.; Dokholyan, R.S.; et al. The Society of Thoracic Surgeons 2008 cardiac surgery risk models: Part 2—Isolated valve surgery. *Ann. Thorac. Surg.* **2009**, *88*, S23–S42. [CrossRef] [PubMed]
3. Grant, S.W.; Hickey, G.L.; Modi, P.; Hunter, S.; Akowuah, E.; Zacharias, J. Propensity-matched analysis of minimally invasive approach versus sternotomy for mitral valve surgery. *Heart* **2019**, *105*, 783–789. [CrossRef] [PubMed]

4. Kang, D.H.; Heo, R.; Lee, S.; Baek, S.; Kim, D.-H.; Song, J.-M.; Song, J.-K.; Lee, J.W. Initial surgery versus conservative management of symptomatic severe mitral regurgitation in the elderly. *Heart* **2018**, *104*, 849–854. [CrossRef] [PubMed]
5. Bonnet, V.; Boisselier, C.; Saplacan, V.; Belin, A.; Gérard, J.-L.; Fellahi, J.-L.; Hanouz, J.-L.; Fischer, M.-O. The role of age and comorbidities in postoperative outcome of mitral valve repair: A propensity-matched study. *Medicine* **2016**, *95*, e3938. [CrossRef]
6. Seeburger, J.; Falk, V.; Garbade, J.; Noack, T.; Kiefer, P.; Vollroth, M.; Mohr, F.W.; Misfeld, M. Mitral valve surgical procedures in the elderly. *Ann. Thorac. Surg.* **2012**, *94*, 1999–2003. [CrossRef]
7. Beckmann, A.; Meyer, R.; Lewandowski, J.; Markewitz, A.; Blassfeld, D.; Boning, A. German Heart Surgery Report 2021: The Annual Updated Registry of the German Society for Thoracic and Cardiovascular Surgery. *Thorac. Cardiovasc. Surg.* **2022**, *70*, 362–376. [CrossRef]
8. Gotte, J.; Zittermann, A.; Hakim-Meibodi, K.; Hata, M.; Schramm, R.; Bleiziffer, S.; Parsa, M.A.; Gummert, J.; Renner, A. Long-Term Clinical Outcome in Elderly Patients Undergoing Mitral Valve Repair. *Thorac. Cardiovasc. Surg.* **2022**, *70*, 93–99. [CrossRef]
9. Kawajiri, H.; Schaff, H.V.; Dearani, J.A.; Daly, R.C.; Greason, K.L.; Arghami, A.; Rowse, P.G.; Viehman, J.K.; Lahr, B.D.; Gallego-Navarro, C.; et al. Clinical Outcomes of Mitral Valve Repair for Degenerative Mitral Regurgitation in Elderly Patients. *Eur. J. Cardiothorac. Surg.* **2022**, *62*, ezac299. [CrossRef]
10. Vollroth, M.; Seeburger, J.; Garbade, J.; Borger, M.A.; Misfeld, M.; Mohr, F.W. Conversion rate and contraindications for minimally invasive mitral valve surgery. *Ann. Cardiothorac. Surg.* **2013**, *2*, 853–854.
11. Doenst, T.; Diab, M.; Sponholz, C.; Bauer, M.; Farber, G. The Opportunities and Limitations of Minimally Invasive Cardiac Surgery. *Dtsch. Arztebl. Int.* **2017**, *114*, 777–784. [CrossRef]
12. Cetinkaya, A.; Geier, A.; Bramlage, K.; Hein, S.; Bramlage, P.; Schönburg, M.; Choi, Y.; Richter, M. Long-term results after mitral valve surgery using minimally invasive versus sternotomy approach: A propensity matched comparison of a large single-center series. *BMC Cardiovasc. Disord.* **2021**, *21*, 314. [CrossRef]
13. Zacharias, J.; Perier, P. Seven Habits of Highly Effective Endoscopic Mitral Surgeons. *Innovations* **2020**, *15*, 11–16. [CrossRef]
14. Oezpeker, U.C.; Barbieri, F.; Hoefer, D.; Bonaros, N.; Grimm, M.; Mueller, L. Partial Upper Sternotomy is a Safe Alternative in Mitral Annulus Decalcification. *Semin. Thorac. Cardiovasc. Surg.* **2022**, *34*, 502–509. [CrossRef]
15. Hage, A.; Hage, F.; Al-Amodi, H.; Gupta, S.; Papatheodorou, S.I.; Hawkins, R.; Ailawadi, G.; Mittleman, M.A.; Chu, M.W.A. Minimally Invasive versus Sternotomy for Mitral Surgery in the Elderly: A Systematic Review and Meta-Analysis. *Innovations* **2021**, *16*, 310–316. [CrossRef]
16. Oezpeker, C.; Barbieri, F.; Hoefer, D.; Schneider, B.; Bonaros, N.; Grimm, M.; Mueller, L. Mitral Valve Surgery via Partial Upper Sternotomy: Closing the Gap between Conventional Sternotomy and Right Lateral Minithoracotomy. *Thorac. Cardiovasc. Surg.* **2019**, *67*, 524–530. [CrossRef]
17. Bonaros, N.; Hoefer, D.; Oezpeker, C.; Gollmann-Tepeköylü, C.; Holfeld, J.; Dumfarth, J.; Kilo, J.; Ruttmann-Ulmer, E.; Hangler, H.; Grimm, M.; et al. Predictors of safety and success in minimally invasive surgery for degenerative mitral disease. *Eur. J. Cardio-Thorac. Surg.* **2022**, *61*, 637–644. [CrossRef]
18. Gaur, P.; Kaneko, T.; McGurk, S.; Rawn, J.D.; Maloney, A.; Cohn, L.H. Mitral valve repair versus replacement in the elderly: Short-term and long-term outcomes. *J. Thorac. Cardiovasc. Surg.* **2014**, *148*, 1400–1406. [CrossRef]
19. Farid, S.; Ladwiniec, A.; Hernandez-Sanchez, J.; Povey, H.; Caruana, E.; Ali, A.; Moorjani, N.; Irons, J.; Ring, L.; Abu-Omar, Y. Early Outcomes after Mitral Valve Repair versus Replacement in the Elderly: A Propensity Matched Analysis. *Heart Lung Circ.* **2019**, *28*, 314–319. [CrossRef]
20. Bonaros, N.; Hofer, D.; Holfeld, J.; Grimm, M.; Muller, L. Cannulation of the Carotid Artery for Minimally Invasive Mitral or Tricuspid Valve Surgery. *Ann. Thorac. Surg.* **2020**, *110*, e517–e519. [CrossRef]
21. Al Otaibi, A.; Gupta, S.; Belley-Cote, E.P.; Alsagheir, A.; Spence, J.; Parry, D.; Whitlock, R.P. Mini-thoracotomy vs. conventional sternotomy mitral valve surgery: A systematic review and meta-analysis. *J. Cardiovasc. Surg.* **2017**, *58*, 489–496. [CrossRef] [PubMed]
22. Oezpeker, C.U.; Barbieri, F.; Hoefer, D.; Bonaros, N.; Grimm, M.; Mueller, L. Upper Hemi-Sternotomy Provides Benefit for Patients with Isolated or Combined Mitral Valve Surgery. *Medicina* **2022**, *58*, 142. [CrossRef] [PubMed]
23. Vlahakes, G.J. Right ventricular failure after cardiac surgery. *Cardiol. Clin.* **2012**, *30*, 283–289. [CrossRef] [PubMed]
24. Zanobini, M.; Loardi, C.; Poggio, P.; Tamborini, G.; Veglia, F.; di Minno, A.; Myasoedova, V.; Mammana, L.F.; Biondi, R.; Pepi, M.; et al. The impact of pericardial approach and myocardial protection onto postoperative right ventricle function reduction. *J. Cardiothorac. Surg.* **2018**, *13*, 55. [CrossRef]
25. Chivasso, P.; Bruno, V.D.; Farid, S.; Malvindi, P.G.; Modi, A.; Benedetto, U.; Ciulli, F.; Abu-Omar, Y.; Caputo, M.; Angelini, G.D.; et al. Predictors of survival in octogenarians after mitral valve surgery for degenerative disease: The Mitral Surgery in Octogenarians study. *J. Thorac. Cardiovasc. Surg.* **2018**, *155*, 1474–1482.e2. [CrossRef]
26. Moscarelli, M.; Emmanuel, S.; Athanasiou, T.; Speziale, G.; Fattouch, K.; Casula, R. The role of minimal access valve surgery in the elderly. A meta-analysis of observational studies. *Int. J. Surg.* **2016**, *33 Pt A*, 164–171. [CrossRef]
27. Loulmet, D.F.; Ranganath, N.K.; Neragi-Miandoab, S.; Koeckert, M.S.; Galloway, A.C.; Grossi, E.A. Advanced experience allows robotic mitral valve repair in the presence of extensive mitral annular calcification. *J. Thorac. Cardiovasc. Surg.* **2019**. *epub ahead of print*. [CrossRef]

28. Helmers, M.R.; Shin, M.; Iyengar, A.; Arguelles, G.R.; Mays, J.; Han, J.J.; Patrick, W.; Altshuler, P.; Hargrove, W.C.; Atluri, P. Permanent pacemaker implantation following mitral valve surgery: A retrospective cohort study of risk factors and long-term outcomes. *Eur. J. Cardiothorac. Surg.* **2021**, *60*, 140–147. [CrossRef]
29. Lukac, P.; Hjortdal, V.; Pedersen, A.K.; Jensen, H.K.; Mortensen, P.T.; Hansen, P.S. The superior transseptal surgical approach to mitral valve creates slow conduction. *Pacing Clin. Electrophysiol.* **2006**, *29*, 719–726. [CrossRef]

Journal of
*Cardiovascular
Development and Disease*

MDPI

Review

Minimal-Access Atrial Septal Defect (ASD) Closure

Gillian Hardman * and Joseph Zacharias

Department of Cardiothoracic Surgery, Blackpool Victoria Hospital, Blackpool FY3 8NR, UK
* Correspondence: g.hardman@nhs.net

Abstract: Progress towards the development and adoption of minimally invasive techniques in cardiac surgery has been slower than that seen in other surgical specialties. Congenital heart disease (CHD) patients represent an important population within cardiac disease, of which atrial septal defect (ASD) is one of the most common diagnoses. Management of ASD encompasses a range of minimal-access and minimally invasive approaches, including transcatheter device closure, mini-sternotomy, thoracotomy, video-assisted, endoscopic, and robotic approaches. In this article, we will discuss the pathophysiology of ASD, along with diagnosis, management, and indications for intervention. We will review the current evidence supporting minimally invasive and minimal-access surgical ASD closure in the adult and paediatric patient, highlighting peri-operative considerations and areas for further research.

Keywords: minimal access; minimally invasive; cardiac surgery; atrial septal defect (ASD); congenital heart disease (CHD); adult congenital heart disease (ACHD); grown-up congenital heart disease (GUCH)

1. Introduction

Minimal-access and minimally invasive approaches to congenital heart disease (CHD) have been adopted, with the development of percutaneous transcatheter device closure and a range of surgical approaches to septal defect closure. For the CHD patient, who is more likely to be younger, of working age or adolescent, the benefits of these approaches, with the potential for safe, effective treatment with good long-term outcomes, a reduction in trauma, fewer post-operative complications, shorter hospital stay, a faster return to functional status and improved cosmesis, cannot be underestimated.

The prevalence of CHD worldwide is approximately 9 per 1000 newborns [1], and while severe congenital heart defects are declining in many developed nations, globally, overall prevalence is increasing. With advances in technology, diagnosis and medical and surgical management, over the last decade, the majority of individuals born with CHD now survive into adulthood [2], with CHD representing a not-insignificant burden of disease in the cardiovascular disease patient population. CHD can be classified into mild, moderate or severe [3], with atrial septal defect (ASD) considered mild or moderate, depending on size, morphology and associated lesions. In this review, we will provide an overview of atrial septal defect pathology, diagnosis and management, including transcatheter and surgical approaches, with a focus on surgical intervention and the evidence base guiding current practice.

1.1. Atrial Septal Defect (ASD)

Atrial septal defect (ASD) is one of the most common congenital heart defects, accounting for 10% to 15% of all forms of congenital cardiac malformations [4]. ASD can remain undiagnosed into adulthood [3] with the majority of patients developing symptoms beyond the fourth decade.

Secundum ASD, located in the region of the fossa ovalis, is the most common defect type, accounting for approximately 80% of all ASDs. Primum ASD is synonymous with partial atrioventricular septal defect (AVSD), with communication at the atrial level only, and accounts for 15% of all ASDs. Superior sinus venosus defects (5% of ASDs) are located near the entry point of the superior vena cava (SVC) within the right atrium and are associated with the partial or complete connection of the right pulmonary veins to the right atrium. Inferior sinus venosus defects are located near the entry of the inferior vena cava (IVC) and account for less than 1% of atrial septal lesions. Finally, an unroofed coronary sinus represents a spectrum of anomalies where part or all of the wall between the coronary sinus and left atrium is absent. Most cases are associated with anomalous systemic venous return, including a persistent left superior vena cava, and represent the most rare form of ASD, at less than 1% [5]. The vascular anomalies and lesions most frequently associated with ASD include anomalous pulmonary venous connection, persistent left SVC, pulmonary valve stenosis, coarctation of the aorta and mitral valve prolapse. Conversely, ASD is frequently a component of other CHD lesions, including the Ebstein anomaly [3].

Pathophysiology is associated with the shunting of blood across the defect, with shunt volume dependent on the compliance of the left and right ventricles, the size of the defect and the pressure difference between the left and right atria. A simple ASD results in a left to right shunt because of the higher compliance of the right ventricle compared with the left ventricle, causing right ventricular volume overload and pulmonary over-circulation. A defect size of $\geq$10 mm is deemed to result in a clinically relevant shunt [3]. Any condition resulting in a reduction in left ventricular compliance or elevation of left atrial pressure, for example, systemic hypertension, ischaemic heart disease, cardiomyopathy or left sided valve lesions (aortic and mitral valve disease) will result in an increase in the left to right shunt. For this reason, an ASD may become more clinically and haemodynamically important with increasing age. Conversely, conditions that decrease right ventricular compliance will reduce the left to right shunt and may eventually cause shunt reversal (Eisenmenger syndrome), with resultant cyanosis [6].

Most commonly, patients develop symptoms associated with reduced functional capacity, including shortness of breath on exertion, palpitations (associated with supraventricular tachyarrhythmias) and less frequently, pulmonary infection and right heart failure. Life expectancy is reduced overall, but survival is better than previously assumed [7]. Pulmonary artery pressure can be normal but typically increases with age in the un-repaired ASD. With increasing age and increasing pulmonary artery pressure, tachyarrhythmias, for example, atrial fibrillation (AF) and atrial flutter, become more common [8]. Systemic embolism may occur due to AF or atrial flutter or, more rarely, paradoxical embolism, which may prompt investigation for ASD in the previously undiagnosed, asymptomatic adult. Clinical findings include fixed splitting of the second heart sound and a systolic pulmonary flow murmur. Electrocardiogram (ECG) classically shows a partial right bundle branch block with right-axis deviation, and an increased pulmonary vascularity may be noted on a plain chest radiograph [3]. Echocardiography is the first-line diagnostic technique.

ASD Closure

The diagnosis and management of ASD in the adult is outlined in the 2020 ESC Guidelines for the management of adult congenital heart disease [3]. Indications for ASD closure include evidence of right ventricular volume overload, and in the absence of pulmonary hypertension (PH) and left ventricular disease, ASD closure is recommended as a Class I, level B indication, regardless of symptoms. In patents with suspicion of paradoxical embolism, ASD closure should be considered, regardless of size, providing there is absence of PH and left ventricular disease (Class IIa, level C).

Percutaneous transcatheter device closure is considered the first-choice treatment for most ASDs however surgical repair is indicated for limited non-secundum ASD, or secundum ASD characterised by large defects, insufficient septal rim or a left atrium that is too small to accommodate a closure device [9]. Surgical repair has low mortality (less than 1% in patients without significant comorbidity) and good long-term outcomes when performed in adolescence and early adulthood, and in the absence of pulmonary hypertension [10,11]. With increasing patient age, surgical ASD repair can still be considered, with low operative risk, however comorbidities may affect operative risk and should be weighed against the potential benefit.

1.2. Device Closure

Device closure for cardiac septal defects (including ASD and ventricular septal defect (VSD)) was developed in the 1990s, with the deployment of the device performed either percutaneously or by mini-thoracotomy approaches. The advantages of transcatheter device closure include less trauma, faster post-procedure recovery and improved cosmesis. Device closure is recommended for the treatment of secundum ASDs, when technically feasible (Class I, level C). Feasibility for device closure depends on the morphology of the defect and includes a stretched diameter ≤38 mm, with a sufficient rim of remaining septum of 5 mm, except towards the aorta [3]. Several studies have reported no mortality following device closure, and serious complications have been observed in less than 1% of cases [12,13]. Complications of device closure include early atrial tachyarrhythmias and, more rarely, erosion of the atrial wall, anterior mitral leaflet or the aorta, as well as thromboembolic events [14,15]. Antiplatelet therapy (a suggested minimum treatment with Aspirin 75 mg once daily) is required for at least 6 months following the procedure. Studies comparing transcatheter intervention and surgical ASD closure have reported similar survival rates. Hospital length of stay and procedure-related complications are lower in the in the catheter intervention group but with slightly higher rates of residual shunt and reintervention compared to the surgical group [12,16–18].

1.3. Surgical Closure

Surgical ASD closure has been previously reviewed [19], and repair via median sternotomy, using cardiopulmonary bypass (CPB) instituted with the cannulation of the ascending aorta and both vena cavae, is considered the standard approach to surgical treatment. For isolated secundum defects, this approach can be performed with excellent results and mortality approaching zero percent [20]. Complications of surgical ASD repair include arrhythmia, pneumothorax, bleeding, pericardial and pleural effusions. As outlined above, the consequences of post-operative complications will be more marked with increasing patient age and comorbidity and with arrhythmia and prolonged intensive care unit (ICU) and hospital stay, and they are more common in adults and older patients [21]. When surgery is performed in the young adult, the long-term results for surgical secundum defect-closure return actuarial survival curves similar to that of the general population [10].

The American Heart Association defined "minimally invasive" as smaller sternotomy or non-sternotomy strategies aided by robotic or video-assisted technologies [22], and a variety of approaches have been described. Access route is a minor component of invasiveness within cardiac surgery, with cardiopulmonary bypass (CPB), aortic cross clamping, cardioplegic arrest and opening of cardiac chambers contributing more to the invasiveness and risk of complications of the procedure, beyond that of the incision [23]. For the surgical treatment of ASD, minimal-access approaches include partial or mini-sternotomy, right anterolateral thoracotomy, right oblique sub-axillary incision, right vertical sub-axillary incision, right posterior mini-thoracotomy, video-assisted thoracoscopy (VATS)/endoscopic and robotic approaches, with peripheral cannulation for cardiopulmonary bypass. Multiple heart centres have reported their experiences of minimal-access surgical ASD closure for both paediatric and adult congenital populations worldwide.

1.3.1. Minimal-Access Surgery versus Median Sternotomy

The mini-sternotomy approach to CHD has been studied, with an associated reduction in post-operative drainage, shorter hospital length of stay and improved cosmesis compared to standard median sternotomy [24]. Right anterolateral mini-thoracotomy has been widely applied as an alternative to median sternotomy, with similar mortality and post-operative morbidity and superior cosmetic results compared to sternotomy. Minimally invasive video-assisted and endoscopic surgical closure have previously been described with detailed outlines of the approach and surgical technique [25,26]. Single-centre reports describing the evolution of practice and decades-long experience with minimal-access approaches to ASD closure in the adult have been reported [27–31], including comparisons of median sternotomy, totally thoracoscopic and axillary thoracotomy access techniques [32]. A recent systematic review and meta-analysis by Lei et al. [33], including 7 publications and 665 patients, compared short-term outcomes between anterolateral mini-thoracotomy and median sternotomy for the surgical treatment of ASD. They concluded that both approaches were equally safe and effective, with similar success and complication rates. Anterolateral mini-thoracotomy was associated with a faster return to function and better cosmetic results compared to the sternotomy group. The cosmetic benefit is amplified with the use of the periareolar incision, which is adopted within our unit, and it is shown in Figure 1.

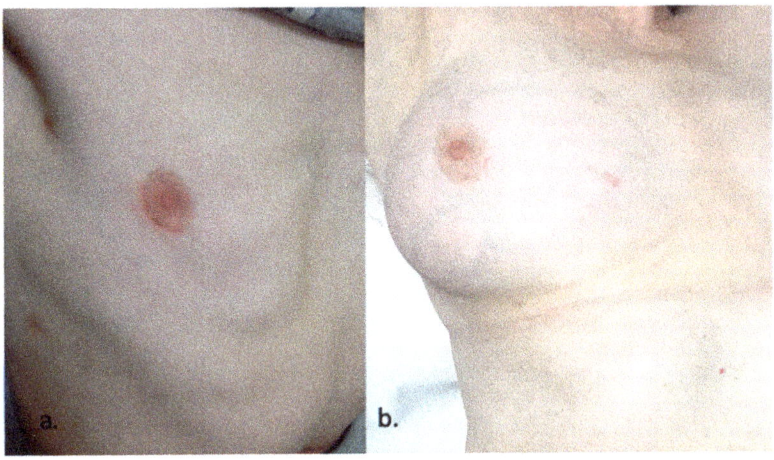

Figure 1. Healed periareolar scars in (**a**) a male patient and (**b**) a female patient 4 months after endoscopic atrial septal defect closure.

As outlined within the guidelines for ASD management, surgical closure is becoming increasingly relevant, compared to transcatheter device closures, for more-complex atrial septal lesions. Clinical case series comparing minimal-access approaches with median sternotomy for adult and paediatric patients with sinus venosus defects and partial anomalous pulmonary venous drainage [34,35], for the treatment of unroofed coronary sinus [36] and more-complex grown-up congenital heart disease [37], have been reported. Although the proportion of patients undergoing minimal-access approaches is relatively small, all conclude that this approach is as safe and effective as conventional median sternotomy.

1.3.2. Minimal-Access Surgery versus Transcatheter Device Closure

A comparison between transcatheter device closure and minimal-access surgical closure for ASD has been made. In single-centre retrospective reviews for secundum ASD closure in adults, a minimally invasive approach was found to achieve a more complete closure compared to transcatheter device closure methods, along with decreased rates of AF and anticoagulation use [38], with another study identifying zero mortality and similar rates of serious complications in both groups [39]. More recently, Goh et al. [40] performed a systematic review and meta-analysis comparing minimally invasive and transcatheter approaches for secundum ASD repair, which included 6 observational studies and a total of 1524 patients. As with the median sternotomy approach, they highlighted that transcatheter closure was associated with shorter hospital length of stay and lower rates of pneumothorax and pericardial effusion, but with higher rates of residual shunt. They concluded that minimally invasive repair had similar outcomes to device closure but recognised the need for further randomised controlled trials comparing the two. Similar meta-analyses have also been reported within the paediatric literature [41]. Finally, a single-centre experience comparing transcatheter device closure and totally endoscopic robotic closure has described similar findings, with shorter hospital and ICU length of stay for the transcatheter group but similar complication risk profiles between the two groups [42].

2. Insights

2.1. Pre-Operative Work-Up and Patient Selection

Echocardiography is the first-line technique in the diagnosis and quantification of ASD. Right ventricular volume overload, which may be the first unexpected finding in a patient with previously undiagnosed ASD, is the key finding and best characterises the haemodynamic relevance of the defect. In general, sinus venosus defects require trans-oesophageal echo (TOE) for accurate diagnosis, with cardiovascular magnetic resonance imaging (CMR) or cardiovascular computed tomography (CCT) alternative modalities in cases of inferior sinus venosus defects. TOE is required for the precise evaluation of secundum defects before device closure, where assessment includes sizing, exploration of the residual septum's morphology, rim size and quality, exclusion of additional defects and confirmation of normal pulmonary venous connection. Other key information includes the estimation of pulmonary artery pressure (PAP) and tricuspid regurgitation (TR).

CMR has become an essential modality in specialist units for the assessment of complex CHD, enabling 3D anatomical reconstruction, which is not restricted by body size or acoustic windows and avoids exposure to radiation [43]. Of note, adults with CHD with conventional pacemakers and defibrillators can undergo CMR where local support is available [44]. CMR is rarely required in the diagnosis and pre-operative planning of ASD repair but may be useful for the assessment of RV volume overload, identification of inferior sinus venosus defects, quantification of pulmonary to systemic flow ratio (Qp:Qs) and evaluation of pulmonary venous connection. CCT can be used to assess ventricular size and function, with inferior temporal resolution compared to CMR and typically higher radiation dose. CCT does, however, benefit MICS ASD repair assessment through high spatial resolution and rapid acquisition time, with the ability to aid pre-operative planning with the assessment of the systemic great vessels, coronary arteries, collateral arterial supply and lung parenchyma. Developments have substantially reduced the amount of radiation exposure for combined CCT coronary, pulmonary and aortic angiograms, making CCT a more attractive option for pre-operative planning in ACHD patients [45].

Cardiac catheterisation is required in the case of non-invasive signs of raised pulmonary artery pressure (PAP) and is used to determine pulmonary vascular resistance (PVR). Pulmonary hypertension (PH) is an important prognostic factor in CHD. PH is now defined as an increase in invasively measured PAP $\geq$ 20 mmHg at rest [46]. Pulmonary hypertension in ASD (and other shunt lesions) typically manifests as pre-capillary PH (PAH), defined as a mean PAP > 20 mmHg, with a pulmonary arterial wedge pressure (PAWP) of $\leq$15 mmHg and a pulmonary vascular resistance of $\geq$3 woods units (WU). The successful management of an ACHD patient with PH requires a multidisciplinary team approach, and where PH is identified, exercise testing should be performed to exclude desaturation. Cardiopulmonary exercise testing (CPET) provides an evaluation of functional capacity and physical fitness prior to surgery, which correlate well with morbidity and mortality in ACHD patients [47]. Pulmonary Function Tests (PFTs) can also be useful in the evaluation of patients for MCS, where single-lung ventilation is planned, in the context of known respiratory disease or significant positive smoking history.

2.2. Anaesthetic Considerations

A recent review of anaesthesia for minimally invasive cardiac surgery has been published [48] outlining the anaesthetic considerations common to all minimally invasive cardiac surgical procedures.

Beyond mini-sternotomy, all other access for surgical ASD closure requires single-lung ventilation prior to cardio-pulmonary bypass, to facilitate right mini-thoracotomy and the placement of utility ports. This can be achieved using a double lumen endotracheal intubation or a single lumen tube with intermittent ventilation or an endobronchial blocker.

To establish cardiopulmonary bypass in the context of right atriotomy for ASD closure, the inferior vena cava (IVA) is cannulated by the surgeon by insertion into the femoral vein, advancing distal to the cavoatrial junction using TOE guidance from the anaesthetist. The SVC cannula is placed in the right internal jugular vein via the Seldinger technique and advanced proximally during anaesthetic induction, using ultrasound guidance. Alternative peripheral perfusion strategies for cardiopulmonary bypass in ASD closure have been reported from a single-centre, retrospective review [49].

As discussed above, patients with raised pulmonary artery pressures and pulmonary hypertension must be carefully evaluated. In patients with PVR < 5 woods units, ASD closure has been shown to be safe and associated with a decrease in PAP and an improvement of symptoms [50–52]. Patients with PVR ≥ 5 woods units are unlikely to improve [52] and more likely to have worse outcomes with complete ASD closure [53]. In patients with impaired left ventricular function (systolic and diastolic), ASD closure may worsen heart failure. Again, careful consideration must be paid to pre-operative evaluation and peri-/post-operative haemodynamic inotropic management. Pre-interventional testing (balloon occlusion with reassessment of haemodynamics) can aid operative decision making with the potential for complete, fenestrated or no closure, considering that an increase in filling pressure due to the ASD closure may worsen symptoms and outcome [54].

2.3. Surgical Technique

The surgical technique, including operating room set-up, positioning, establishing cardiopulmonary bypass and pericardial patch closure, for minimally invasive ASD repair via right mini-thoracotomy, is well described by Nagendran et al. [26] and mirrors the approach taken within our centre. Approaches to myocardial protection during minimally invasive mitral valve surgery have been summarized by Garbade et al. [55] and are applicable to minimally invasive ASD repair. Intra-operative views of the endoscopic right mini-thoracotomy pericardial patch ASD repair are shown in Figure 2.

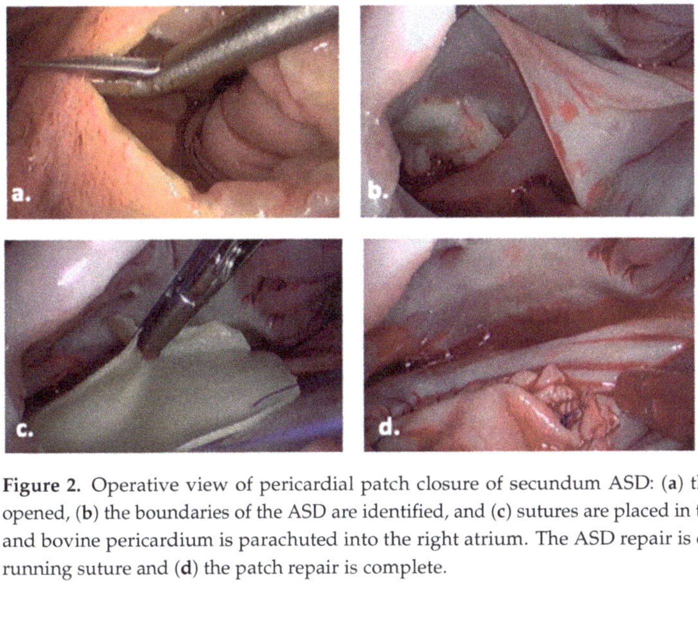

Figure 2. Operative view of pericardial patch closure of secundum ASD: (**a**) the right atrium is opened, (**b**) the boundaries of the ASD are identified, and (**c**) sutures are placed in the rim of the ASD and bovine pericardium is parachuted into the right atrium. The ASD repair is continued using a running suture and (**d**) the patch repair is complete.

Beyond these technical considerations, specific issues relating to minimal-access surgical ASD repair include the persistent left SVC, anomalous pulmonary venous connections, and other associated anomalies, including valve lesions and atrial arrhythmias. In patients with atrial flutter/AF, cryo- or radio-frequency ablation (modified maze procedure) should be considered at the time of surgery [3]. Here, surgical ASD closure benefits the patient, as device closure may restrict access to the left atrium and limit the potential for electrophysiology (EP) interventions at a later date. Evidence for the surgical or interventional treatment of adult patients with ASD and AF suggests that there is a reduction in the prevalence of AF after ASD closure alone. This is more likely for paroxysmal AF but less successful for persistent or long-standing AF. The reduction in recurrence rate for AF, post-ablation, is highest with bi-atrial surgical ablation [56]. For the patient with persistent AF in the context of ASD, these factors may influence decision making and surgical approach.

Anomalous pulmonary venous connections do not only occur in association with ASD (typically sinus venosus defects) but can also be isolated. Pathophysiologically, these connections result in volume overload of the right heart, with a physiological effect similar to that of an ASD. Most common are the connection of the right pulmonary vein(s) to the IVC ("scimitar vein", which might be associated with sequestration of the right lower lobe), the left upper pulmonary vein(s) to the left innominate vein, and the right upper pulmonary vein(s) connecting high on the SVC. A case report of an anomalous left hepatic vein to coronary sinus in a patient with ASD is also reported [57]. Here, the anomalous connection was repaired using a minimally invasive approach. Surgical repair can be challenging, and low-velocity venous flow imparts the risk of thrombosis of the surgically operated vein, particularly in scimitar syndrome. Indications for surgery follow the principles of recommendations for ASD closure, but technical suitability for the repair and operative risk must be weighed against the potential benefit of intervention [3]. Anomalous venous connections and systemic vascular anomalies can prove technically challenging within minimal-access surgery due to the inability to maintain adequate venous drainage, flooding of the operative field and ventricular distension. These vascular anomalies should be identified pre-operatively, with a careful review of imaging and a high index of suspicion in appropriate patients.

2.4. Post-Operative Care

Immediate post-operative care of the minimal-access ASD closure patient does not differ significantly from that of the adult patient undergoing standard sternotomy closure. After weaning from CPB, the pericardium is loosely closed with the placement of a small pericardial drain. A second drain is placed in the right pleura. Following transfer to the cardiac ICU, a post-operative chest radiograph is performed to ensure right lung expansion and confirm the position of the right pleural drain. Drain removal typically occurs within 24 to 48 h post-surgery, once drainage has ceased and residual pneumothorax is excluded.

As per ESC and AHA guidelines, evaluation following ASD closure is the same, regardless of closure method, and should include an assessment of residual shunt, RV size and function, presence of tricuspid regurgitation and PAP measurement using echocardiography. Patients should be assessed for the presence of arrhythmias by history, ECG and, if suspected, Holter monitor. For patients who undergo ASD closure aged over 40 years, the prevalence of atrial arrhythmias is up to 60%. Anticoagulation should be considered for patients with persisting atrial arrhythmias, and in the absence of arrhythmia, antiplatelet medication can be considered for at least six months following surgical repair, although guidance around dose and duration of treatment is limited. Patients repaired below the age of 25 years, without relevant sequelae or residual disease (no residual shunt, normal PAP, normal right ventricular volume and function, no arrhythmias) do not require regular follow-up. However, patients should be informed of the possibility of late-occurrence tachyarrhythmias. Patients with residual shunt, elevated PAP or arrhythmias (before or after repair) and those repaired at adult age (particularly >40 years) should be followed up on a regular basis [3].

As with the adult congenital population more widely, specific guidance should be given to those patients following ASD closure, with regards to future pregnancy, which, in the absence of pulmonary hypertension, can be considered low risk in this patient population.

The risk of infective endocarditis (IE) in ACHD patients is higher than that of the general population, with marked variation between lesions. The 2015 ESC Guidelines on IE maintain that antibiotic prophylaxis for invasive procedures should be restricted to the highest-risk patients for the highest-risk procedures [58]. High-risk conditions include any CHD repaired with prosthetic material, up to 6 months after the procedure, or lifelong if residual shunt or valvular regurgitation remains. All un-repaired and repaired ACHD patients should be counselled around good oral and cutaneous hygiene, aseptic measures during invasive procedures, the avoidance of unnecessary invasive procedures, such as piercings or tattoos and the signs and symptoms of IE, along with the promotion of health-seeking behaviour during any episodes of infection.

3. Robotic ASD Closure

As minimal-access and minimally invasive cardiac surgical techniques advance, the role for robotic surgery is increasingly considered. The use of robotic surgery for ASD closure has been reported for a cohort of 54 adult and paediatric cases with secundum ASD using the da Vinci robotic system, with the cannulation of the femoral vessels and right internal jugular vein [59]. As with all developing techniques, significant learning curves were reported, evidenced by cross-clamp time, cardiopulmonary bypass time and operative duration, with the authors concluding that ASD closure can be safely and effective performed using a totally endoscopic approach and robotic surgery. More recently, robotically assisted congenital cardiac surgery has been retrospectively reviewed in a single centre, including 242 procedures for secundum ASD, sinus venosus ASD, partial anomalous pulmonary venous drainage and unroofed coronary sinus, as well as other CHDs, in adult patients. Conversion to larger thoracic incision was required in 0.8% of cases, and a mean hospital stay of 3.5 ($\pm$1.1) days was reported [60].

3.1. Minimal-Access Surgery and the Paediatric Patient

Although the focus of this review is on the adult ASD population, minimal-access surgical approaches to ASD closure in the paediatric population have been reported. The development of transcatheter device closure in children is well described [61], and the use of lower mini-sternotomy approaches to surgical management, in order to improve cosmesis, are also reported [62]. The range of minimal-access approaches to ASD closure in the paediatric population, including details of the operative approach and technical considerations, has previously been reviewed [63]. In 2011, Wang et al. reported on 28 patients, with a mean age of 5.8 years and a mean weight of 15 kg, undergoing totally thoracoscopic surgery for ASD closure, with no mortality or re-intervention and of New York Heart Association (NYHA) functional class I, at 6-month follow-up [64]. Similar outcomes have since been described by other groups [65], with Sabzi et al. comparing conventional median sternotomy and modified anterior mini-thoracotomy in 54 children [66]. Here, again, the benefit of a minimal-access approach to surgical closure compared to sternotomy for more-complex ASDs was emphasised.

3.2. Patient Perspectives

In contrast to general surgery, where laparoscopic approaches have been widely and rapidly implemented, the adoption of minimal-access approaches to cardiac surgery have been much slower. As highlighted in the evidence presented within this review, median sternotomy is a well-tolerated incision, and the invasiveness of a cardiac surgical procedure extends beyond that of access alone. With high success rates and low procedural risk and mortality across all approaches to ASD closure, including transcatheter devices, conventional median sternotomy and minimal-access surgical approaches, the assessment of other patient-related outcome measures takes on increasing significance. Within the paediatric population, health-related quality of life (HRQL) has been compared for children undergoing interventional closure and minimally invasive surgical closure for both ASD and VSD repair [67]. The group concluded that HRQL continuously improved post-procedure, regardless of the type of intervention; however, catheter-based intervention was associated with better HRQL in the early post-procedure period.

Patient reported outcome measures (PROMS) and patient reported experience measures (PREMS) are standardised tools used to collect data about the subjective assessment of medical care from the perspective of the patient and are increasingly implemented across of range of health care settings. A recent letter from Kent [68] summarises the importance of qualitative outcome measures in the assessment of minimally invasive techniques, including measures such as pain scores, functional disability and return to daily activities. These factors are likely to be a priority to patients, beyond mortality and post-operative complications, particularly when a range of safe and effective management options are available to them. The ability to adequately describe the impact of a procedure for a given patient is fundamental to informed consent and shared decision making. Within minimally invasive robotic cardiac surgery, across a range of procedures, the study of patient body image, self-esteem and cosmetic result identified benefits in comparison to conventional sternotomy [69]. For the CHD population, who are younger and more likely to be in adolescence or of working age, these factors potentially take on increased significance.

3.3. Team Working and Safe Implementation

The importance of a heart team approach to the management of ASD, and ACHD more widely, should not be underestimated. With the range of approaches to ASD closure all proving to be safe, effective and with low to minimal risk, individualised patient decision making, including shared decision-making models based on the patients' priorities, should be implemented, particularly as expertise and volume for minimal-access approaches grow. For all minimally invasive cardiac surgical programmes more generally, widespread implementation requires careful consideration and a team-based approach to ensure the safe delivery of care, including adequate training for the operative team, provision of post-operative care and patient follow-up. This approach has recently been highlighted in the UK [70] and has been described in our own centre [71].

4. Conclusions

A minimal-access surgical approach to closure of atrial septal defects should be considered for all patients discussed at an ACHD multi-disciplinary team meeting. Patients do benefit from this approach when it is performed in experienced centres, and the advantages extend to both the patient and the institution. Access to minimal-access and minimally invasive ASD closure likely requires increased collaboration between ACHD centres and cardiac surgical centres with expertise in endoscopic or robotic cardiac surgery procedures. We hope this review gives confidence to both physicians and patients considering the surgical closure of an ASD to find an experienced team to offer a minimally invasive, cosmetically superior option.

Author Contributions: Conceptualization, J.Z. and G.H.; writing—original draft preparation, G.H.; writing—review and editing, J.Z.; visualization, J.Z.; supervision, J.Z. All authors have read and agreed to the published version of the manuscript.

Funding: This research received no external funding.

Institutional Review Board Statement: Not applicable.

Informed Consent Statement: Not applicable.

Conflicts of Interest: G Hardman declares no conflict of interest. J Zacharias declares the following conflicts of interest: Speaker and advisory fees from Edwards Life Sciences, Medtronic, Cambridge Medical Robotics, Terumo and Ethicon.

References

1. Liu, Y.; Chen, S.; Zühlke, L.; Black, G.C.; Choy, M.K.; Li, N.; Keavney, B.D. Global birth prevalence of congenital heart defects 1970–2017: Updated systematic review and meta-analysis of 260 studies. *Int. J. Epidemiol.* **2019**, *48*, 455–463. [CrossRef] [PubMed]
2. Moons, P.; Bovijn, L.; Budts, W.; Belmans, A.; Gewillig, M. Temporal trends in survival to adulthood among patients born with congenital heart disease from 1970 to 1992 in Belgium. *Circulation* **2010**, *122*, 2264–2272. [CrossRef]
3. Baumgartner, H.; De Backer, J.; Babu-Narayan, S.V.; Budts, W.; Chessa, M.; Diller, G.-P.; lung, B.; Kluin, J.; Lang, I.M.; Meijboom, F.; et al. 2020 ESC Guidelines for the management of adult congenital heart disease: The Task Force for the management of adult congenital heart disease of the European Society of Cardiology (ESC). Endorsed by: Association for European Paediatric and Congenital Cardiology (AEPC), International Society for Adult Congenital Heart Disease (ISACHD). *Eur. Heart J.* **2021**, *42*, 563–645. [CrossRef] [PubMed]
4. Hoffman, J.I.; Kaplan, S. The incidence of congenital heart disease. *J. Am. Coll. Cardiol.* **2002**, *39*, 1890–1900. [CrossRef] [PubMed]
5. Murli, L.; Ranjit, M.S.; Shah, P. Unroofed coronary sinus: An unusual interatrial communication and a rare childhood entity. *Ann. Pediatr. Cardiol.* **2019**, *12*, 64–65. [CrossRef]
6. Forlemu, A.N.; Ajmal, M.; Saririan, M. Atrial Septal Defect with Eisenmenger Syndrome: A Rare Presentation. *Case Rep. Cardiol.* **2020**, *2020*, 8681761. [CrossRef]
7. Nyboe, C.; Karunanithi, Z.; Nielsen-Kudsk, J.E.; Hjortdal, V.E. Long-term mortality in patients with atrial septal defect: A nationwide cohort-study. *Eur. Heart J.* **2018**, *39*, 993–998. [CrossRef]
8. Gatzoulis, M.A.; Freeman, M.A.; Siu, S.C.; Webb, G.D.; Harris, L. Atrial arrhythmia after surgical closure of atrial septal defects in adults. *N. Engl. J. Med.* **1999**, *340*, 839–846. [CrossRef]
9. Turner, D.R.; Owada, C.Y.; Sang, C.J., Jr.; Khan, M.; Lim, D.S. Closure of Secundum Atrial Septal Defects With the AMPLATZER Septal Occluder: A Prospective, Multicenter, Post-Approval Study. *Circ. Cardiovasc. Interv.* **2017**, *10*, e004212. [CrossRef]
10. Murphy, J.G.; Gersh, B.J.; McGoon, M.D.; Mair, D.D.; Porter, C.J.; Ilstrup, D.M.; McGoon, D.C.; Puga, F.J.; Kirklin, J.W.; Danielson, G.K. Long-term outcome after surgical repair of isolated atrial septal defect. Follow-up at 27 to 32 years. *N. Engl. J. Med.* **1990**, *323*, 1645–1650. [CrossRef]
11. Roos-Hesselink, J.W.; Meijboom, F.J.; Spitaels, S.E.; van Domburg, R.; van Rijen, E.H.; Utens, E.M.; Bogers, A.J.; Simoons, M.L. Excellent survival and low incidence of arrhythmias, stroke and heart failure long-term after surgical ASD closure at young age. A prospective follow-up study of 21–33 years. *Eur. Heart J.* **2003**, *24*, 190–197. [CrossRef] [PubMed]
12. Butera, G.; Carminati, M.; Chessa, M.; Youssef, R.; Drago, M.; Giamberti, A.; Pomè, G.; Bossone, E.; Frigiola, A. Percutaneous versus surgical closure of secundum atrial septal defect: Comparison of early results and complications. *Am. Heart J.* **2006**, *151*, 228–234. [CrossRef]
13. Fischer, G.; Stieh, J.; Uebing, A.; Hoffmann, U.; Morf, G.; Kramer, H.H. Experience with transcatheter closure of secundum atrial septal defects using the Amplatzer septal occluder: A single centre study in 236 consecutive patients. *Heart* **2003**, *89*, 199–204. [CrossRef] [PubMed]
14. Amin, Z.; Hijazi, Z.M.; Bass, J.L.; Cheatham, J.P.; Hellenbrand, W.E.; Kleinman, C.S. Erosion of Amplatzer septal occluder device after closure of secundum atrial septal defects: Review of registry of complications and recommendations to minimize future risk. *Catheter. Cardiovasc. Interv.* **2004**, *63*, 496–502. [CrossRef]
15. Krumsdorf, U.; Ostermayer, S.; Billinger, K.; Trepels, T.; Zadan, E.; Horvath, K.; Sievert, H. Incidence and clinical course of thrombus formation on atrial septal defect and patient foramen ovale closure devices in 1000 consecutive patients. *J. Am. Coll. Cardiol.* **2004**, *43*, 302–309. [CrossRef]
16. Du, Z.D.; Hijazi, Z.M.; Kleinman, C.S.; Silverman, N.H.; Larntz, K. Comparison between transcatheter and surgical closure of secundum atrial septal defect in children and adults: Results of a multicenter nonrandomized trial. *J. Am. Coll. Cardiol.* **2002**, *39*, 1836–1844. [CrossRef] [PubMed]
17. Butera, G.; Biondi-Zoccai, G.; Sangiorgi, G.; Abella, R.; Giamberti, A.; Bussadori, C.; Sheiban, I.; Saliba, Z.; Santoro, T.; Pelissero, G.; et al. Percutaneous versus surgical closure of secundum atrial septal defects: A systematic review and meta-analysis of currently available clinical evidence. *EuroIntervention* **2011**, *7*, 377–385. [CrossRef] [PubMed]
18. Villablanca, P.A.; Briston, D.A.; Rodés-Cabau, J.; Briceno, D.F.; Rao, G.; Aljoudi, M.; Shah, A.M.; Mohananey, D.; Gupta, T.; Makkiya, M.; et al. Treatment options for the closure of secundum atrial septal defects: A systematic review and meta-analysis. *Int. J. Cardiol.* **2017**, *241*, 149–155. [CrossRef]
19. Liava'a, M.; Kalfa, D. Surgical closure of atrial septal defects. *J. Thorac. Dis.* **2018**, *10*, S2931–S2939. [CrossRef] [PubMed]
20. Zhu, J.; Zhang, Y.; Bao, C.; Ding, F.; Mei, J. Individualized strategy of minimally invasive cardiac surgery in congenital cardiac septal defects. *J. Cardiothorac. Surg.* **2022**, *17*, 5. [CrossRef]
21. Nyboe, C.; Fenger-Grøn, M.; Nielsen-Kudsk, J.E.; Hjortdal, V. Closure of secundum atrial septal defects in the adult and elderly patients. *Eur. J. Cardiothorac. Surg.* **2013**, *43*, 752–757. [CrossRef] [PubMed]
22. Rosengart, T.K.; Feldman, T.; Borger, M.A.; Vassiliades, T.A., Jr.; Gillinov, A.M.; Hoercher, K.J.; Vahanian, A.; Bonow, R.O.; O'Neill, W. Percutaneous and minimally invasive valve procedures: A scientific statement from the American Heart Association Council on Cardiovascular Surgery and Anesthesia, Council on Clinical Cardiology, Functional Genomics and Translational Biology Interdisciplinary Working Group, and Quality of Care and Outcomes Research Interdisciplinary Working Group. *Circulation* **2008**, *117*, 1750–1767. [CrossRef] [PubMed]

23. Ali, J.M.; Abu-Omar, Y. Minimally invasive cardiac surgery-a Fad or the Future? *J. Thorac. Dis.* **2021**, *13*, 1882–1885. [CrossRef]
24. Luo, W.; Chang, C.; Chen, S. Ministernotomy versus full sternotomy in congenital heart defects: A prospective randomized study. *Ann. Thorac. Surg.* **2001**, *71*, 473–475. [CrossRef] [PubMed]
25. Burkhart, H.M.; Suri, R.M. Minimally invasive video assisted surgical closure of secundum atrial septal defect. *Ann. Cardiothorac. Surg.* **2017**, *6*, 60–63. [CrossRef]
26. Nagendran, J.; Habib, H.F.; Kiaii, B.; Chu, M.W. Minimally invasive endoscopic repair of atrial septal defects via right minithoracotomy. *Multimed. Man Cardiothorac. Surg.* **2016**, *2016*, mmv042. [CrossRef]
27. Vistarini, N.; Aiello, M.; Mattiucci, G.; Alloni, A.; Cattadori, B.; Tinelli, C.; Pellegrini, C.; D'Armini, A.M.; Viganò, M. Port-access minimally invasive surgery for atrial septal defects: A 10-year single-center experience in 166 patients. *J. Thorac. Cardiovasc. Surg.* **2010**, *139*, 139–145. [CrossRef]
28. Ak, K.; Aybek, T.; Wimmer-Greinecker, G.; Ozaslan, F.; Bakhtiary, F.; Moritz, A.; Dogan, S. Evolution of surgical techniques for atrial septal defect repair in adults: A 10-year single-institution experience. *J. Thorac. Cardiovasc. Surg.* **2007**, *134*, 757–764. [CrossRef]
29. Baharestani, B.; Rezaei, S.; Jalili Shahdashti, F.; Omrani, G.; Heidarali, M. Experiences in surgical closure of atrial septal defect with anterior mini-thoracotomy approach. *J. Cardiovasc. Thorac. Res.* **2014**, *6*, 181–184. [CrossRef]
30. Chu, M.W.; Losenno, K.L.; Fox, S.A.; Adams, C.; Al-Habib, H.; Guo, R.; Menkis, A.H.; Kiaii, B. Clinical outcomes of minimally invasive endoscopic and conventional sternotomy approaches for atrial septal defect repair. *Can. J. Surg.* **2014**, *57*, E75–E81. [CrossRef]
31. Vida, V.L.; Zanotto, L.; Zanotto, L.; Tessari, C.; Padalino, M.A.; Zanella, F.; Pittarello, D.; Stellin, G. Minimally invasive surgery for atrial septal defects: A 20-year experience at a single centre. *Interact. Cardiovasc. Thorac. Surg.* **2019**, *28*, 961–967. [CrossRef] [PubMed]
32. Luo, H.; Wang, J.; Qiao, C.; Zhang, X.; Zhang, W.; Song, L. Evaluation of different minimally invasive techniques in the surgical treatment of atrial septal defect. *J. Thorac. Cardiovasc. Surg.* **2014**, *148*, 188–193. [CrossRef] [PubMed]
33. Lei, Y.Q.; Liu, J.F.; Xie, W.P.; Hong, Z.N.; Chen, Q.; Cao, H. Anterolateral minithoracotomy versus median sternotomy for the surgical treatment of atrial septal defects: A meta-analysis and systematic review. *J. Cardiothorac. Surg.* **2021**, *16*, 266. [CrossRef] [PubMed]
34. Amirghofran, A.A.; Nirooei, E.; Edraki, M.; Ramsheh, A.R.; Ajami, G.; Amoozgar, H.; Arabi, H.; Hemmati, R. Minimally invasive versus sternotomy approach for double-patch repair of partial anomalous pulmonary venous connection and sinus venosus defect in pediatric and adult patients: Mid to long-term outcomes. *J. Card. Surg.* **2022**, *37*, 4808–4815. [CrossRef] [PubMed]
35. Bozso, S.J.; Evans, B.; Chu, M.W.A. Minimally invasive periareolar approach to repair sinus venosus atrial septal defect with partial anomalous pulmonary venous connection. *J. Card. Surg.* **2020**, *35*, 1653–1656. [CrossRef]
36. Bozso, S.J.; Grant, A.; Iglesias, I.; Chu, M.W.A. Minimally Invasive Periareolar Approach to Unroofed Coronary Sinus Atrial Septal Defect Repair. *Ann. Thorac. Surg.* **2016**, *102*, e223–e225. [CrossRef]
37. Barbero, C.; Marchetto, G.; Pace Napoleone, C.; Calia, C.; Cura Stura, E.; Pocar, M.; Rinaldi, M.; Boffini, M. Right mini-thoracotomy approach for grown-up congenital heart disease. *J. Card. Surg.* **2021**, *36*, 1917–1921. [CrossRef]
38. Schneeberger, Y.; Schaefer, A.; Conradi, L.; Brickwedel, J.; Reichenspurner, H.; Kozlik-Feldmann, R.; Detter, C. Minimally invasive endoscopic surgery versus catheter-based device occlusion for atrial septal defects in adults: Reconsideration of the standard of care. *Interact. Cardiovasc. Thorac. Surg.* **2017**, *24*, 603–608. [CrossRef]
39. Kodaira, M.; Kawamura, A.; Okamoto, K.; Kanazawa, H.; Minakata, Y.; Murata, M.; Shimizu, H.; Fukuda, K. Comparison of Clinical Outcomes After Transcatheter vs. Minimally Invasive Cardiac Surgery Closure for Atrial Septal Defect. *Circ. J.* **2017**, *81*, 543–551. [CrossRef]
40. Goh, E.; Mohammed, H.; Salmasi, M.Y.; Ho, S.; Benedetto, U.; Caputo, M.; Angelini, G.; Vohra, H.A. Minimally invasive versus transcatheter closure of secundum atrial septal defects: A systematic review and meta-analysis. *Perfusion* **2022**, *37*, 700–710. [CrossRef]
41. Mylonas, K.S.; Ziogas, I.A.; Evangeliou, A.; Hemmati, P.; Schizas, D.; Sfyridis, P.G.; Economopoulos, K.P.; Bakoyiannis, C.; Kapelouzou, A.; Tzifa, A.; et al. Minimally Invasive Surgery vs. Device Closure for Atrial Septal Defects: A Systematic Review and Meta-analysis. *Pediatr. Cardiol.* **2020**, *41*, 853–861. [CrossRef] [PubMed]
42. Kadirogullari, E.; Onan, B.; Timur, B.; Birant, A.; Reyhancan, A.; Basgoze, S.; Aydin, U. Transcatheter closure vs. totally endoscopic robotic surgery for atrial septal defect closure: A single-center experience. *J. Card. Surg.* **2020**, *35*, 764–771. [CrossRef] [PubMed]
43. Di Salvo, G.; Miller, O.; Babu Narayan, S.; Li, W.; Budts, W.; Valsangiacomo Buechel, E.R.; Frigiola, A.; van den Bosch, A.E.; Bonello, B.; Mertens, L.; et al. Imaging the adult with congenital heart disease: A multimodality imaging approach-position paper from the EACVI. *Eur. Heart J. Cardiovasc. Imaging* **2018**, *19*, 1077–1098. [CrossRef] [PubMed]
44. Brignole, M.; Auricchio, A.; Baron-Esquivias, G.; Bordachar, P.; Boriani, G.; Breithardt, O.A.; Cleland, J.; Deharo, J.C.; Delgado, V.; Elliott, P.M.; et al. 2013 ESC Guidelines on cardiac pacing and cardiac resynchronization therapy: The Task Force on cardiac pacing and resynchronization therapy of the European Society of Cardiology (ESC). Developed in collaboration with the European Heart Rhythm Association (EHRA). *Eur. Heart J.* **2013**, *34*, 2281–2329. [CrossRef] [PubMed]

45. Kilner, P.; Nichol, E.; Rubens, M. ESC Textbook of Cardiovascular Imaging. Oxford univeristy Press: Oxford, UK, 2015; pp. 563–600.
46. Simonneau, G.; Montani, D.; Celermajer, D.S.; Denton, C.P.; Gatzoulis, M.A.; Krowka, M.; Williams, P.G.; Souza, R. Haemodynamic definitions and updated clinical classification of pulmonary hypertension. *Eur. Respir. J.* **2019**, *53*, 1801913. [CrossRef]
47. Diller, G.P.; Dimopoulos, K.; Okonko, D.; Li, W.; Babu-Narayan, S.V.; Broberg, C.S.; Johansson, B.; Bouzas, B.; Mullen, M.J.; Poole-Wilson, P.A.; et al. Exercise intolerance in adult congenital heart disease: Comparative severity, correlates, and prognostic implication. *Circulation* **2005**, *112*, 828–835. [CrossRef]
48. White, A.; Patvardhan, C.; Falter, F. Anesthesia for minimally invasive cardiac surgery. *J. Thorac. Dis.* **2021**, *13*, 1886–1898. [CrossRef]
49. Kitahara, H.; Okamoto, K.; Kudo, M.; Yoshitake, A.; Ito, T.; Hayashi, K.; Inaba, Y.; Akamatsu, Y.; Shimizu, H. Alternative peripheral perfusion strategies for safe cardiopulmonary bypass in atrial septal defect closure via a right minithoracotomy approach. *Gen. Thorac. Cardiovasc. Surg.* **2016**, *64*, 131–137. [CrossRef]
50. Humenberger, M.; Rosenhek, R.; Gabriel, H.; Rader, F.; Heger, M.; Klaar, U.; Binder, T.; Probst, P.; Heinze, G.; Maurer, G.; et al. Benefit of atrial septal defect closure in adults: Impact of age. *Eur. Heart J.* **2011**, *32*, 553–560. [CrossRef]
51. Yong, G.; Khairy, P.; De Guise, P.; Dore, A.; Marcotte, F.; Mercier, L.A.; Noble, S.; Ibrahim, R. Pulmonary arterial hypertension in patients with transcatheter closure of secundum atrial septal defects: A longitudinal study. *Circ. Cardiovasc. Interv.* **2009**, *2*, 455–462. [CrossRef]
52. Steele, P.M.; Fuster, V.; Cohen, M.; Ritter, D.G.; McGoon, D.C. Isolated atrial septal defect with pulmonary vascular obstructive disease–long-term follow-up and prediction of outcome after surgical correction. *Circulation* **1987**, *76*, 1037–1042. [CrossRef] [PubMed]
53. Manes, A.; Palazzini, M.; Leci, E.; Bacchi Reggiani, M.L.; Branzi, A.; Galiè, N. Current era survival of patients with pulmonary arterial hypertension associated with congenital heart disease: A comparison between clinical subgroups. *Eur. Heart J.* **2014**, *35*, 716–724. [CrossRef]
54. Tadros, V.X.; Asgar, A.W. Atrial septal defect closure with left ventricular dysfunction. *EuroIntervention* **2016**, *12* (Suppl. X), X13–X17. [CrossRef] [PubMed]
55. Garbade, J.; Davierwala, P.; Seeburger, J.; Pfannmueller, B.; Misfeld, M.; Borger, M.A.; Mohr, F.W. Myocardial protection during minimally invasive mitral valve surgery: Strategies and cardioplegic solutions. *Ann. Cardiothorac. Surg.* **2013**, *2*, 803–808. [CrossRef] [PubMed]
56. Wu, S.J.; Fan, Y.F.; Chien, C.Y. Surgical or interventional treatment for adult patients with atrial septal defect and atrial fibrillation: A systemic review and meta-analysis. *Asian J. Surg.* **2022**, *45*, 62–67. [CrossRef]
57. Rao, R.K.; Varadaraju, R.; Girish, B.; Singh, N. Anomalous left hepatic vein to coronary sinus in a patient with atrial septal defect: Minimally invasive approach; technical challenges. *J. Card. Surg.* **2021**, *36*, 4390–4392. [CrossRef] [PubMed]
58. Habib, G.; Lancellotti, P.; Antunes, M.J.; Bongiorni, M.G.; Casalta, J.P.; Del Zotti, F.; Dulgheru, R.; El Khoury, G.; Erba, P.A.; Iung, B.; et al. 2015 ESC Guidelines for the management of infective endocarditis: The Task Force for the Management of Infective Endocarditis of the European Society of Cardiology (ESC). Endorsed by: European Association for Cardio-Thoracic Surgery (EACTS), the European Association of Nuclear Medicine (EANM). *Eur. Heart J.* **2015**, *36*, 3075–3128. [CrossRef]
59. Onan, B.; Onan, I.S. Early Results of Robotically Assisted Congenital Cardiac Surgery: Analysis of 242 Patients. *Ann. Thorac. Surg.* **2021**, *112*, 2020–2027. [CrossRef]
60. Xiao, C.; Gao, C.; Yang, M.; Wang, G.; Wu, Y.; Wang, J.; Wang, R.; Yao, M. Totally robotic atrial septal defect closure: 7-year single-institution experience and follow-up. *Interact. Cardiovasc. Thorac. Surg.* **2014**, *19*, 933–937. [CrossRef]
61. Bennhagen, R.G.; McLaughlin, P.; Benson, L.N. Contemporary management of children with atrial septal defects: A focus on transcatheter closure. *Am. J. Cardiovasc. Drugs* **2001**, *1*, 445–454. [CrossRef]
62. Konstantinov, I.E.; Buratto, E. Atrial Septal Defect Closure via Ministernotomy in Children. *Heart Lung Circ.* **2021**, *30*, e98–e100. [CrossRef] [PubMed]
63. Konstantinov, I.E.; Kotani, Y.; Buratto, E.; Schulz, A.; Ivanov, Y. Minimally invasive approaches to atrial septal defect closure. *JTCVS Tech.* **2022**, *14*, 184–190. [CrossRef] [PubMed]
64. Wang, F.; Li, M.; Xu, X.; Yu, S.; Cheng, Z.; Deng, C.; Yi, D. Totally thoracoscopic surgical closure of atrial septal defect in small children. *Ann. Thorac. Surg.* **2011**, *92*, 200–203. [CrossRef] [PubMed]
65. Sabate Rotes, A.; Burkhart, H.M.; Suri, R.M.; Grogan, M.; Taggart, N.W.; Li, Z.; Schaff, H.V.; Dearani, J.A. Minimally invasive video-assisted surgical closure of atrial septal defects: A safe approach. *World J. Pediatr. Congenit. Heart Surg.* **2014**, *5*, 527–533. [CrossRef]
66. Sabzi, F.; Faraji, R.; Kazeminasab, M. Minimal Invasive Technique in Atrial Septal Defect Surgery. *Cardiol. Res.* **2018**, *9*, 90–93. [CrossRef]
67. Yuan, Y.; Pan, B.; Liang, X.; Lv, T.; Tian, J. Health-related quality of life in children with congenital heart disease following interventional closure versus minimally invasive closure. *Front. Cardiovasc. Med.* **2022**, *9*, 974720. [CrossRef]
68. Kent, W.D.T.; Fedak, P.W.M. Minimally invasive cardiac surgery and the importance of qualitative patient-centered metrics to guide innovations. *J. Thorac. Cardiovasc. Surg.* **2019**, *157*, e356–e357. [CrossRef]

69. İyigün, T.; Kaya, M.; Gülbeyaz, S.; Fıstıkçı, N.; Uyanık, G.; Yılmaz, B.; Onan, B.; Erkanlı, K. Patient body image, self-esteem, and cosmetic results of minimally invasive robotic cardiac surgery. *Int. J. Surg.* **2017**, *39*, 88–94. [CrossRef]
70. Vohra, H.A.; Salmasi, M.Y.; Chien, L.; Caputo, M.; Baghai, M.; Deshpande, R.; Akowuah, E.; Ahmed, I.; Tolan, M.; Bahrami, T.; et al. BISMICS consensus statement: Implementing a safe minimally invasive mitral programme in the UK healthcare setting. *Open Heart* **2020**, *7*, e001259. [CrossRef]
71. Kirmani, B.H.; Knowles, A.; Saravanan, P.; Zacharias, J. Establishing minimally invasive cardiac surgery in a low-volume mitral surgery centre. *Ann. R. Coll. Surg. Engl.* **2021**, *103*, 444–451. [CrossRef]

Journal of
Cardiovascular
Development and Disease

MDPI

Article

Minimally Invasive Surgery for Simple Congenital Heart Defects: Preserving Aesthetics without Jeopardizing Patient Safety

Mauro Lo Rito [1,*], Ylenia Claudia Maria Brindicci [1], Mario Moscatiello [1], Alessandro Varrica [1], Matteo Reali [1], Antonio Saracino [2], Massimo Chessa [2], Tommaso Aloisio [3], Giuseppe Isgrò [3] and Alessandro Giamberti [1]

1 Department of Congenital Cardiac Surgery, IRCCS Policlinico San Donato, San Donato Milanese, 20097 Milan, Italy; ylenia.brindicci@gmail.com (Y.C.M.B.); alessandro.varrica@grupposandonato.it (A.V.); matteo.reali@grupposandonato.it (M.R.); alessandro.giamberti@grupposandonato.it (A.G.)
2 Department of Pediatric and Adult Congenital Cardiology, IRCCS Policlinico San Donato, San Donato Milanese, 20097 Milan, Italy; antonio.saracino@grupposandonato.it (A.S.); massimo.chessa@grupposandonato.it (M.C.)
3 Department of Cardiothoracic and Vascular Anesthesia and Intensive Care Unit (ICU), IRCCS Policlinico San Donato, San Donato Milanese, 20097 Milan, Italy; tommaso.aloisio@grupposandonato.it (T.A.); giuseppe.isgro@grupposandonato.it (G.I.)
* Correspondence: mauro.lorito@grupposandonato.it; Tel.: +39-025-277-4511

Abstract: Minimally invasive surgeries for pediatric patients have been proposed for decades, with different approaches in mind. Minimal right axillary thoracotomy (MRAT), proposed two decades ago, allows the preservation of patients' safety alongside faster aesthetic and functional recovery. The MRAT did not become widely adopted due to the prejudice that to follow a minimally invasive approach, safety and efficacy must be compromised. With this study, we aim to compare MRAT to the standard median sternotomy approach with a focus on safety and clinical outcomes. Between January 2017 and April 2021, 216 patients diagnosed with ASD, pAVSD, or PAPVD underwent surgical repair with different approaches in the same period. MRAT was used for 78 patients, and median sternotomy was used for 138 patients. In this last group, standard median sternotomy (SMS) was used for 116 patients, while a minimal skin incision (SMS mini) was used for 22 patients. There were no major complications overall nor in each specific approach. MRAT enabled the successful repair of simple heart defects, providing similar post-operative and cardiological recovery. MRAT does not compromise patients' safety and does not prolong the duration of surgery once the learning curve is overcome, which is generally after 15–20 consecutive operations.

Keywords: atrial septal defect; partial anomalous venous return; partial atrioventricular septal defect; minimally invasive surgery; right anterior thoracotomy; congenital heart defect; surgery

1. Introduction

Surgical repair of simple congenital heart defects, such as atrial septal defects (ASD), partial atrioventricular septal defect (pAVSD), and partial anomalous pulmonary venous return (PAPVD), using standard median sternotomy (SMS) has excellent results, with low mortality and morbidity [1,2]. We aim to specify that the treated PAPVD was, above all, with a return to SVC and occasionally to IVC, and the surgical approach was sometimes in minimal right axillary thoracotomy. Still, more often, we treated PAPVD in sternotomy or mini-sternotomy. Considering that we were establishing a program, we decided to use MRAT primarily for ASD for the first few years.

In the last decade [3–5], different minimally invasive approaches have been proposed to enhance patients' recovery and provide better cosmetic results [3–7]. Surgical approaches, such as right anterolateral thoracotomy, posterolateral thoracotomy, and partial sternotomy, may carry the risk of suboptimal results [8–11] in a growing number of patients. Possible complications related to the approach can be scoliosis and asymmetrical breast development, which are fundamental to patients' appearance and satisfaction [11,12]. To overcome these drawbacks, the technique of minimal right axillary thoracotomy (MRAT) was developed and introduced as a variation of Denis Browne's original right thoracotomy [13], allowing correction of simple congenital heart defects while avoiding chest wall deformities and anomalous breast development and hiding surgical scar beneath the right arm. With this study, we aim to assess the results of the introduction of MRAT for simple defects compared to standard approaches (SMS and SMS mini) in terms of surgical outcomes and early results.

2. Materials and Methods

In this retrospective single-center study, we included all patients with the diagnosis of atrial septal defect (ASD), partial atrial septal defect (pAVSD), and partial anomalous pulmonary venous return (PAPVD) operated using MRAT or SMS between January 2017 and April 2021 at the IRCCS Policlinico San Donato. All subjects with other diagnoses or those who were treated with other approaches were excluded. Clinical and operative data were obtained from medical records, operative notes, and follow-up reports. Outcomes of interest were operative parameters, post-operative course, incidence of complications, and wound-related complications. We included 216 patients divided according to the approach in the following groups: MRAT (n = 78 pts) and sternotomy (n = 138 pts). In this last group, SMS was used in 116, and in the other 22, we adopted a minimal cosmetic skin incision (SMS mini).

Statistical Analysis

We expressed continuous variables as median with interquartile range (IQR), considering a non-normal distribution that was assessed with the Shapiro–Wilk test. The differences between groups were assessed with Kruskal–Wallis Test and Dunn's test with Bonferroni correction to evaluate differences among the three groups. Categorical and ordinal variables were reported as frequencies and percentages, and differences were assessed with Chi-squared or Fisher exact test according to group size. We investigated the improvement or worsening of echocardiographic parameters (intended as a shift from the starting value) between pre-operative and discharge using symmetry test (Bowker's test and the Stuart–Maxwell test). The Bowker's test is a symmetry test, and the Stuart–Maxwell test is marginal homogeneity test; if both tests provide significant p-value, then a significant shift has occurred. p-value was considered significant when <0.05. Data analyses were performed with Stata Statistical Software (Release 17; StataCorp 2022, College Station, TX, USA: StataCorp LP).

3. Results

Among the 216 patients, there were 128 females (59.3%) and 88 males (40.7%) with a median age at surgery of 6.1 years (IQR: 4–14.5). The most frequent diagnoses were ASD (n = 149 pts), PAPVD (n = 54), and pAVSD (n = 13). At the pre-operative echocardiogram, the left ventricular function was preserved; meanwhile, the right ventricle had moderate or severe dilatation in 88.8% (see Table 1). Mitral and tricuspid valves presented severe regurgitation in a minority of the population, as described in Table 1.

Table 1. Pre-operative and discharge echocardiographic data. Pre-operative and discharge data comparisons for each single approach (intended as a shift from the pre-operative to the post-operative value) were assessed with symmetry test (Bowker's test and the Stuart–Maxwell test). A significant *p*-value indicates that there has been a significant shift between categories of the variable.

Variable	MRAT (n = 78 pts)					Sternotomy (n = 138 pts)				
	Pre-Operative n (%)		Post-Operative n (%)		*p*-Value	Pre-Operative n (%)		Post-Operative n (%)		*p*-Value
Left ventricle EF					ns					0.1573
Normal	78	100%	78	100%		138	100%	138	100%	
Right ventricle EF					0.0009					0.0009
Normal	78	100%	33	42%		138	100%	61	44%	
Right ventricle dilatation					0.0009					0.0009
No	1	1%	26	33%		9	7%	36	26%	
Mild	6	8%	17	22%		8	6%	41	30%	
Moderate	61	78%	34	44%		97	70%	60	43%	
Severe	10	13%	1	1%		24	17%	0	0%	
Pulmonary artery pressure increment					0.0558					0.0001
Normal	67	86%	75	96%		101	73%	126	91%	
Mild	7	9%	3	4%		24	17%	10	7%	
>Moderate	4	5%	0	0%		13	9%	1	1%	
Tricuspid valve regurgitation degree					0.2719					0.0009
No	15	19%	23	29%		13	9%	36	26%	
Mild	57	73%	51	65%		107	78%	100	72%	
Moderate	5	6%	4	5%		16	12%	2	1%	
Severe	0	0%	0	0%		2	1%	0	0%	
Mitral valve regurgitation degree					0.2035					0.1395
Normal	69	88%	66	85%		119	86%	124	90%	
Mild	4	5%	11	14%		12	9%	13	9%	
Moderate	4	5%	1	1%		7	5%	1	1%	

3.1. Surgical Technique Description

All operations, independent from the surgical approach, were monitored similarly with arterial access (preferably right radial artery), right jugular internal central venous catheter, transesophageal echocardiography, and defibrillating external pads for MRAT and SMS mini. The use of external defibrillating pads is indicated for the minimal approaches because it is possible that internal defibrillating palettes may not be used. The cardiopulmonary bypass strategy was similar in all approaches with aortic cross-clamp, cardioplegic arrest, and operation conducted in normothermia or mild hypothermia. We administered antegrade hematic or crystalloid cardioplegia that provided long myocardial protection, avoiding the need for repetition. The SMS approach was prepared as routinely performed. In 2018, we started the program for CHD minimally invasive treatment, and, with regard to MRAT, we adopted the approach described by Prêtre et al. [14] for the patients with partial left lateral decubitus and a 3–5 cm incision in the right anterior axillary line that needed to be hidden beneath the right arm (Figure 1A–C). We usually entered the chest cavity in the fourth intercostal space for ASD and small-size patients (<20 kg) and the third intercostal space for PAVD and larger patients that required direct aortic cannulation (>20 and <50). We modified the Prêtre approach by adding the Alexis wound protector/retractor (Applied Medical) that fit well with different pediatric chest conformations (Figure 1D). We used size S for pediatric cases and size M for adolescent/adult patients. The soft tissue retractor was placed after the opening of the intercostal space and allowed gentle retraction of the wound's surrounding tissues; the finocchietto spreader was then placed to enlarge the intercostal space (Figure 1D). The soft tissue retractor could not be used by adding a second finocchietto spreader in orthogonal direction to retract the soft tissues. The remaining preparation technique does not differ from the already published method [14]. The cannulation strategy needs to be planned ahead of the case, with proper device selection. In particular, we prefer central cannulation (aortic/bicaval) for all cases weighing <30 kg, a hybrid strategy for cases weighing between 30 and 50 kg, and complete peripheral cannulation for cases >50 kg. In particular, for patients weighing between 30 and 50 kg, the cannulation strategies were personalized to patients, height, and size, considering femoral artery and vein cannulation in patients that already had a developed "adult" body conformation. For adult-sized patients, peripheral cannulation consisted of a typical setting for minimally invasive surgeries, with percutaneous neck right SVC cannulation and surgically isolated femoral vessel direct cannulation. After decannulation, the femoral artery, especially for adolescents or borderline weight cases, was reconstructed with a pericardial patch to avoid stenosis related to purse string closure.

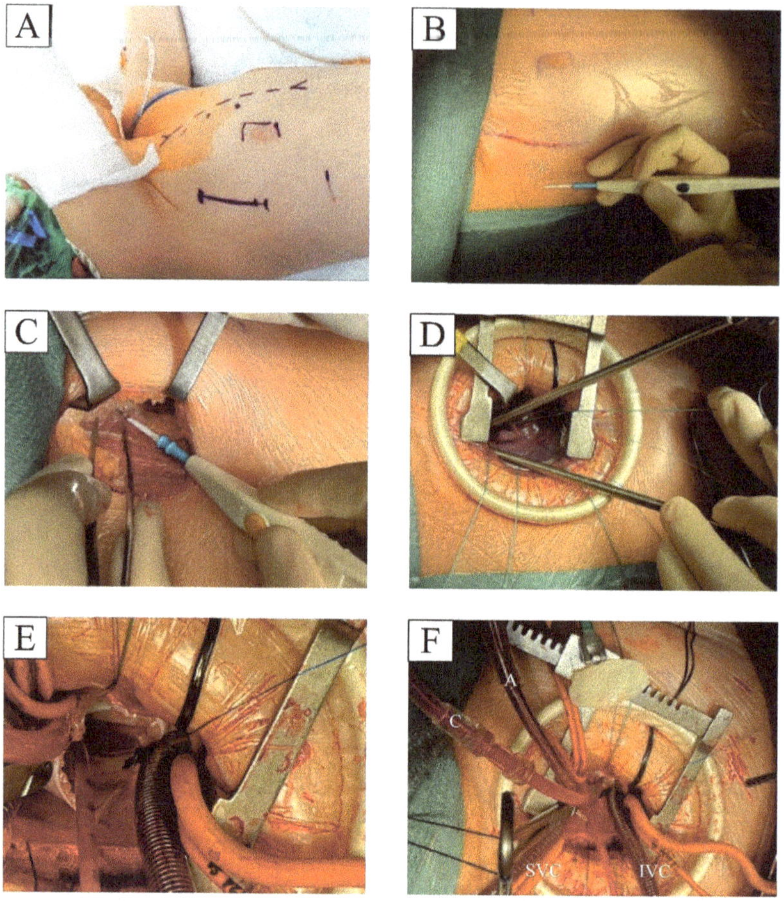

Figure 1. Patient preparation and surgically relevant steps: (**A**) Patient reference marking for MRAT incision, right nipple, and potential bail-out sternotomy; the patient is placed in partial left decubitus with the right arm lifted gently above the head. (**B**,**C**) limited skin incision and muscle sparing with preservation of the long thoracic nerve. (**D**) Soft tissue and finocchietto exposure with pericardial suspension. (**E**) atrial septal defect visualization with central cannulation. (**F**) atrial septal defect patch closure.

3.2. Demographic Data and Operative Results

The sternotomy (SMS) was the approach most frequently used (63.9%) with a subgroup of patients in which we made a 5 cm skin incision (22/138) but performed a full sternotomy (SMS mini). The most frequent operation performed with SMS was ASD patch closure (56%), followed by PAPVD repair (36%) and pAVSD correction (8%). We used SMS mini only for ASD closure (n = 17) and PAPVD repair (n = 5), and we did not treat any case of pAVSD. Main echocardiographic preoperative findings showed typical characteristics for an interatrial shunt with a volume overload of the right ventricle with moderate-to-severe dilatation in 89% of the cases and moderate-to-severe tricuspid valve regurgitation in 11% of the population. Detailed information on the population according to the approach is illustrated in Table 1.

We began a minimally invasive structured program in 2018 with the adoption of the MRAT approach. The minimally invasive program was planned with the aim of abolising the surgical learning curve and eliminating any potential complications. We invited an experienced surgeon (R. Prêtre) to perform the first cases, teaching everyone relevant methods and warning us of potential pitfalls. The first year of the program focused on only performing ASD cases in the weight range of (<20 kg), which allowed central cannulation to maintain a homogeneous and replicable method among the four surgeons of the team who received equal and regular case exposure. After the first year, we widened our indications including differents diagnosis and patients' weight, and the MRAT rapidly outgrew the SMS cases (34 vs. 24) in the second year of the program. The cannulation strategies adopted are detailed in Table 2. In the MRAT group, the most frequent defect repaired was ASD (85.9%—n = 67), with few cases of PAPVD (8.9%—n = 7) and pAVSD (5.1%—n = 4). Due to this initial program plan, the adoption of MRAT was significantly more frequent for ASD (85.9% vs. 77% vs. 56% $p < 0.001$) compared to the SMS that was preferred in PAVPD and pAVSD.

Table 2. Type of cannulation according to different approaches.

	Type of Cannulation				
	MRAT (n)	**SMS (n)**	**SMS Mini (n)**	**Total n (%)**	
Central	65	116	21	202	(93.5%)
Peripheral	7	0	1	8	(3.7%)
Mixed	6	0	0	6	(2.8%)
Total	78	116	22	216	(100%)

In terms of operative details, the patients of the MRAT group were significantly younger and were lighter in weight and smaller in height compared to the SMS (Table 3). There was no significant difference in relation to cardiopulmonary bypass (Figure 2) and aortic cross-clamp, although surgical times were significantly longer for the MRAT compared to SMS (190 vs. 170 min, $p = 0.0013$). Accounting for the learning curve, the analysis of surgical times among the four surgeons showed that for MRAT, the surgical operative times become comparable to SMS after 15–20 procedures (Figure 3), indicating that longer surgeries were due to initial experience with this new approach. The majority of MRAT patients had only one chest drain (75/78), draining both the pleural and pericardial spaces. Meanwhile, in the SMS patients, a minority had only one drain (27/116) and SMS mini (15/22). The median ICU stay was 1 day for every approach without any significant differences. The overall median hospital stay was 7 days (IQR: 6–9) with no differences among the three approaches [MRAT 7 days (IQR: 6–7)–SMS 7 days (IQR: 6–10) days, SMS mini: 6 days (IQR: 6–7 days)]. The pericardial effusion of any entity occurred more frequently in the SMS compared to the MRAT (18.8% vs. 2.6%, $p = 0.001$), although all were treated medically except for four cases in the SMS that required subxiphoid pericardial drainage before discharge. In 1 MRAT case, we observed, at pre-discharge echo, the presence of a para right atrial clot without hemodynamic impact that gradually resolved in the follow-up.

Table 3. Population demographic, operative and post-operative. Data expressed as median and (IQR). *p*-values calculated with Kruskal–Wallis test and, if significant, * Dunn's test with Bonferroni adjustment for differences among subgroups with significant difference only between MRAT vs. SMS.

Variable	MRAT (n = 78)	SMS (n = 116)	SMS Mini (n = 22)	Total	*p*-Value	MRAT vs. SMS *
Age (years)	5.0 (4)	9.5 (18.5)	6.5 (6)	6.1 (10)	0.0001	0.00009
Weight (kg)	18.3 (13)	30 (40)	23 (22)	22 (35)	0.0002	0.0001
Height (cm)	110 (24)	140 (54)	122 (40)	122 (52)	0.0001	0.00009
CPB time (min)	55 (23)	49 (32)	45.5 (20)	52 (28)	0.06	n.s.
Aortic cross-clamp (min)	27 (14)	29 (25)	24 (13)	27 (19)	0.6741	n.s.
Surgical Time (min)	190 (61)	170 (60)	170 (34)	178 (64)	0.0133	0.0062
ICU stay (days)	1 (0)	1 (0)	1 (0)	1 (0)	0.7265	n.s.
Hospital stay (days)	7 (1)	7 (4)	6 (1)	7 (3)	0.0036	0.0057
CPB lowest HTC (%)	28 (5)	29 (4)	29 (4)	28 (5)	0.0062	0.0027
CPB lowest temp (C)	34.6 (1)	34.2 (1.2)	34.0 (1.6)	34.3 (1)	0.8304	n.s.
CPB highest Lactate	1.1 (0.4)	1.0 (0.5)	1.1 (0.5)	1.1 (0.4)	0.995	n.s.

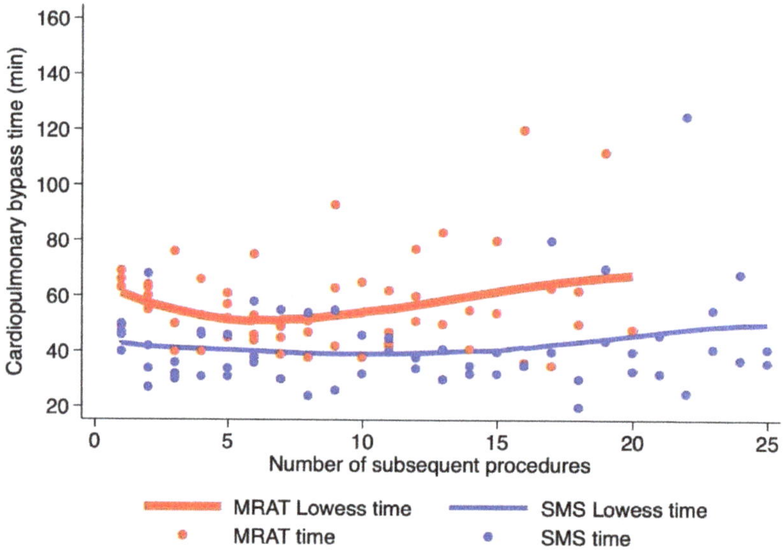

Figure 2. Time of cardiopulmonary bypass time according to the number of procedures starting from the first operation. MRAT (in red dot and line) vs. SMS (in blue dot and line). Lines represent Lowess cardiopulmonary bypass time for each approach (locally weighted scatterplot smoothing).

3.3. Echo at Discharge

A minimal, insignificant residual defect was observed in 10 cases (4.6%). After PAVPD double patch repair, five patients (SMS = 3, MRAT = 2) had isolated non-significant gradients (<5 mmHg) between the superior vena cava and right atrium and did not require any intervention during the follow-up. Trivial residual interatrial shunts on the ecodoppler were seen, pre-discharge, in four MRAT cases and were not appreciable at the first echocardiography follow-up. In one SMS mini case, a significant SVC to right atrium gradient was observed after the Warden operation for PAPVD that required balloon dilatation and did not require any further intervention.

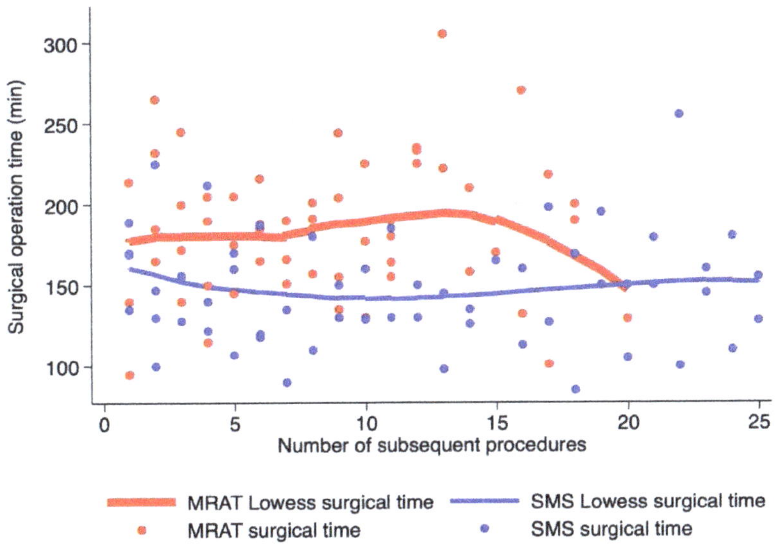

Figure 3. Time of surgical operation, determined as skin-to-skin time (min), according to the number of procedures starting from the first operation. MRAT (in red dot and line) vs. SMS (in blue dot and line). Lines represent Lowess surgical time for each approach.

The post-operative echocardiography showed a typical trend of repaired ASD and PAVPD with a reduced degree of RV dilatation (p-value > 0.001), improvement in the degree of TV regurgitation (p-value > 0.001), and reduced pulmonary artery pressure measurements (p-value > 0.001) (see Table 1). In particular, the right ventricle reduced in volume, with a significant reduction in the population with moderate-to-severe dilatation (from 89% to 44%) with a respective increase to the proportion of normal volumes (from 11% to 56%). The acute right ventricular volume reduction affected the function that was mildly reduced in 68% of the population. The tricuspid valve regurgitation was moderate in 11% of the population and decreased to 3% after repair. The improvement in echocardiographic parameters was significant and similar to all three approaches used (Table 1), suggesting equal efficacy in the surgical repair of the MRAT compared to SMS. All patients were discharged in good clinical condition, without significant intracardiac defects or extracardiac impairment; no significant surgical wound infections were observed.

4. Discussion

In recent years, interest in improving cosmetics and reducing the psychological implications of cardiac surgery has assumed increased importance, with particular attention paid to young patients [11,15]. As a result, a variety of minimally invasive surgical techniques have been developed for cardiac surgery in the pediatric population, including right mini-thoracotomy [12]. In the current era, the trans-catheter approach has evolved and gained more importance in ASD closure as a great alternative to surgery because of the short post-procedural recovery and the cosmetic outcomes [16,17]. Many recent studies have reported no mortality and a very low rate of major complications (<1% of patients) [18,19]. Recently, the device closure of ASD has become the first choice for the correction of ASDs, but the lack of an anatomical device landing border or the presence of other associated lesions may not allow percutaneous treatment. Minimally invasive techniques provide good repair results with an early return to normal daily activity and a physically and psychologically high-quality life after surgery [3,16]. Many studies showed that the minimally invasive approach is safe and represents a good option for correcting simple congenital heart defects, providing better cosmetic results and non-inferior clinical outcomes compared to the conventional approach to median sternotomy [7,8,15]. Although minimally invasive functional advantages are widely recognized, some of these approaches have limited indications in the pediatric field due to suboptimal cosmetic results (i.e., mini-sternotomy, right anterolateral thoracotomy). For example, in the long-term follow-up, the right anterolateral thoracotomy was associated with reduced volume in the right breast compared to median sternotomy. Therefore, right anterolateral thoracotomy has been limited only to adult female patients whose breasts have already developed [20,21].

The MRAT allows the concealment of the incision beneath the right arm and avoid the spares of the sternum. The lateralization of the incision offers other advantages because it does not involve the breast tissue, abolishes mammary gland lesions in prepubescent women, and prevents the impairment of breast development and chest wall deformities [22]. An efficient adoption of the MRAT requires a standardized program that reduces the learning curve, guarantees low morbidity, and maintains patient safety. For this reason, in 2017, we decided to start the MRAT program with the supervision and tutoring of an expert in the field to provide insights to achieve immediate good results and excellent safety. With this program, we were able to reduce learning curves at about 15 consecutive procedures per surgeon to reach the cardiopulmonary bypass and surgical operative times similar to median sternotomy. In terms of efficacy, despite being a newly started program, there were no major post-operative complications or major cases of morbidity compared to sternotomy or minimal sternotomy.

We conduct yearly follow-ups for patients with simple CHD, such as the ones treated in this study. Considering this, to assess the full advantage of the esthetical impacts on patients, we need to wait adolescents age, especially young females who still have not completed their breast development. So far, we have collected reports of parents' satisfaction that are all positive, although patient satisfaction can not be fully comprehended due to different factors, such as the patients' young ages and incomplete development in the majority of the population. In the future, we aim to conduct a questionnaire directed to patients to investigate satisfaction with the approach and the psychological impact of scarring below the arm or in the middle of the sternum. Finally, surgical repair of ASD, pAVSD, or PAPVD through MRAT allows safe repair of the defect with similar echocardiographic recovery of the heart compared to SMS. In particular, MRAT, similarly to SMS, guarantees post-surgical reduction of the right volume overload, reduces right ventricle dilatation, and guarantees similar atrioventricular valve improvement. Therefore, the MRAT is not only comparable to SMS in terms of surgical safety but is also comparable in terms of patient clinical and instrumental post-operative recovery. It is fundamental to note that, although such data were not collected directly, parents and patients expressed great satisfaction regarding the cosmetic results due to the fact that skin incisions were not immediately visible.

5. Conclusions

The surgical repair of simple congenital heart anomalies, such as atrial septal defects or partial anomalous pulmonary venous returns, can be achieved through minimal right axillary thoracotomies, which guarantee safety and efficacy without increasing surgical risk or the duration of surgery. Minimal right axillary thoracotomy preserves the sternum from surgical fractures and allows the concealment of surgical scars beneath the arm, preserving the patient's aesthetic qualities.

Author Contributions: M.L.R.: study design, formal analysis, writing—review and editing; Y.C.M.B. and M.M.: writing—original draft, data collection, and analysis; A.V., A.S. and M.R.: conceptualization, data curation; M.C.: supervision; T.A. and G.I.: conceptualization; A.G.: writing—review and editing, supervision. All authors have read and agreed to the published version of the manuscript.

Funding: This study was supported by the IRCCS Policlinico San Donato, a Clinical Research Hospital rec-ognized and partially supported by the Italian Ministry of Health.

Institutional Review Board Statement: The study was submitted to the Ethical Committee, and consent was waived due to the retrospective nature of the study.

Informed Consent Statement: Informed consent was waived due to the retrospective nature of the study.

Data Availability Statement: The raw data supporting the conclusions of this article will be made available in an online platform (Zenodo) and made available upon request.

Conflicts of Interest: The authors declare no conflict of interest.

References

1. RoseRosengart, T.K.; Stark, J.F. Repair of atrial septal defect through a right thoracotomy. *Ann. Thorac. Surg.* **1993**, *55*, 1138–1140. [CrossRef] [PubMed]
2. Hopkins, R.A.; Bert, A.A.; Buchholz, B.; Guarino, K.; Meyers, M. Surgical patch closure of atrial septal defects. *Ann. Thorac. Surg.* **2004**, *77*, 2144–2149. [CrossRef] [PubMed]
3. Yaliniz, H.; Topcuoglu, M.S.; Gocen, U.; Atalay, A.; Keklik, V.; Basturk, Y.; Gunes, Y.; Turktan, M.; Salih, O.K. Comparison between minimal right vertical infra-axillary thoracotomy and standard median sternotomy for repair of atrial septal defects. *Asian J. Surg.* **2015**, *38*, 199–204. [CrossRef]
4. Heinisch, P.P.; Wildbolz, M.; Beck, M.J.; Bartkevics, M.; Gahl, B.; Eberle, B.; Erdoes, G.; Jenni, H.-J.; Schoenhoff, F.; Pfammatter, J.-P.; et al. Vertical Right Axillary Mini-Thoracotomy for Correction of Ventricular Septal Defects and Complete Atrioventricular Septal Defects. *Ann. Thorac. Surg.* **2018**, *106*, 1220–1228. [CrossRef]
5. Dietl, C.A.; Torres, A.R.; Favaloro, R.G. Right submammarian thoracotomy in female patients with atrial septal defects and anomalous pulmonary venous connections. Comparison between the transpectoral and subpectoral approaches. *J. Thorac. Cardiovasc. Surg.* **1992**, *104*, 723–727. [CrossRef]
6. Yi, K.; Guo, X.; You, T.; Wang, Y.; Ding, F.; Hou, X.; Zhou, L. Standard median sternotomy, right minithoracotomy, totally thoracoscopic surgery, percutaneous closure, and transthoracic closure for atrial septal defects in children. *Medicine* **2019**, *98*, e17270. [CrossRef]
7. Vida, V.L.; Zanotto, L.; Zanotto, L.; Tessari, C.; Padalino, M.A.; Zanella, F.; Pittarello, D.; Stellin, G. Minimally invasive surgery for atrial septal defects: A 20-year experience at a single centre. *Interact. Cardiovasc. Thorac. Surg.* **2019**, *28*, 961–967. [CrossRef] [PubMed]
8. Luo, Z.-R.; Chen, Q.; Yu, L.-L.; Chen, L.-W.; Huang, Z.-Y. Comparative Study between Surgical Repair of Atrial Septal Defect via Median Sternotomy, Right Submammary Thoracotomy, and Right Vertical Infra-Axillary Thoracotomy. *Braz. J. Cardiovasc. Surg.* **2020**, *35*, 285–290. [CrossRef]
9. Nicholson, I.A.; Bichell, D.P.; Bacha, E.A.; del Nido, P.J. Minimal sternotomy approach for congenital heart operations. *Ann. Thorac. Surg.* **2001**, *71*, 469–472. [CrossRef]
10. Mishaly, D.; Ghosh, P.; Preisman, S. Minimally Invasive Congenital Cardiac Surgery Through Right Anterior Minithoracotomy Approach. *Ann. Thorac. Surg.* **2008**, *85*, 831–835. [CrossRef]
11. Yoshimura, N.; Yamaguchi, M.; Oshima, Y.; Oka, S.; Ootaki, Y.; Yoshida, M. Repair of atrial septal defect through a right posterolateral thoracotomy: A cosmetic approach for female patients. *Ann. Thorac. Surg.* **2001**, *72*, 2103–2105. [CrossRef]
12. Isik, O.; Ayik, M.F.; Akyuz, M.; Daylan, A.; Atay, Y. Right Anterolateral Thoracotomy in the Repair of Atrial Septal Defect: Effect on Breast Development. *J. Card. Surg.* **2015**, *30*, 714–718. [CrossRef]
13. Dave, H.H.; Comber, M.; Solinger, T.; Bettex, D.; Dodge-Khatami, A.; Prêtre, R. Mid-term results of right axillary incision for the repair of a wide range of congenital cardiac defects. *Eur. J. Cardiothorac. Surg.* **2009**, *35*, 864–869, discussion 869–870. [CrossRef]
14. Prêtre, R.; Kadner, A.; Dave, H.; Dodge-Khatami, A.; Bettex, D.; Berger, F. Right axillary incision: A cosmetically superior approach to repair a wide range of congenital cardiac defects. *J. Thorac. Cardiovasc. Surg.* **2005**, *130*, 277–281. [CrossRef] [PubMed]
15. Giamberti, A.; Mazzera, E.; Di Chiara, L.; Ferretti, E.; Pasquini, L.; Di Donato, R.M. Right submammary minithoracotomy for repair of congenital heart defects. *Eur. J. Cardiothorac. Surg.* **2000**, *18*, 678–682. [CrossRef]
16. Butera, G.; Romagnoli, E.; Saliba, Z.; Chessa, M.; Sangiorgi, G.; Giamberti, A.; Cappato, R.; Bussadori, C.; Abella, R.; Pelissero, G.; et al. Percutaneous closure of multiple defects of the atrial septum: Procedural results and long-term follow-up. *Catheter. Cardiovasc. Interv.* **2010**, *76*, 121–128. [CrossRef] [PubMed]
17. Butera, G.; Carminati, M.; Chessa, M.; Youssef, R.; Drago, M.; Giamberti, A.; Pomè, G.; Bossone, E.; Frigiola, A. Percutaneous versus surgical closure of secundum atrial septal defect: Comparison of early results and complications. *Am. Hear. J.* **2006**, *151*, 228–234. [CrossRef] [PubMed]
18. Fischer, G.; Stieh, J.; Uebing, A.; Hoffmann, U.; Morf, G.; Kramer, H.H. Experience with transcatheter closure of secundum atrial septal defects using the Amplatzer septal occluder: A single centre study in 236 consecutive patients. *Heart* **2003**, *89*, 199–204. [CrossRef]
19. Du, Z.-D.; Hijazi, Z.M.; Kleinman, C.S.; Silverman, N.H.; Larntz, K. Comparison between transcatheter and surgical closure of secundum atrial septal defect in children and adults: Results of a multicenter nonrandomized trial. *J. Am. Coll. Cardiol.* **2002**, *39*, 1836–1844. [CrossRef] [PubMed]
20. Bleiziffer, S.; Schreiber, C.; Burgkart, R.; Regenfelder, F.; Kostolny, M.; Libera, P.; Holper, K.; Lange, R. The influence of right anterolateral thoracotomy in prepubescent female patients on late breast development and on the incidence of scoliosis. *J. Thorac. Cardiovasc. Surg.* **2004**, *127*, 1474–1480. [CrossRef] [PubMed]

21. Mavroudis, C.; Backer, C.L.; Stewart, R.D.; Heraty, P. The case against minimally invasive cardiac surgery. *Semin. Thorac. Cardiovasc. Surg. Pediatr. Card. Surg. Annu.* **2005**, *8*, 193–197. [CrossRef] [PubMed]
22. Vida, V.L.; Padalino, M.A.; Motta, R.; Stellin, G. Minimally invasive surgical options in pediatric heart surgery. *Expert Rev. Cardiovasc. Ther.* **2011**, *9*, 763–769. [CrossRef] [PubMed]

Journal of
Cardiovascular
Development and Disease

MDPI

Article

Less (Transfusion) Is More—Enhancing Recovery through Implementation of Patient Blood Management in Cardiac Surgery: A Retrospective, Single-Centre Study of 1174 Patients

Mihai Ștefan [1,*], Dana Tomescu [2,3], Cornelia Predoi [1,2], Raluca Goicea [1,2], Mihai Perescu [1], Mihai Popescu [2,3], Dan Dorobanțu [4,5,6], Gabriela Droc [2,7], Ștefan Andrei [7,8], Ovidiu Știru [9,10], Șerban-Ion Bubenek Turconi [2,11] and Daniela Filipescu [1,2]

1 2nd Department of Anaesthesiology and Intensive Care, "Prof Dr CC Iliescu" Emergency Institute for Cardiovascular Diseases, 022322 Bucharest, Romania; cornelia-elena.florescu@drd.umfcd.ro (C.P.)
2 Discipline of Anaesthesiology and Intensive Care, "Carol Davila" University of Medicine and Pharmacy, 419291 Bucharest, Romania
3 3rd Department of Anaesthesiology and Intensive Care, Fundeni Clinical Institute, 022328 Bucharest, Romania
4 Children's Health and Exercise Research Center, University of Exeter, Exeter EX4 4QJ, UK
5 Faculty of Health Sciences, University of Bristol, Bristol BS8 1TH, UK
6 Congenital Heart Unit, Bristol Royal Hospital for Children and Heart Institute, Bristol BS2 8ED, UK
7 1st Department of Anaesthesiology and Intensive Care, Fundeni Clinical Institute, 022322 Bucharest, Romania
8 Department of Anaesthesiology and Critical Care Medicine, Dijon University Medical Centre, 21000 Dijon, France
9 Department of Cardiovascular Surgery, "Prof Dr CC Iliescu" Emergency Institute for Cardiovascular Diseases, 419291 Bucharest, Romania
10 Discipline of Cardiovascular Surgery, "Carol Davila" University of Medicine and Pharmacy, 419291 Bucharest, Romania
11 1st Department of Anaesthesiology and Intensive Care, "Prof Dr CC Iliescu" Emergency Institute for Cardiovascular Diseases, 022322 Bucharest, Romania
* Correspondence: mihai.steph@gmail.com

Abstract: Introduction: The implementation of Patient Blood Management (PBM) in cardiac surgery has been shown to be effective in reducing blood transfusions and associated complications, as well as improving patient outcomes. Despite the potential benefits of PBM in cardiac surgery, there are several barriers to its successful implementation. **Objectives:** The main objectives of this study were to ascertain the impact of the national Romanian PBM recommendations on allogeneic blood product transfusion in cardiac surgery and identify predictors of perioperative packed red blood cell transfusion. **Methods:** As part of the Romanian national pilot programme of PBM, we performed a single-centre, retrospective study in a tertiary centre of cardiovascular surgery, including patients from two time periods, before and after the implementation of the national recommendations. Using coarsened exact matching, from a total of 1174 patients, 157 patients from the before group were matched to 169 patients in the after group. Finally, we built a multivariate regression model from the entire cohort to analyse independent predictors of PRBC transfusion in the perioperative period. **Results:** Although there was a trend towards a lower proportion of patients requiring PRBC transfusion in the "after" group compared to the "before" group (44.9%vs. 50.3%), it was not statistically significant. There was a significant difference between the "after" group and the "before" group in terms of fresh-frozen plasma (FFP) transfusion rates, with a lower percentage of patients requiring FFP transfusion in the "after" group compared to "before" (14.2%, vs. 22.9%, $p = 0.04$). This difference was also seen in the total perioperative FFP transfusion (mean transfusion 0.7 units in the "before" group, SD 1.73 vs. 0.38 units in the "after" group, SD 1.05, $p = 0.04$). In the multivariate regression analysis, age > 64 years (OR 1.652, 95% CI 1.17–2.331, $p = 0.004$), female sex (OR 2.404, 95% CI 1.655–3.492, $p < 0.001$), surgery time (OR 1.295, 95% CI 1.126–1.488, $p < 0.001$), Hb < 13 g/dl (OR 3.611, 95% CI 2.528–5.158, $p < 0.001$), re-exploration for bleeding (OR 3.988, 95% CI 1.248–12.738, $p = 0.020$), viscoelastic test use (OR 2.18, 95% CI 1.34–3.544, $p < 0.001$), FFP transfusion (OR 4.023, 95% CI 2.426–6.671, $p < 0.001$), and use of a standardized pretransfusion checklist (OR

8.875, 95% CI 5.496–14.332, $p < 0.001$) remained significantly associated with PRBC transfusion. The use of a preoperative standardized haemostasis questionnaire was independently associated with a decreased risk of perioperative PRBC transfusion (0.565, 95% CI 0.371–0.861, $p = 0.008$). **Conclusions:** Implementation of national PBM recommendations led to a reduction in FFP transfusion in a cardiac surgery centre. The use of a preoperative standardized haemostasis questionnaire is an independent predictor of a lower risk for PRBC transfusion in this setting.

Keywords: transfusion; anaemia; cardiac surgery; patient blood management

1. Introduction

Cardiac surgery is a complex and high-risk procedure that often requires the use of blood products to replace blood loss and support the patient's cardiovascular system [1,2]. However, blood transfusions are not without risks, including transfusion reactions, infections, and immunological complications [3,4]. Additionally, transfusions can be costly and may not always be necessary [5,6].

PBM is a methodical and evidence-based approach that prioritizes the patient and aims to enhance their outcomes by safeguarding and utilizing their own blood. This approach also emphasizes patient safety and empowerment [7]. PBM is proactive, multidisciplinary, and multimodal, and it includes anaemia detection and treatment, haemostasis optimisation, blood loss minimisation, the rational use of blood products, and the optimisation of anaemia tolerance to strengthen and to preserve patients' own blood mass, to enable the safe handling of donor blood, and to improve the patient's outcome/prognosis [8,9].

The implementation of PBM in cardiac surgery has been shown to be effective in reducing blood transfusions and associated complications, as well as improving patient outcomes such as mortality, morbidity, and length of hospital stay [10]. However, the implementation of PBM requires a multidisciplinary approach and significant changes in clinical practice, which can be challenging.

Despite the potential benefits of implementing PBM in cardiac surgery, there are several barriers to its successful implementation [11,12]. Some of the most common include a lack of knowledge and awareness among healthcare providers, resistance to change, inadequate resources, and inadequate communication and collaboration among different healthcare disciplines [13]. In addition, there may be cultural and institutional barriers, as well as differences in local landscape, that can make it difficult to implement PBM programs and lead to significant variability [14,15]. Overcoming these barriers requires a concerted effort from all stakeholders, including hospital administrators, healthcare providers, and patients [16]. By addressing these challenges, PBM can be successfully implemented in cardiac surgery, leading to improved patient outcomes and reduced healthcare costs [17].

In Romania, a multidisciplinary initiative group endorsed by the Ministry of Health has developed national recommendations for PBM, aimed at improving patient outcomes and reducing the use of allogeneic blood transfusions, which are a precious but insufficient resource in the elective surgical setting [18,19]. The recommendations cover a range of areas, including the preoperative optimization of haemoglobin (Hb) levels and haemostasis, intraoperative haemostasis management and protocols, and postoperative monitoring and management of anaemia. They also emphasize the importance of individualizing transfusion decisions based on patient characteristics and clinical factors, rather than relying on fixed transfusion thresholds. The implementation of these recommendations has the potential to reduce the risks associated with blood transfusions, such as transfusion reactions and infections, while improving patient outcomes and optimizing the use of healthcare resources. Previous papers have been published as part of the programme [20,21].

The main objectives of this study were to ascertain the impact of the national PBM recommendations on allogeneic blood product transfusion and identify predictors of perioperative packed red blood cell (PRBC) transfusion in a tertiary care cardiac surgery academic centre.

2. Materials and Methods

2.1. Patient Population and Data Collection

As part of the Romanian national pilot programme of PBM [19], we performed a single-centre, retrospective study in a tertiary centre of cardiovascular surgery. Data were recorded using a pre-approved protocol, available in Supplementary Table S1.

We included consecutive patients who underwent non-emergent cardiac surgery with cardio-pulmonary bypass (CPB) during two distinct periods: 1 January 2017–30 June 2017 and 1 July 2018–31 December 2018, referred to as the "before" group, and 1 January 2020–31 December 2020, referred to as the "after" group, following the implementation of the Romanian PBM recommendations. These periods of data collection were selected as representing the periods before publishing the recommendations, right at the beginning of the implementation and one year after, respectively. Patients who underwent emergency surgery and those for whom research information could not be adequately collected (incomplete observation sheets) were excluded from the study.

The data were recorded according to the directives of the Order of the Minister of Health no. 1251 of 2018 and their statistical processing for publication was approved by the ethics and study approval committee of the Emergency Institute for Cardiovascular Diseases "Prof. Dr. C. C. Iliescu", Bucharest, nr. 15324/ 03.06.2021.

All data were recorded retrospectively, based on written observation sheets and electronic logs.

2.2. Clinical Management

The surgical procedure was performed under general anaesthesia with intravenous (iv) induction and volatile-based maintenance, utilizing sevoflurane. During CPB, total iv anaesthesia was administered using either propofol or midazolam, and analgesia was achieved through a fentanyl infusion. The CPB was conducted using crystalloid priming and cardioplegia, which involved either a 4:1 mix of blood and crystalloid or Custodiol solution, based on the surgeon's preference and the anticipated surgery duration. Heparin was administered before bypass at a dose of 350 units per kilogram of body weight and supplemented, if necessary, to achieve an activated clotting time above 480 s, and protamine was used to antagonize heparin at a ratio of 0.8 of the initial heparin doses. Cell saver and intraoperative hemofiltration were used only in complex cases, at the attending anaesthesiologist's discretion. Point-of-care viscoelastic haemostasis monitoring was available and primarily used in high-risk patients, utilizing rotation thromboelastometry (ROTEM) and an institutional bleeding management algorithm that included allogeneic blood products and factor concentrates. All patients received tranexamic acid prophylactically. The decision to administer PRBC transfusions was based on a restrictive-oriented approach, with Hb triggers of 7 g/dL during CPB and 8 g/dL during the rest of the perioperative period, while considering other factors such as patient characteristics, (mixed venous blood saturation of oxygen) SvO2, and lactate level. The recorded outcomes included the duration of surgery; hospital stay; surgical re-exploration due to bleeding; PRBC transfusion pre-, intra-, and postoperatively; the use of ROTEM and cell saver; and FFP and platelet (PLT) transfusion. Haemoglobin (Hb) values were recorded at four distinct time points: Hb1—at hospital admission, Hb 2—last Hb recorded preoperatively, Hb3—first Hb recorded postoperatively, and Hb4—at hospital discharge. Anaemia was defined as an Hb value < 13 g/dl, regardless of sex, for the analysis.

2.3. Statistical Analysis

Data analysis involved the use of Microsoft Excel® (Microsoft Corporation, Redmond, WA, USA), STATA® (StataCorp. 2021. Stata Statistical Software: Release 17. StataCorp LLC, College Station, TX, USA College Station, TX, USA), and Wizard 2 (Wizard–Statistics

& Analysis®, Raipur, Chattisgarh, India). A p-value < 0.05 was considered statistically significant a priori.

Quantitative data were expressed as medians with [25–75%] interquartile ranges (IQR). Normal distribution for continuous variables was evaluated by histograms and the Shapiro–Wilk test. Student's t-test or Mann–Whitney U-test were used as appropriate for comparisons of continuous variables. Qualitative data were expressed as numbers (percentages). Chi-square or Fisher's exact test was used to compare categorical variables, as appropriate.

To determine the impact of the adoption of the PBM recommendations on intrahospital transfusion, we performed a coarsened exact matching between patients in the "before" group and those in the "after" group, using age, sex, hospital length of stay (LOS), ICU LOS, the type of surgery, surgery time, preoperative anaemia, preoperative Hb, and the use of ROTEM and cell saver as co-variates and compared the selected cohorts with appropriate statistical tests, as above.

To investigate the association between perioperative variables and transfusion risk, we built a multivariable logistic regression model, using the perioperative transfusion requirement as the dependent variable, and predictors selected by univariate analysis with a p-value less than 0.05.

3. Results

This is a before and after study in a non-emergent cardiac surgery population that compared two cohorts, one before the implementation of the PBM national guidelines and the other after. The cohorts have been matched using coarsened exact matching. The study flowchart is available in Figure 1. In total, 710 patients were included in the before group and 464 in the after group. After performing the coarsened exact matching, 157 patients from the before group were matched to 169 patients in the after group.

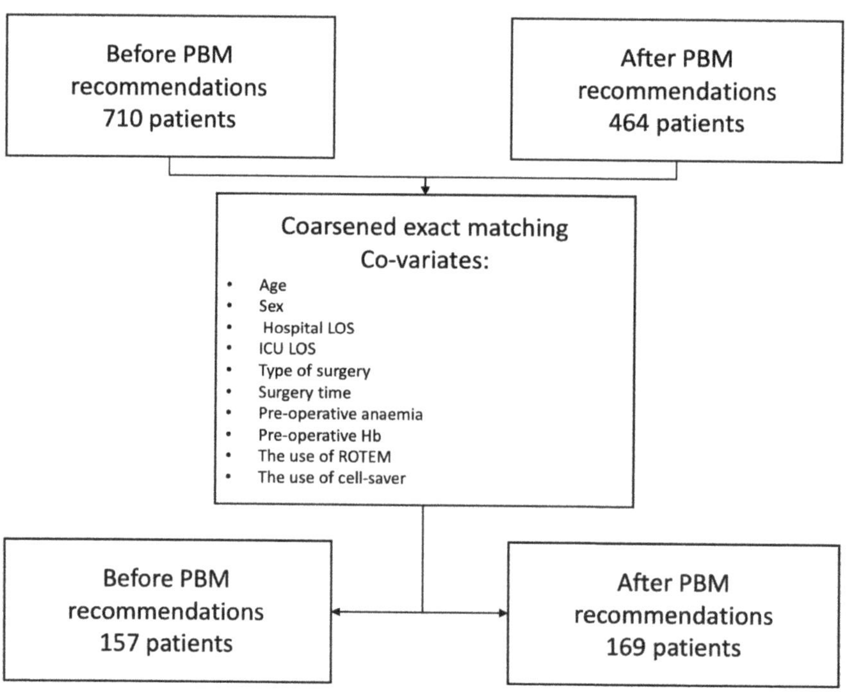

Figure 1. Study flowchart.

Demographic Characteristics and Outcomes

Before matching, there were 710 patients in the "before" group and 464 patients in the "after" group, who had a median age of 64 years (IQR 58–69 vs. 56–69, $p = 0.643$) and were predominantly male (66.1% vs. 65.9%, $p = 0.970$).

Table 1 shows the types of surgeries performed in each time period.

Table 1. Types of surgeries performed in each analysed period.

Type of Surgery	Before (Number and Percentage)	After (Number and Percentage)
CABG	252 (35.5%)	171 (36.9%)
One valve replacement/repair	256 (36.1%)	144 (31%)
Two or more valves replacement/repair	59 (8.3%)	42 (9.1%)
Valve(s) and CABG	69 (9.7%)	52 (11.4%)
Surgery on thoracic aorta	44 (6.2%)	32 (6.9%)
Other	29 (4.1%)	23 (4.9%)

Legend: CABG—coronary artery bypass grafting.

The perioperative co-variates used in the model are available in Table 2. The only statistical differences found between the groups after matching are lower ICU LOS in the "before" group compared to "after" (2 days, IQR 2–3 vs. 3 days, IQR 3–3), and a higher Hb 2 in the "before" group compared to "after" (13.6 g/d, IQR 12.6–14.5, vs. 13.2, IQR 12.1–14.2). There were no significant differences between groups in regard to age, sex, hospital LOS, surgery time, prevalence of preoperative anaemia, Hb1, or the use of ROTEM or cell saver.

Table 2. Perioperative outcomes used as co-variates in the coarsened exact matching model.

Variable	Before	After	$p =$	Matched Before	Matched After	$p =$
Number	710	464		157	169	
Age	64 (58–69)	64 (56–69)	0.643	66 (60–69)	65 (59–69)	0.504
Sex (M)	469 (66.1%)	306 (65.9%)	0.970	111 (70.7%)	117 (69.2%)	0.772
Hospital LOS (days)	13 (10–16)	14 (11–18)	0.037	12 (9–15)	12 (10–15)	0.412
ICU LOS (days)	2 (2–4)	3 (3–4)	<0.001	2 (2–3)	3 (3–3)	<0.001
Surgical re-exploration n (%)	45 (6.3%)	53 (11.4%)	0.002	0	0	
Surgery time (mins)	270 (220–330)	245 (210–290)	<0.001	240 (210–300)	245 (210–280)	0.987
Hb < 13 g/dl	288 (40.5%)	183 (39.4%)	0.701	49 (31.1%)	55 (32.5%)	0.796
Hb1 (g/dl)	13.4 (12.3–14.4)	13.4 (12.3–14.3)	0.863	13.6 (12.6–14.5)	13.6 (12.7–14.5)	0.844
Hb2 (g/dl)	13.3 (12.2–14.4)	13 (11.7–14.1)	<0.001	13.6 (12.6–14.5)	13.2 (12.1–14.2)	0.004
ROTEM use n (%)	123 (17.3%)	98 (21.5%)	0.822	6 (3.8%)	7 (4.1%)	0.883
Cell saver n (%)	7 (1.2%)	7 (1.5%)	0.657	0	0	

Legend: LOS—length of stay, ICU—intensive care unit, Hb—haemoglobin, ROTEM—rotational thromboelastometry.

Perioperative transfusion outcomes, as well as the implementation of specific guideline measures, such as the standardized preoperative haemostasis questionnaire (Supplementary Figure S1) and the standardized pretransfusion checklist (Supplementary Figure S2), are presented in Table 3.

Although there was a trend towards a lower proportion of patients requiring PRBC transfusion in the "after" group (44.9% vs. 50.3%), it was not statistically significant. Similarly, there was no significant difference between the groups in terms of perioperative PRBC units transfused (1 vs. 0 units per patient, $p = 0.424$). The findings reveal that in the "after" group, there was a decrease in median Hb levels compared to the "before" group, both at point 3–10.1 g/dl (IQR 9.1–11.1) vs. 9.4 (IQR 8.7–10.1) and at point 4–9.8 g/dl (IQR 9.2–10.7) vs. 9.3 g/dl (IQR 8.5–9.9).

Table 3. Perioperative study outcomes.

Variable	Before	After	*p* =	Matched Before	Matched After	*p* =
PRBC transfusion, n patients (%)	369 (52%)	266 (57.3%)	0.072	79 (50.3%)	78 (44.9%)	0.334
Perioperative PRBC transfusion (units, medians, and IQR)	1 (0–2)	1 (0–3)	0.009	1 (0–2)	0 (0–1)	0.424
Perioperative PRBC transfusion (units, means, and SD)	1.39 (2.26)	2.04 (3.88)	<0.001	0.94 (1.32	0.89 (1.32)	0.705
Intraoperative PRBC transfusion (units, medians, and IQR)	0 (0–1)	0 (0–1)	0.802	0 (0–1)	0 (0–1)	0.283
Intraoperative PRBC transfusion (units, means, and SD)	0.84 (1.46)	0.82 (1.46)	0.797	0.6 (1.01)	0.47 (0.85)	0.190
Postoperative PRBC transfusion (units, medians, and IQR)	0 (0–1)	0 (0–1)	0.021	0 (0–1)	0 (0–1)	0.960
Postoperative PRBC transfusion (units, means, and SD)	0.67 (1.56)	1.2 (3.4)	<0.001	0.36 (0.64)	0.41 (0.8)	0.529
Hb3 (g/dl)	9.9 (8.9–10.8)	9.3 (8.6–10.2)	<0.001	10.1 (9.1–11.1)	9.4 (8.7–10.1)	<0.001
Hb4 (g/dl)	9.7 (9–10.6)	9.2 (8.5–9.9)	<0.001	9.8 (9.2–10.7)	9.3 (8.5–9.9)	<0.001
Perioperative FFP transfusion (units, medians, and IQR)	0 (0–2)	0 (0–2)	0.348	0 (0–0)	0 (0–0)	0.04
Perioperative FFP transfusion (units, means, and SD)	1.02 (2.34)	1.83 (5.27)	<0.001	0.7 (1.73)	0.38 (1.05)	0.04
Intraoperative FFP transfusion (units, medians, and IQR)	0 (0–0)	0 (0–0)	0.387	0 (0–0)	0 (0–0)	0.004
Intraoperative FFP transfusion (units, means, and SD)	0.76 (1.7)	0.77 (1.92)	0.933	0.59 (1.31)	0.23 (0.79)	0.003
Postoperative FFP transfusion (units, medians, and IQR)	0 (0–0)	0 (0–0)	0.002	0 (0–0)	0 (0–0)	0.481
Postoperative FFP transfusion (units, means, and SD)	0.29 (1.23)	1.05 (4.38)	<0.001	0.11 (0.73)	0.15 (0.74)	0.591
PLT transfusion, n patients (%)	65 (9.3%)	40 (8,6%)	0.748	10 (6.3%)	6 (3.5%)	0.239
Preoperative anaesthetic consultation (days before surgery, median with IQR)	1 (1–1)	1 (0–1)	<0.001	1 (1–1)	1 (1–1)	0.005
Preoperative anaesthetic consultation (days before surgery, mean, SD)	1.32	0.96	<0.001	1.3 (1.4)	0.9 (0.7)	0.002
Standardised haemostasis questionnaire, n patients (%)	72 (10.14%)	332 (71.8%)	<0.001	19 (12.1%)	128 (75.7%)	<0.001
Standardized pretransfusion checklist, n patients (%)	0	301 (65.1%)		0	93 (55%)	

Legend: PRBC—packed red blood cells, FFP—fresh-frozen plasma, PLT—platelets.

There was a significant difference between the "after" group and the "before" group in terms of FFP transfusion rates, with a lower percentage of patients requiring FFP transfusion in the "after" group (14.2%, vs. 22.9%, $p = 0.04$). This difference was also seen in the total number of perioperative FFP units transfused (mean transfusion 0.7 units, SD 1.73 vs. 0.38 units, SD 1.05, $p = 0.04$) and intraoperative FFP transfusion (mean transfusion 0.59 units, SD 1.31, vs. 0.23 units, SD 0.79, $p = 0.003$).

The interval between the preoperative anaesthetic consultation and surgery was statistically different between the groups, but the clinical significance was negligible (median 1 day in both groups, $p = 0.005$, mean 1.3 days, SD 1.4 vs. 0.9 days, SD 0.7, $p = 0.002$).

There was an increase in the utilization of the standardized haemostatic questionnaire, with 75.7% of patients in the "after" group compared to 12.1% of patients in the "before" group ($p < 0.001$).

The standardised pretransfusion checklist was only used in the "after" period.

PLT transfusion rate was not statistically different between the two groups, 6.3% vs. 3.5%, $p = 0.239$.

In the univariate analysis (Table 4), we selected age >64 years (OR 2.31, 95% CI 1.825–2.922, $p < 0.001$), female sex (OR 2.645, 95% CI 2.048–3.415, $p < 0.001$), hospital LOS (OR 1.037, 95% CI 1.021–1.054, $p < 0.001$), ICU LOS (OR 1.168, 95% CI 1.097–1.243, $p < 0.001$), surgery time (OR 1.348, 95% CI 1.219–1.489, $p < 0.001$), Hb < 13 g/dl (OR 4.315, 95% CI 3.34–5.576, $p < 0.001$), re-exploration for bleeding (OR 6.879, 95% CI 3.717–12.733, $p < 0.001$), ROTEM use (OR 4.401, 95% CI 3.053–6.344, $p < 0.001$), FFP transfusion (OR 7.898, 95% CI 5.601–11.135, $p < 0.001$), PLT transfusion (OR 3.32, 95% CI 2.059–5.354, $p < 0.001$), and use of a standardized pretransfusion checklist (OR 8.151, 95% CI 5.73–11.596, $p < 0.001$), which were significantly associated with PRBC transfusion, while the use of a standardized haemostasis questionnaire was inversely associated with PRBC transfusion (OR 0.766, 95% CI 0.6–0.976, $p = 0.031$).

Table 4. Univariate and multivariate analyses of the association between perioperative variables and transfusion risk.

Variables	*Univariate*		*Multivariate*	
	OR (95% CI)	***p***	**OR (95% CI)**	***p***
Age > 64 years	2.31 (1.825–2.922)	<0.001	1.652 (1.17–2.331)	0.004
Female sex	2.645 (2.048–3.415)	<0.001	2.404 (1.655–3.492)	<0.001
Hospital LOS (days)	1.037 (1.021–1.054)	<0.001	1.02 (0.994–1.047)	0.138
ICU LOS (days)	1.168 (1.097–1.243)	<0.001	1.065 (0.995–1.14)	0.067
Surgery time (hours)	1.348 (1.219–1.489)	<0.001	1.295 (1.126–1.488)	<0.001
Hb < 13 g/dl	4.315 (3.34–5.576)	<0.001	3.611 (2.528–5.158)	<0.001
Re-exploration for bleeding	6.879 (3.717–12.733)	<0.001	3.988 (1.248–12.738)	0.020
ROTEM use	4.401 (3.053–6.344)	<0.001	2.18 (1.34–3.544)	<0.001
FFP transfusion	7.898 (5.601–11.135)	<0.001	4.023 (2.426–6.671)	<0.001
PLT transfusion	3.32 (2.059–5.354)	<0.001	0.951 (0.478–1.892)	0.887
Standardised haemostasis questionnaire use	0.766 (0.6–0.976)	0.031	0.565 (0.371–0.861)	0.008
Standardized pretransfusion checklist use	8.151 (5.73–11.596)	<0.001	8.875 (5.496–14.332)	<0.001

Using these variables as predictors and perioperative transfusion as the dependent variable, we built a multivariate model, and logistic regression analysis showed that age > 64 years (OR 1.652, 95% CI 1.17–2.331, $p = 0.004$), female sex (OR 2.404, 95% CI 1.655–3.492, $p < 0.001$), surgery time (OR 1.295, 95% CI 1.126–1.488, $p < 0.001$), Hb < 13 g/dl (OR 3.611, 95% CI 2.528–5.158, $p < 0.001$), re-exploration for bleeding (OR 3.988, 95% CI 1.248–12.738, $p = 0.020$), ROTEM use (OR 2.18, 95% CI 1.34–3.544, $p < 0.001$), FFP transfusion (OR 4.023, 95% CI 2.426–6.671, $p < 0.001$), and standardized pretransfusion checklist use (OR 8.875, 95% CI 5.496–14.332, $p < 0.001$) remained significantly associated with PRBC transfusion. The use of a preoperative standardized haemostasis questionnaire was independently associated with a decreased risk of perioperative PRBC transfusion (0.565, 95% CI 0.371–0.861, $p = 0.008$).

4. Discussion

In this before and after retrospective study, we showed that the implementation of the PBM national recommendations in a cardiac surgery population led to a decrease in FFP transfusion rates and an increase in the utilization of the standardized haemostatic questionnaire, with no significant difference in perioperative PRBC and PLT transfusion rates.

There was a predictable decrease in Hb concentration throughout hospital stay in both cohorts. This decrease in Hb has been previously shown in other trials in cardiac surgery and is arguably pluri-factorial, due to blood loss, inflammation, and haemodilution [20,22]. Although there was a trend towards a lower proportion of patients requiring PRBC transfusion in the "after" group, this difference was not statistically significant. It is possible that the sample size was not large enough to detect a significant difference, or that other unmeasured factors influenced the results. This finding is atypical in comparison to other results from the literature, where transfusion is reduced after the implementation of PBM measures, despite controversial results regarding other outcomes [23]. This can be explained by a significant barrier to implementation identified in our cohort, which is the short time between the pre-anaesthetic visit and surgery, which was, on average, 1.3 days (SD 1.4) in the "before" group, vs. 0.9 days (SD 0.7) in the "after" group. This is a particularity of the medical system of the country, where there is no systematic ambulatory pre-anaesthetic evaluation with sufficient time before elective surgery. This proves to be a significant barrier to the implementation of preoperative treatment for anaemia, in the absence of a functional pre-hospital care. Furthermore, the worsening during the "after" period is explained by the beginning of the pandemic in 2020 and the associated pressure of minimizing the contact between the patient and the medical system.

Notably, there is a high PRBC transfusion rate in both groups. However, previous studies of large cohorts have reported a large variability in transfusion practice in national and international registries, ranging from 22 to 67% of patients being transfused with at least one unit of PRBC [24,25]. This is not ideal, but these are real-world data from a country where allogeneic blood is not paid for by hospitals, so the incentives to reduce transfusion rates come from scientific societies and practice guidelines, sometimes at odds with hospital administrators, who, at first, pay more for blood conservation measures.

Postoperative Hb was lower in the after group, both in the immediate postoperative period as well as at hospital discharge. This suggests a better compliance of physicians with the rational use of PRBC and adherence to a restrictive transfusion protocol. This approach is supported by several studies in the literature and has been shown to be non-inferior in terms of perioperative outcome in cardiac surgery [26–28] and is endorsed by recent guidelines [29].

Although the numerical reduction in PRBC transfusion after matching is not significant, we interpret the results as an encouragement to further add measures in the implemented PBM armamentarium, such as the treatment of anaemia before surgery and the systematic use of cell saver. Future data and regular benchmarking will be necessary to validate this hypothesis.

Fresh-frozen plasma transfusion is a common intervention in cardiac surgery and can lead to significant morbidity, as each unit has a cumulative detrimental effect on perioperative outcomes [30,31]. Therefore, any reduction in FFP transfusion rates is clinically relevant, as it can lead to improved patient outcomes and reduced healthcare costs. The reduction in FFP transfusion rates seen in this study is consistent with previous studies that have reported a decrease in blood product utilization following the implementation of PBM [32]. The decrease in FFP transfusion in the matched cohorts is potentially attributable to more evidence-based transfusion practice, as well as better access to single-factor concentrates (fibrinogen and prothrombin complex concentrates—PCC). This has not been recorded and is a limitation in our study.

PLT was not different between the two groups, but it is to be noted that there is a very low PLT transfusion rate in both groups. This is explainable by the frequent blood product shortage in a system where donation is voluntary, but remains very low, compared to other healthcare systems in Europe [33].

The increase in the utilization of the standardized haemostatic questionnaire is also noteworthy, as it suggests that the implementation of PBM guidelines can lead to changes in clinical practice and improved adherence to evidence-based protocols. The use of standardized questionnaires and checklists has been shown to improve patient safety and reduce medical errors in other areas of anaesthesiology [34]. Our study provides further evidence of their effectiveness in the context of blood management.

The use of a standardized haemostatic questionnaire is independently associated with a reduction in PRBC use in the multivariate regression model. This suggests that, had there been a better uptake of the questionnaire (the implementation was for only 75.7% of patients), it is likely to have led to a reduction in PRBC transfusion in the matched "after" cohort. The result is coherent with the aim of the questionnaire [19], which not only triages patients with a potentially undetected bleeding disorder, but also signals to the physician to adequately adjust or discuss with the multidisciplinary team the management of antiplatelet and anticoagulant agents. In other published data, various risk scores and questionnaires have performed differently in cardiac surgery, so there is no consensus on the best risk assessment score [35].

The positive predictors of transfusion identified in the multivariable analysis confirm our previous study [20].

Age > 64 years was an independent predictor of PRBC transfusion, and this may be explained by the perceived lower tolerance to anaemia of elderly patients, due to expected additional co-morbidities in elderly, frail patients. However, recent data suggest that restrictive transfusion in elderly patients could lead to better outcomes [28].

Female sex was a strong predictor of perioperative PRBC transfusion. This is explained by the smaller blood volume in females and consequently greater haemodilution during CPB. This has been previously reported in other, larger cohorts, where it could have also been linked to the different definition of anaemia between sexes according to the World Health Organization (WHO) [36–38].

However, we used a uniform definition of anaemia in this cohort, of Hb < 13 g/dl, irrespective of sex, as recommended by recent consensus papers and expert reviews [39]. Using this definition, preoperative anaemia was still a strong independent predictor of perioperative PRBC transfusion, adding to the data which suggest that the WHO classification might be obsolete.

Fresh-frozen plasma transfusion was independently associated with PRBC transfusion, which seems counterintuitive as our institution does not have a fixed-ration transfusion protocol but rather includes FFP and a staged algorithm as an alternative to PCC in the institutional protocol for the management of acute haemorrhage (Supplementary Figure S3). This association of FFP with PRBC transfusion confirms the previous paper from our group [20], and could be related to the non-compliance with guidelines but also potential residual confounders in our analysis.

This study has several limitations. Firstly, it is a retrospective study which uses observational data, and the possibility of residual confounding despite the use of coarsened exact matching remains. Additionally, the study was conducted in a single centre, which may limit the generalizability of the results. Furthermore, the Romanian PBM recommendations were followed in collecting data, but are not specific to cardiac surgery. Additionally, since the systematic treatment of preoperative anaemia was not yet in place at our institution and was rather anecdotal, data on this aspect were considered not pertinent for our analysis. Finally, most of the patients included in the analysis from the year 2020 were operated on after March 11, when the WHO declared the COVID-19 health crisis as a pandemic, which altered patient management hospital logistics worldwide. This is why, when building the matching model, we included hospital and ICU LOS as potential confounders, and not as outcomes.

5. Conclusions

Our before and after study provides further evidence of the effectiveness of PBM l recommendations in reducing blood product utilization and improving adherence to evidence-based protocols in the context of cardiac surgery. Implementing national PBM recommendations was associated with a reduction in FFP transfusion after coarsened exact matching. The adherence to a standardized preoperative bleeding risk questionnaire was independently associated with less PRBC transfusion. Age > 64 years, female sex, FFP transfusion, preoperative anaemia, surgery time, re-exploration for bleeding, ROTEM use, and standardized pretransfusion checklist use were independently associated with PRBC transfusion. Future studies with larger sample sizes and randomized designs are needed to further evaluate the impact of PBM programs on patient outcomes.

Supplementary Materials: The following supporting information can be downloaded at: https://www.mdpi.com/article/10.3390/jcdd10070266/s1, Figure S1: Standardized pre-operative haemostasis questionnaire, Figure S2: Standardized pre-transfusion checklist, Figure S3: Bleeding management standardized procedure, Table S1: PBM report form.

Author Contributions: Conceptualization, M.Ș., C.P. and D.F.; Methodology, M.Ș., D.T., R.G., M.P. (Mihai Perescu), M.P. (Mihai Popescu) and Ș.-I.B.T.; Software, D.F.; Validation, M.Ș., D.T., C.P., R.G., M.P. (Mihai Popescu), D.D., G.D., Ș.A., O.Ș. and Ș.-I.B.T.; Formal analysis, M.Ș., D.D., Ș.A. and D.F.; Investigation, M.Ș. and D.T.; Resources, O.Ș. and D.F.; Data curation, M.Ș. and M.P. (Mihai Perescu); Writing—original draft, M.Ș. and D.F.; Writing—review & editing, M.Ș., D.T., C.P., R.G., M.P. (Mihai Perescu), M.P. (Mihai Popescu), D.D., G.D., Ș.A., O.Ș., Ș.-I.B.T. and D.F.; Visualization, M.Ș., R.G., M.P. (Mihai Popescu), G.D., O.Ș. and Ș.-I.B.T.; Supervision, M.Ș. and D.F.; Project administration, M.Ș. and D.F. All authors have read and agreed to the published version of the manuscript.

Funding: This research received no external funding.

Institutional Review Board Statement: The study was conducted according to the guidelines of the Declaration of Helsinki and approved by the Institutional Review Board.

Informed Consent Statement: Patient consent was waived due to the retrospective, non-interventional nature of the study, as well as the legal obligation of data gathering as per the Order of the Romanian Ministry of Health, number 1251/2018.

Data Availability Statement: Restrictions apply to the availability of these data. The data presented in this study are available on reasonable request from the corresponding author.

Conflicts of Interest: The authors declare no conflict of interest.

References

1. Gombotz, H.; Rehak, P.H.; Shander, A.; Hofmann, A. The second Austrian benchmark study for blood use in elective surgery: Results and practice change: The Second Austrian Benchmark Study. *Transfusion* **2014**, *54*, 2646–2657. [CrossRef]
2. Bennett-Guerrero, E.; Zhao, Y.; O'Brien, S.M.; Jr, T.B.F.; Peterson, E.D.; Gammie, J.S.; Song, H.K. Variation in Use of Blood Transfusion in Coronary Artery Bypass Graft Surgery. *JAMA* **2010**, *304*, 1568–1575. [CrossRef]
3. Mazzeffi, M.A.; Holmes, S.; Taylor, B.; Ghoreishi, M.; McNeil, J.; Kertai, M.; Bollen, B.; Tanaka, K.; Raphael, J.; Glance, L. Red Blood Cell Transfusion and Postoperative Infection in Patients Having Coronary Artery Bypass Grafting Surgery: An Analysis of the Society of Thoracic Surgeons Adult Cardiac Surgery Database. *Anesth. Analg.* **2022**, *135*, 558–566. [CrossRef] [PubMed]
4. Tauriainen, T.; Kinnunen, E.-M.; Laitinen, I.; Anttila, V.; Kiviniemi, T.; Airaksinen, J.K.E.; Biancari, F. Transfusion and blood stream infections after coronary surgery. *Interact. Cardiovasc. Thorac. Surg.* **2018**, *26*, 325–327. [CrossRef]
5. Cataife, G.; Pagano, M.B. How much does a blood transfusion cost?: EDITORIAL. *Transfusion* **2018**, *58*, 833–835. [CrossRef]
6. Stokes, M.E.; Ye, X.; Shah, M.; Mercaldi, K.; Reynolds, M.W.; Rupnow, M.F.; Hammond, J. Impact of bleeding-related complications and/or blood product transfusions on hospital costs in inpatient surgical patients. *BMC Health Serv. Res.* **2011**, *11*, 135. [CrossRef] [PubMed]
7. Shander, A.; Hardy, J.-F.; Ozawa, S.; Farmer, S.L.; Hofmann, A.; Frank, S.M.; Kor, D.J.; Faraoni, D.; Freedman, J. Collaborators A Global Definition of Patient Blood Management. *Anesth. Analg.* **2022**, *135*, 476–488. [CrossRef] [PubMed]
8. Tibi, P.; McClure, R.S.; Huang, J.; Baker, R.A.; Fitzgerald, D.; Mazer, C.D.; Stone, M.; Chu, D.; Stammers, A.H.; Dickinson, T.; et al. STS/SCA/AmSECT/SABM Update to the Clinical Practice Guidelines on Patient Blood Management. *Ann. Thorac. Surg.* **2021**, *112*, 981–1004. [CrossRef] [PubMed]
9. Boer, C.; Meesters, M.I.; Milojevic, M.; Benedetto, U.; Bolliger, D.; Von Heymann, C.; Jeppsson, A.; Koster, A.; Osnabrugge, R.L.; Ranucci, M.; et al. 2017 EACTS/EACTA Guidelines on patient blood management for adult cardiac surgery. *J. Cardiothorac. Vasc. Anesth.* **2018**, *32*, 88–120. [CrossRef]
10. Dhir, A.; Tempe, D.K. Anemia and Patient Blood Management in Cardiac Surgery—Literature Review and Current Evidence. *J. Cardiothorac. Vasc. Anesth.* **2018**, *32*, 2726–2742. [CrossRef]
11. Baron, D.M.; Metnitz, P.G.H.; Fellinger, T.; Metnitz, B.; Rhodes, A.; Kozek-Langenecker, S.A. Evaluation of clinical practice in perioperative patient blood management. *Br. J. Anaesth.* **2016**, *117*, 610–616. [CrossRef]

12. Hofmann, A.; Spahn, D.R.; Holtorf, A.-P.; PBM Implementation Group; Isbister, J.; Hamdorf, J.; Campbell, L.; Benites, B.; Duarte, G.; Rabello, G.; et al. Making patient blood management the new norm(al) as experienced by implementors in diverse countries. *BMC Health Serv. Res.* **2021**, *21*, 634. [CrossRef]
13. Rancati, V.; Scala, E.; Ltaief, Z.; Gunga, M.Z.; Kirsch, M.; Rosner, L.; Marcucci, C. Challenges in Patient Blood Management for Cardiac Surgery: A Narrative Review. *J. Clin. Med.* **2021**, *10*, 2454. [CrossRef] [PubMed]
14. Klein, A.; Agarwal, S.; Cholley, B.; Fassl, J.; Griffin, M.; Kaakinen, T.; Mzallassi, Z.; Paulus, P.; Rex, S.; Siegemund, M.; et al. A survey of patient blood management for patients undergoing cardiac surgery in nine European countries. *J. Clin. Anesth.* **2021**, *72*, 110311. [CrossRef] [PubMed]
15. Van Der Linden, P.; Hardy, J.-F. Implementation of patient blood management remains extremely variable in Europe and Canada: The NATA benchmark project An observational study. *Eur. J. Anaesthesiol.* **2016**, *33*, 913–921. [CrossRef]
16. World Health Organization. *The Urgent Need to Implement Patient Blood Management: Policy Brief*; World Health Organization: Geneva, Switzerland, 2021. Available online: https://apps.who.int/iris/handle/10665/346655 (accessed on 27 April 2023).
17. Blaudszun, G.; Butchart, A.; Klein, A.A. Blood conservation in cardiac surgery. *Transfus. Med.* **2017**, *28*, 168–180. [CrossRef] [PubMed]
18. *Order of the Romanian Ministry of Health, no 1251/2018 for the Approval of the Guideline for Patient Blood Management during the Peri-Operative Period*; published in the Official Gazette of Romania no 877; Romanian Ministry of Health: Bucharest, Romania, 2018.
19. Filipescu, D.; Banateanu, R.; Beuran, M.; Burcos, T.; Corneci, D.; Cristian, D.; Diculescu, M.; Dobrota, A.; Droc, G.; Isacoff, D.; et al. Perioperative Patient Blood Management Programme. Multidisciplinary recommendations from the Patient Blood Management Initiative Group. *Rom. J. Anaesth. Intensive Care* **2017**, *24*, 139–157. [CrossRef] [PubMed]
20. Stefan, M.; Lupu, A.R.; Andrei, Ș.; Văleanu, L.; Știru, O.; Robu, C.; Bute, T.; Moroșanu, B.; Dumitrescu, A.; Stegaru, A.; et al. Perioperative trajectory of haemoglobin, predictors of blood transfusion and tailoring targets for patient blood management interventions: A single-centre, retrospective study of non-emergent cardiac surgery patients. *Rom. J. Anaesth. Intensive Care* **2022**, *28*, 47–56. [CrossRef]
21. Ristescu, I.; Pintilie, G.; Filip, D.; Jitca, M.; Fecheta, R.; Florescu, I.; Scripcariu, V.; Filipescu, D.; Grigoraş, I. Perioperative Anemia and Transfusion in Colorectal Cancer Patients. *Chirurgia* **2019**, *114*, 234. [CrossRef]
22. Ranucci, M.; Conti, D.; Castelvecchio, S.; Menicanti, L.; Frigiola, A.; Ballotta, A.; Pelissero, G. Hematocrit on Cardiopulmonary Bypass and Outcome After Coronary Surgery in Nontransfused Patients. *Ann. Thorac. Surg.* **2010**, *89*, 11–17. [CrossRef]
23. Roman, M.A.; Abbasciano, R.G.; Pathak, S.; Oo, S.; Yusoff, S.; Wozniak, M.; Qureshi, S.; Lai, F.Y.; Kumar, T.; Richards, T.; et al. Patient blood management interventions do not lead to important clinical benefits or cost-effectiveness for major surgery: A network meta-analysis. *Br. J. Anaesth.* **2021**, *126*, 149–156. [CrossRef] [PubMed]
24. Snyder-Ramos, S.A.; Mhnle, P.; Weng, Y.-S.; Bttiger, B.W.; Kulier, A.; Levin, J.; Mangano, D.T. Investigators of the Multicenter Study of Perioperative Ischemia; MCSPI Research Group The ongoing variability in blood transfusion practices in cardiac surgery. *Transfusion* **2008**, *48*, 1284–1299. [CrossRef] [PubMed]
25. McQuilten, Z.K.; Andrianopoulos, N.; Wood, E.M.; Cole-Sinclair, M.F.; McNeil, J.J.; Cameron, P.A.; Reid, C.M.; Newcomb, A.E.; Smith, J.A.; Phillips, L.E. Transfusion practice varies widely in cardiac surgery: Results from a national registry. *J. Thorac. Cardiovasc. Surg.* **2014**, *147*, 1684–1690.e1. [CrossRef] [PubMed]
26. Shehata, N.; Mistry, N.; Da Costa, B.R.; Pereira, T.V.; Whitlock, R.; Curley, G.F.; Scott, D.A.; Hare, G.M.T.; Jüni, P.; Mazer, C.D. Restrictive compared with liberal red cell transfusion strategies in cardiac surgery: A meta-analysis. *Eur. Heart J.* **2019**, *40*, 1081–1088. [CrossRef]
27. Mazer, C.D.; Whitlock, R.P.; Fergusson, D.A.; Hall, J.; Belley-Cote, E.; Connolly, K.; Khanykin, B.; Gregory, A.J.; De Médicis, É.; McGuinness, S.; et al. Restrictive or Liberal Red-Cell Transfusion for Cardiac Surgery. *N. Engl. J. Med.* **2017**, *377*, 2133–2144. [CrossRef]
28. Mazer, C.D.; Whitlock, R.P.; Fergusson, D.A.; Belley-Cote, E.; Connolly, K.; Khanykin, B.; Gregory, A.J.; De Médicis, É.; Carrier, F.M.; McGuinness, S.; et al. Six-Month Outcomes after Restrictive or Liberal Transfusion for Cardiac Surgery. *N. Engl. J. Med.* **2018**, *379*, 1224–1233. [CrossRef]
29. Mueller, M.M.; Van Remoortel, H.; Meybohm, P.; Aranko, K.; Aubron, C.; Burger, R.; Carson, J.L.; Cichutek, K.; De Buck, E.; Devine, D.; et al. Patient Blood Management: Recommendations From the 2018 Frankfurt Consensus Conference. *JAMA* **2019**, *321*, 983. [CrossRef]
30. Ad, N.; Massimiano, P.S.; Rongione, A.J.; Taylor, B.; Schena, S.; Alejo, D.; Fonner, C.E.; Salenger, R.; Whitman, G.; Metkus, T.S.; et al. Number and Type of Blood Products Are Negatively Associated With Outcomes After Cardiac Surgery. *Ann. Thorac. Surg.* **2022**, *113*, 748–756. [CrossRef]
31. Ming, Y.; Liu, J.; Zhang, F.; Chen, C.; Zhou, L.; Du, L.; Yan, M. Transfusion of Red Blood Cells, Fresh Frozen Plasma, or Platelets Is Associated With Mortality and Infection After Cardiac Surgery in a Dose-Dependent Manner. *Anesth. Analg.* **2020**, *130*, 488–497. [CrossRef]
32. Kaserer, A.; Rössler, J.; Braun, J.; Farokhzad, F.; Pape, H.-C.; Dutkowski, P.; Plass, A.; Horisberger, T.; Volbracht, J.; Manz, M.G.; et al. Impact of a Patient Blood Management monitoring and feedback programme on allogeneic blood transfusions and related costs. *Anaesthesia* **2019**, *74*, 1534–1541. [CrossRef]

33. *An EU-Wide Overview of the Market of Blood, Blood Components and Plasma Derivatives Focusing on Their Availability for Patients*; Creative Ceutical Report, Revised by the Commission, to Include Stakeholders' Comments; European Commission: Brussels, Belgium, 2015.
34. Saxena, S.; Krombach, J.W.; Nahrwold, D.A.; Pirracchio, R. Anaesthesia-specific checklists: A systematic review of impact. *Anaesth. Crit. Care Pain Med.* **2020**, *39*, 65–73. [CrossRef] [PubMed]
35. Gunertem, E.; Urcun, S.; Pala, A.A.; Budak, A.B.; Ercisli, M.A.; Gunaydin, S. Predictiveness of different preoperative risk assessments for postoperative bleeding after coronary artery bypass grafting surgery. *Perfusion* **2021**, *36*, 277–284. [CrossRef] [PubMed]
36. Hung, M.; Besser, M.; Sharples, L.D.; Nair, S.K.; Klein, A.A. The prevalence and association with transfusion, intensive care unit stay and mortality of pre-operative anaemia in a cohort of cardiac surgery patients*: Pre-operative anaemia in a cohort of cardiac surgery patients. *Anaesthesia* **2011**, *66*, 812–818. [CrossRef] [PubMed]
37. Domenica Cappellini, M.; Motta, I. Anemia in Clinical Practice—Definition and Classification: Does Hemoglobin Change With Aging? *Semin. Hematol.* **2015**, *52*, 261–269. [CrossRef] [PubMed]
38. Stammers, A.H.; Tesdahl, E.A.; Mongero, L.B.; Stasko, A. Gender and intraoperative blood transfusion: Analysis of 54,122 non-reoperative coronary revascularization procedures. *Perfusion* **2019**, *34*, 236–245. [CrossRef]
39. Muñoz, M.; Acheson, A.G.; Auerbach, M.; Besser, M.; Habler, O.; Kehlet, H.; Liumbruno, G.M.; Lasocki, S.; Meybohm, P.; Rao Baikady, R.; et al. International consensus statement on the peri-operative management of anaemia and iron deficiency. *Anaesthesia* **2017**, *72*, 233–247. [CrossRef]

Journal of
Cardiovascular Development and Disease

MDPI

Article

Postoperative Weight Gain within Enhanced Recovery after Cardiac Surgery

Alexandra Krüger [1,†], Anna Flo Forner [2,†], Jörg Ender [2], Aniruddha Janai [2], Youssef Roufail [3], Wolfgang Otto [4], Massimiliano Meineri [2,‡] and Waseem Z. A. Zakhary [2,*,‡]

1 Heart Center Leipzig, University of Leipzig, Strümpellstraße 39, 04289 Leipzig, Germany; ak85qape@studserv.uni-leipzig.de
2 Department of Anesthesiology and Intensive Care Medicine, Heart Center Leipzig, Strümpellstraße 39, 04289 Leipzig, Germany; anna.floforner@helios-gesundheit.de (A.F.F.); joerg.ender@helios-gesundheit.de (J.E.); aniruddha.janai@helios-gesundheit.de (A.J.); massimiliano.meineri@helios-gesundheit.de (M.M.)
3 Health Sciences, Faculty of Science, Waterloo Campus, Wilfrid Laurier University, Waterloo, ON N2L 3C5, Canada; rouf6200@mylaurier.ca
4 Department of Cardiac Surgery, Heart Center Leipzig, Strümpellstraße 39, 04289 Leipzig, Germany; wolfgang.otto@helios-gesundheit.de
* Correspondence: waseemzakariaaziz.zakhary@helios-gesundheit.de
† These authors contributed equally to this work.
‡ These authors contributed equally to this work.

Abstract: Optimal fluid therapy during perioperative care as part of enhanced recovery after cardiac surgery (ERACS) should improve the outcome. Our objective was finding out the effects of fluid overload on outcome and mortality within a well-established ERACS program. All consecutive patients undergoing cardiac surgery between January 2020 and December 2021 were enrolled. According to ROC curve analysis, a cut-off of ≥7 kg (group M, n = 1198) and <7 kg (group L, n = 1015) was defined. A moderate correlation was shown between weight gain and fluid balance r = 0.4, and a simple linear regression was significant $p < 0.0001$, $R^2 = 0.16$. Propensity score matching showed that increased weight gain was associated with a longer hospital length of stay (LOS) (L 8 [3] d vs. M 9 [6] d, $p < 0.0001$), an increased number of patients who received pRBCs (L 311 (36%) vs. M 429 (50%), $p < 0.0001$), and a higher incidence of postoperative acute kidney injury (AKI) (L 84 (9.8%) vs. M 165 (19.2%), $p < 0.0001$). Weight gain can easily represent fluid overload. Fluid overload after cardiac surgery is common and is associated with prolonged hospital LOS and increases the incidence of AKI.

Keywords: ERACS enhanced recovery after cardiac surgery; weight gain; fluid overload; postoperative outcome

1. Introduction

Fluid overload after cardiac surgery (CABG) is common and increases postoperative complications [1]. To date, its impact within an Enhanced Recovery after Cardiac Surgery (ERACS) program has not been well studied. We can expect less fluid overload by applying ERACS elements such as liberal preoperative oral fluid intake, early extubation, early postoperative oral intake, and early mobilization.

Goal directed fluid therapy (GDT) has been recommended during ERACS [2] within the early postoperative period, between 8 h [3] and 24 h [4]; however, it has only shown weak impact on mortality through reduced morbidity and hospital length of stay [5]. Nevertheless, GDT was not consistently associated with a reduction in fluid intake [3].

Fluid overload could be minimized using a restrictive fluid therapy protocol. However, studies comparing liberal versus restrictive fluid therapy in cardiac [4] and non-cardiac surgeries [6,7] showed non-superiority in fluid-restricted groups.

Postoperative fluid overload can be quantified either by calculating the fluid balance or by measuring postoperative weight gain. The fluid balance calculation seems to be more precise but time consuming and less reliable due to charting errors and gaps [8]. Conversely, weight gain is more robust and easier to interpret [9].

The aim of this retrospective study was to assess the impact of fluid overload on outcome and mortality in a well-established ERACS program.

The primary endpoints are the incidence of weight gain after cardiac surgery and the correlation between postoperative weight gain and fluid balance. The secondary endpoints are the effects of fluid overload on hospital length of stay (LOS), fast track failure (FTF), acute and chronic kidney injury (AKI), postoperative pulmonary complications, packed red blood cells (pRBCs) transfusion, and mortality.

2. Materials and Methods

This retrospective observational study was performed at a university affiliated Heart Center and began after approval by the local ethics committee (registration number 552/20-ek).

We selected all consecutive patients who followed the Leipzig ERACS protocol from January 2020 to December 2021 undergoing elective or emergency cardiac surgery. Exclusion criteria were: patients ineligible for ERACS, younger than 18 years, non-cardiac surgery patients (e.g., PM, ICD, TAVR), and incomplete data.

Patients without any complications were transferred to the postanesthetic care unit (PACU) directly from the operating room (OR). Once in the PACU, they were stabilized and extubated, hereafter transferred to the intermediate care unit (IMC) on the same day (POD 0). Patients were then transferred to the ward at the earliest on POD 1. The definition of a fast-track failure (FTF) is the unplanned transfer from the ward to the ICU or IMC at any time during the same hospital stay (Figure 1).

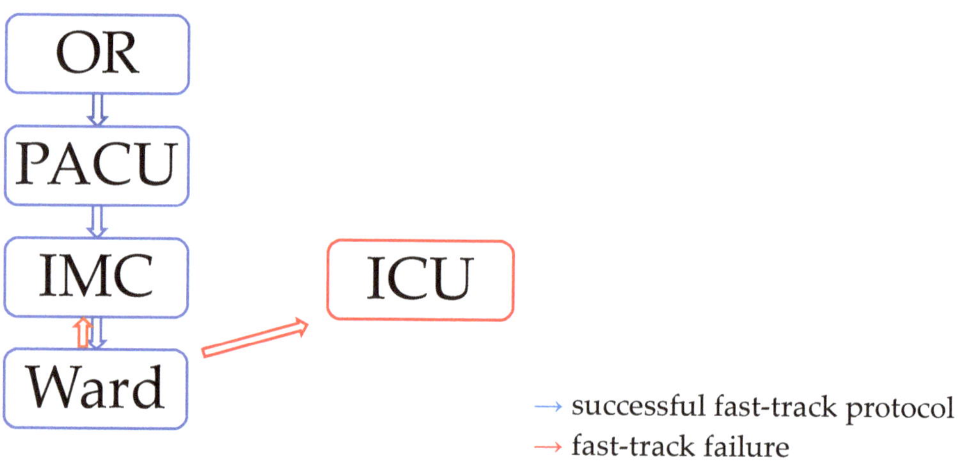

Figure 1. Fast-track pathway. OR = operating room, PACU = postanesthetic care unit, IMC = intermediate care unit, ICU = intensive care unit.

2.1. Pre-and Intraoperative Management

Patients were allowed to drink clear fluids, e.g., water, clear juices, and tea up to 2 h before surgery.

After anesthesia induction, a three-lumen central venous catheter and an 8.5 F introducer sheath were placed in the internal jugular vein under ultrasound guidance, and an arterial catheter was inserted for blood pressure monitoring. Body temperature was measured through a nasopharyngeal temperature probe and core temperature through a urinary catheter. Arterial and central venous blood gas analysis including hemoglobin (Hb), hematocrit (Hct), serum lactate, and central venous oxygen saturation ($ScvO_2$) were collected every 30 min. A transesophageal echocardiography (TOE) probe was inserted in all patients, if not contraindicated (esophageal pathology). Swan-Ganz catheters were spared to patients with a low ejection fraction (EF) of $\leq$35% or impaired right ventricle (RV) function or tricuspid valve (TV) surgery. More details regarding anesthesia and postoperative analgesia were published previously [10,11].

The blood transfusion threshold was a hematocrit less than 20% during CBP and less than 25% after weaning from CBP and during off-pump surgery. Cell saver CATSmart® (Fresenius Kabi AG, Bad Homburg, Germany) was used in all patients.

The following data were routinely collected intraoperatively: the amount of crystalloid/colloid infusion, packed red blood cells (pRBCs), fresh frozen plasma (FFP), platelets, cell saver, and fluid volume of the heart-lung machine during surgery (priming, cardioplegia). The outputs included urine output, remaining volume of the heart-lung machine, and ultrafiltration.

2.2. Perioperative Fluid Management

Patients were treated with a specific fluid management algorithm starting intraoperatively and until transfer to the ward (Figure 2). The Swan-Ganz catheter (if indicated) was removed in the PACU if the patient had normal parameters; otherwise, the patient would have been transferred to ICU. Fluid therapy was monitored by the mean blood pressure (BP), heart rate (HR), urinary output (UOP), serum lactate, central venous oxygen saturation ($ScvO_2$), TOE, transthoracic echocardiography (TTE), lung ultrasound (LUS), and hematocrit level (Hct). Swan-Ganz parameters were added for patients with reduced EF. The passive leg raising (PLR) maneuver, Trendelenburg position, or fluid challenge test using 200 mL of electrolyte crystalloids solution, e.g., Jonosteril® (Fresenius Kabi, Bad Homburg, Germany), are used if the TTE, TOE, and LUS results are not conclusive (Figure 2).

2.3. Postanesthetic Care Unit (PACU) and Intermediate Care Unit (IMC) Management

Criteria for PACU eligibility were: hemodynamic stability (±low-dose inotropic support), no severe bleeding, core temperature $\geq$ 36 °C, and clinical judgement and communication between anesthesiologist and surgeon [12,13].

The PACU, managed by the department of anesthesia, includes 8 beds and is staffed with a physician to patient ratio of 1:4 and a nurse-to-patient ratio of 1:3. The PACU opening hours were from 10:00 a.m. to 10:30 p.m. only during weekdays.

Intraoperative fluid therapy monitoring continued in the PACU. Arterial and venous blood gas analysis and UOP were documented hourly. Combined transthoracic echocardiography (TTE) and lung ultrasound (LUS) imaging were performed for all patients at least twice in the PACU (before extubation and before transfer to the IMC) and if otherwise indicated (e.g., hemodynamic instability).

Patients were extubated after fulfilling the predefined extubation criteria [11], and thereafter, a noninvasive ventilation was performed for half an hour. Transfer to the Intermediate Care Unit (IMC) was usually done after monitoring the patient 2–3 h after extubation. The transfer criteria were: a fully awake and alert patient without neurologic deficit, hemodynamically stable with no or minimal inotropic support, acceptable blood gas analysis (PaO_2 > 90 mmHg and $PaCO_2$ < 46 mmHg, SpO_2 > 96% on O_2 flow 2–6 L/min), urinary output $\geq$ 0.5 mL/kg/h, no significant bleeding (<50 mL/h), normal serum lactate, normal SvO_2, cardiac enzymes, and chest X-ray [12].

In the IMC, patients are fully monitored including invasive BP. Blood gas analysis was assessed every 3 h and POCUS (point of care ultrasound) if indicated.

Postoperative fluid intake (crystalloids/colloids, pRBCs, FFP, platelets, oral intake, medications) and output (blood loss, urine output (UOP), feces) were collected until discharge from the IMC to the ward, where the first postoperative weight was measured, which mostly represented the maximum recorded postoperative weight.

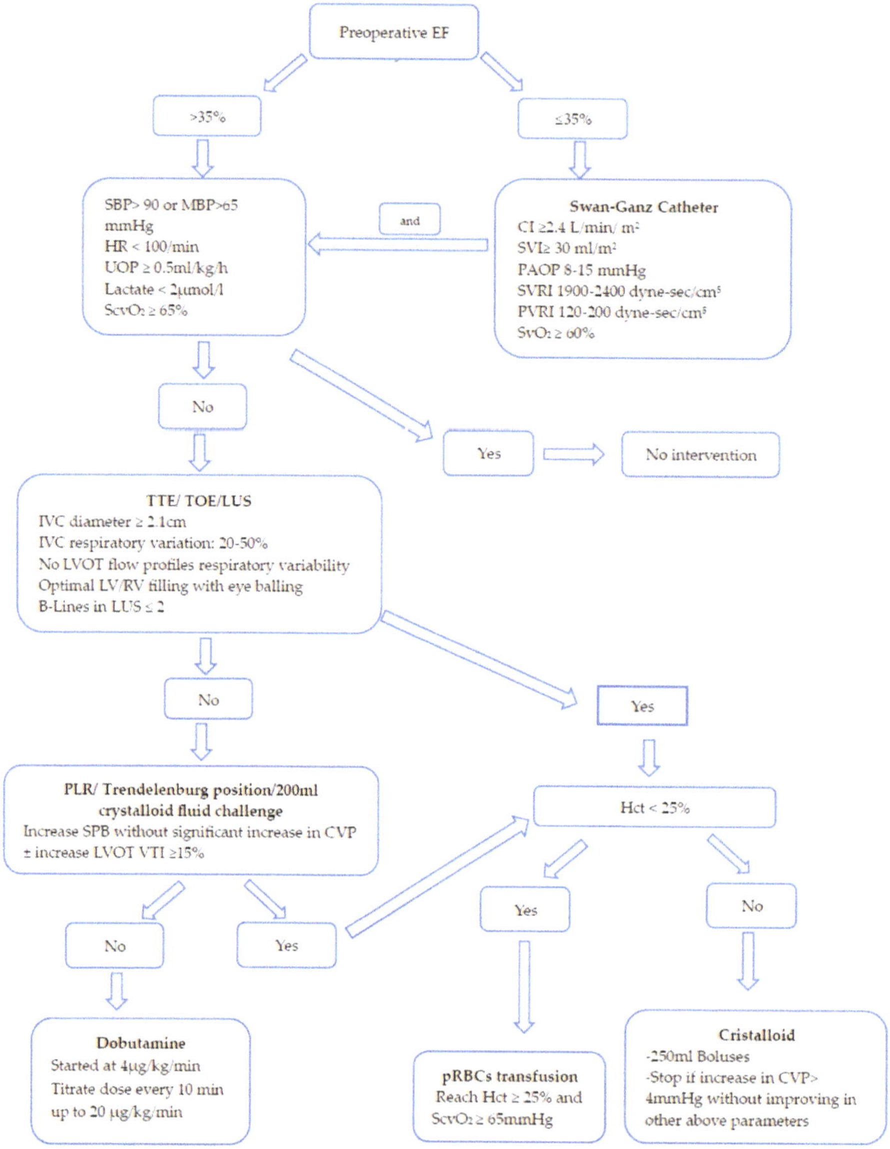

Figure 2. Fluid management algorithm. EF—ejection fraction; SBP—systolic blood pressure; MBP—mean blood pressure; UOP—urinary output; $ScvO_2$—central venous oxygen saturation; SvO_2—mixed venous oxygen saturation; IVC—inferior vena cava; PAOP—pulmonary artery occlusion pressure; SVRI—systemic vascular resistance index; PVRI—pulmonary vascular resistance index; CI—cardiac index; SVI—stroke volume index; TTE—transthoracic echocardiography; TOE—transesophageal echocardiography; LUS—lung ultrasound; PLR—passive leg raising; LVOT—left ventricular outflow tract.

2.4. ERACS Protocol

We started with the fast-track protocol in November 2005 with 3 beds in the PACU completely separated from the ICU. The early experimental results were published in 2008 [13]. Many aspects of this concept were tested and published [10–12,14–17]. This protocol was dynamically developed to match ERACS evolution over the time. Fourteen from the 21 elements of perioperative ERACS bundles, guidelines by Engelman et al. [2] were already applied in our protocol (tranexamic acid; perioperative glycemic control; a care bundle to reduce surgical site infections; goal-directed therapy; a multimodal, opioid-sparing, pain management plan; avoid hypothermia after CBP; active maintenance of chest tube patency; post-operative systematic delirium screening; an ICU liberation bundle; early extubation strategies; chemical thromboprophylaxis; a clear liquid diet may be considered to be continued up until 4 hours before general anesthesia; routine stripping of chest tubes is not recommended; hyperthermia (>37.9 °C) should be avoided). Many of the preoperative elements are still not adequately applied. We were also applying some non-graded elements suggested by Zaouter et al. [18]. Yearly, we are adding more elements to the protocol. We used to use the Vigileo® system (Edwards Lifesciences Corporation, Irvine, CA, USA) for all off-pump CABG for continuous stroke volume variation and cardiac index monitoring. Since 2018, intraoperative TOE, with certain indications for a Swan-Ganz catheter (see above), replaced Vigileo®.

2.5. Variables

The patients' body weight was measured preoperatively as the baseline value and after transfer from the IMC to the ward.

Weight gain is defined as the difference between the preoperative weight and maximum postoperative weight.

Complex surgery is defined as any surgery including more than one procedure, e.g., CABG + Valve/s or 2 or more valves.

Postoperative respiratory complications included any cause of pneumonia, ARDS, and severe airway edema. The categorization of acute kidney injury follows the KDIGO stadium classification [19]. According to the KDIGO guidelines, chronic kidney disease was used to define persistence of kidney damage for more than 3 months.

Calculated fluid balance is defined as the mathematical subtraction of every single fluid output from every single fluid input. Measured fluid balance is the sum of all fluid balances documented in the nursing documentation sheet.

2.6. Statistical Analysis

Data were retrieved from the clinical information system iMedOne® (Deutsche Telekom Healthcare and Security Solutions GmbH, Bonn, Germany) and the machine-readable patient's chart Medlinq® (Medlinq Softwaresysteme GmbH, Hamburg, Germany). Anesthesia and PACU observation sheets were corrected manually by the anesthesiologist directly after scanning. Data of cardiopulmonary bypass were documented by a special machine operator in the Connect Manager (LivaNova; London, UK). SPSS (SPSS® Statistics 25.0; Chicago, IL, USA) and StatsDirect (StatsDirect® version 3.3.5, StatsDirect Ltd., Cheshire, UK) were used for statistics.

Due to a number of studies with a difference in the time of collecting postoperative weight [1,8,9,20–24], ROC curve analysis for postoperative acute renal injury was used to determine the cut-off point of weight gain between both groups. Continuous variables were assessed for normal distribution using the Shapiro–Wilk test. The continuous data are expressed as mean ± SD and compared using a Student's paired t-test in case of normal distribution or a Mann–Whitney U test for data not normally distributed. Categorical data were expressed as numbers (proportion) and compared using the X^2 test or Fisher's exact test where appropriate. Means of maximum weight gain for each postoperative day (POD) were compared with a one-way ANOVA with a Tukey–Kramer post-hoc test to show the differences between each pair. A p-value < 0.05 was considered statistically significant. A Pearson correlation coefficient (r) and simple linear regression was used for the relationship between weight gain and fluid balance.

According to our sample size analysis, 1538 patients had to be included if the hospital length of stay would have been shorter by one day (15 days vs. 14 days) ± 7 with a power of 80% and $p = 0.05$.

Propensity score matching was performed to minimize the bias that might result from differences in demographic, preoperative, and intraoperative data, especially for the complexity of the surgeries. The variables used for the logistic regression model were: age, gender, day of maximum recorded weight, EuroScore II, surgery complexity, x-clamp time, CPB time, and length of surgery. We used one to one matching, paring each subject to the closest propensity score subject from the other group. Based on the pre-matching range of baseline variable differences, the maximum caliper width for pair-matching was defined as 0.2 of the pooled logit score standard deviation.

3. Results

A total of 6437 patients were operated between January 2020 to December 2021. In total, 3754 were admitted to the PACU. We included 2213 patients with complete data and who completed the ideal fast-track pathway from the PACU to the IMC and thereafter to the ward (Figure 3).

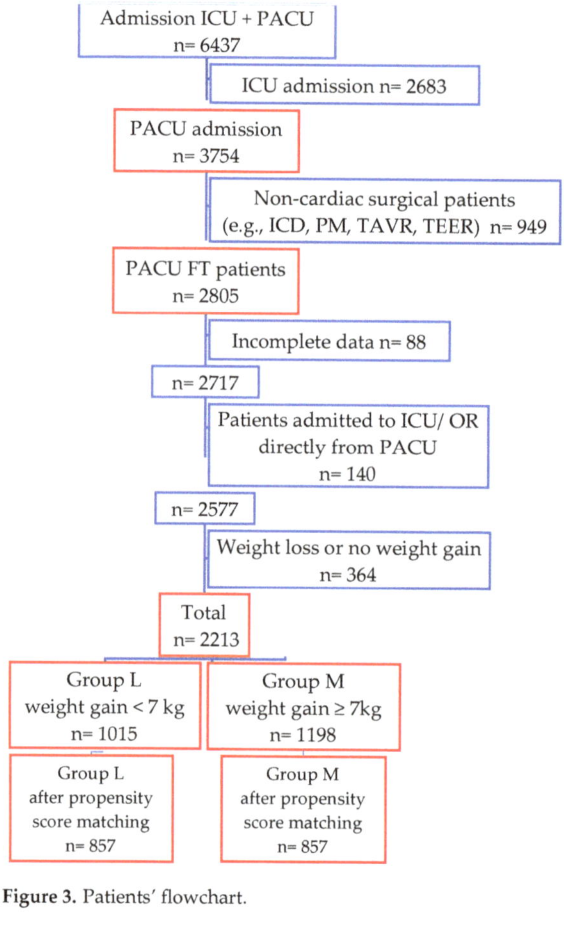

Figure 3. Patients' flowchart.

According to ROC curve analysis (see Appendix A, Figure A1), a cut-off point of ≥7 kg (area under ROC curve = 0.601, PPV = 0.19, NPV = 0.88, sensitivity (95% CI) = 0.66, specificity (95% CI) = 0.48) was defined. Accordingly, patients were divided into 2 groups:

group (L) with less weight gain (<7 kg, n = 1015 (46%)) and group (M) with more weight gain (≥7 kg, n = 1198 (54%)). After propensity score matching, each group included 857 patients.

Demographic data, baseline characteristics, and type of surgery before and after PSM are summarized in Table 1.

Table 1. Baseline characteristics and demographic data; values in mean ± SD or median [IQR] or number (%); {propensity score matching (PSM) results}.

	L **n = 1015** **{after PSM n = 857}**	**M** **n = 1198** **{after PSM n = 857}**	***p* Value**
Age (y)	62.7 ± 11.6 {63 ± 11.5}	64.3 ± 11.8 {64 ± 11.6}	0.02 {0.129}
Female gender	238 (23) {207 (24)}	331 (27) {234 (27)}	0.02 {0.15}
NYHA III and IV	353 (34) {311 (36)}	453 (37) {315 (37)}	0.1 {0.92}
Preoperative weight (kg)	85 ± 17 {85.3 ± 16.9}	84 ± 17 {84.3 ± 17.1}	0.137 {0.255}
BMI (kg/m^2)	28.2 ± 4.7 {28 ± 4.7}	28 ± 5 {28.1 ± 5.1}	0.249 {0.486}
EuroSCORE II	1.82 ± 2.0 {1.6 ± 2.1}	2.0 ± 2.1 {1.6 ± 2}	0.547 {0.949}
Complex surgeries (CABG + Valve/s or 2 or more x Valve)	149 (14.6) {143 (16.6)}	283 (23.6) {153 (17.8)}	<0.0001 {0.565}
On-pump CABG	271 (26.6) {226 (26)}	221 (18.4) {165 (19.2)}	<0.0001 {0.0006}
OPCAB/MIDCAB	237 (23.3) {167 (19.5)}	155 (13) {149 (17.3)}	<0.0001 {0.289}
Isolated AVR	170 (16.7) {150 (17.5)}	314 (26) {210 (24.5)}	<0.0001 {0.005}
Isolated MVR	106 (10.4) {100 (11.6)}	147 (12) {98 (11.4)}	0.20 {0.939}
Minimal invasive approaches (Thoracotomy or partial sternotomy)	255 (25) {237 (27.5)}	317 (26.3) {227 (26.4)}	0.504 {0.624}
Thoracotomy approach	170 (16.7) {156 (18.2)}	169 (14) {129 (15)}	0.096 {0.091}
Partial sternotomy (superior)	85 (8.3) {81 (9.4)}	148 (12.3) {98 (11.4)}	0.003 {0.20}
Emergency surgery	127 (12.6) {101 (12)}	153 (12.9) {106 (12.5)}	0.905 {0.76}
Re-do operations	60 (6.2) {53 (6)}	83 (7.2) {56 (6.5)}	0.375 {0.781}
Preoperative ejection fraction (%)	56 ± 10.5 {56 ± 10.5}	57 ± 10.4 {57 ± 10.5}	0.082 {0.148}
Hypertension	761 (78.3) {643 (77.5)}	852 (75) {625 (73)}	0.47 {0.349}

Table 1. *Cont.*

	L n = 1015 {after PSM n = 857}	M n = 1198 {after PSM n = 857}	*p* Value
DM	244 (24) {205 (24)}	276 (23) {196 (23)}	0.614 {0.648}
Preoperative hematocrit (%)	40.8 ± 5.4 {38.9 ± 4.9}	40.1 ± 5.8 {38.3 ± 4.9}	0.161 {0.001}
Preoperative hemoglobin (g/dl)	12.5 ± 2 {12.5 ± 1.6}	12.2 ± 2 {12.3 ± 1.6}	0.09 {0.001}
Minimal intraoperative hemoglobin (g/dl)	10.7 ± 4.8 {10.7 ± 5}	10.1 ± 3.2 {10.1 ± 2}	<0.0001 {<0.001}
Preoperative creatinine (mg/dl)	0.96 ± 0.02 {0.97 ± 0.69}	0.91 ± 0.01 {0.92 ± 0.3}	0.642 {0.02}
CPB duration (min)	71 ± 56 {76 ± 51}	87 ± 51 {78 ± 49}	<0.0001 {0.322}
x-clamp time (min)	40 ± 41 {46 ± 41}	55 ± 40 {47 ± 40}	<0.0001 {0.574}
Length of surgery (min)	183 ± 61 {184 ± 60}	192 ± 55 {188 ± 53}	0.002 {0.06}
Postoperative ventilation time (min)	106 ± 54 {106 ± 55}	115 ± 60 {115 ± 60}	0.015 {0.004}
PACU LOS (min)	240 [90] {235 [95]}	245 [90] {255 [85]}	0.006 {<0.001}
IMC LOS (h)	27.5 [47] {25 [46]}	23.1 [45] {24 [47]}	0.008 {0.625}
Weight gain (kg)	4.1 ± 1.8 {4.2 ± 1.8}	10.6 ± 3.1 {10.4 ± 3}	<0.0001 {<0.0001}

LOS—length of stay; CABG—coronary artery bypass graft; OPCAB—off-pump coronary artery bypass; MIDCAB—minimal invasive coronary artery bypass; AVR—aortic valve replacement; MVR—mitral valve replacement; DM—diabetes mellitus; CPB—cardiopulmonary bypass.

3.1. Weight Gain vs. Fluid Balance

The mean increase in weight was +7.6 ± 4.1 kg, while the mean intra- and postoperative fluid balance was +8.6 ± 3.7 L and the mean of the difference between fluid balance and weight gain was 1.0 ± 4.3 kg. Group L had a weight gain of 4.1 ± 1.8 kg, whereas group M had an average weight gain of 10.6 ± 3.1 kg. Only a moderate correlation was shown between weight gain and fluid balance (r = 0.4). A simple linear regression for weight change and fluid balance was significant ($p < 0.001$, $R^2 = 0.16$). A total of 1675 patients was included in the fluid balance analysis (538 patients were excluded because of incomplete data). Inconsistency between the measured and calculated fluid balance was found in 26% of the patients.

3.2. Day of Maximum Collected Weight

Figure 4 shows the proportion of patients for the first day of recorded weight and the day of maximum weight gain for each postoperative day (POD). Weight could be collected in 43% of the patients on POD1 and 23% on POD2. The maximum postoperative weight gain was concomitant to the first collected weight in 75% of patients weighed on POD1.

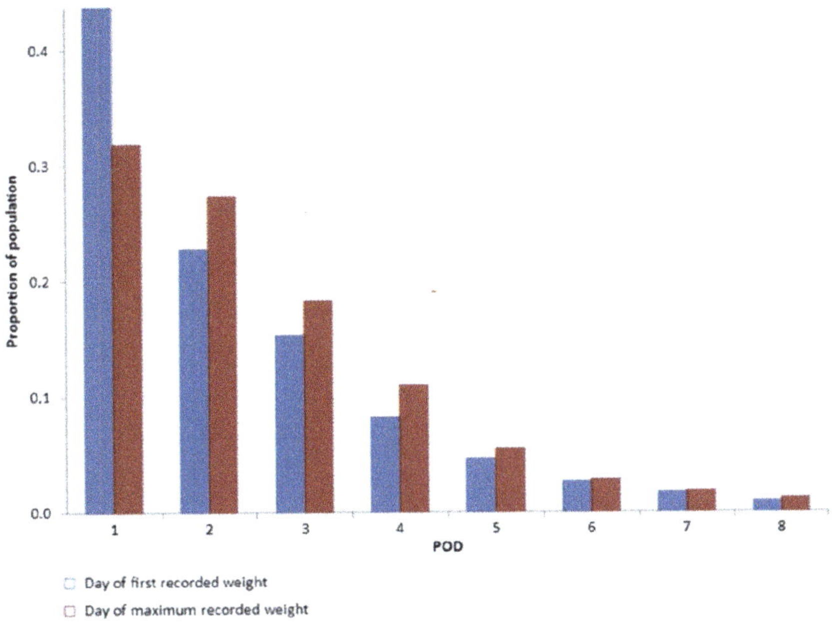

Figure 4. Day of first recorded weight vs. day of maximum recorded weight.

The mean of maximum weight gain is comparable for patients weighed from POD1 to POD4 (7.6–7.8 kg) (Figure 5) with a drop in the mean on POD5 ($p < 0.05$ when compared with each day from POD1 to POD4).

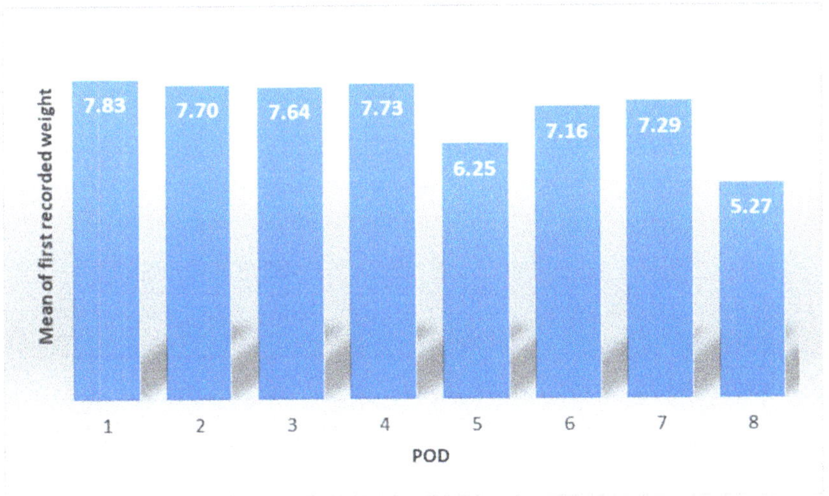

Figure 5. Mean of maximum weight gain.

Figure 6 shows a significant difference ($p < 0.001$) in the day of maximum recorded weight. After PSM, no significant difference ($p = 0.3$) was found between groups (Figure 7).

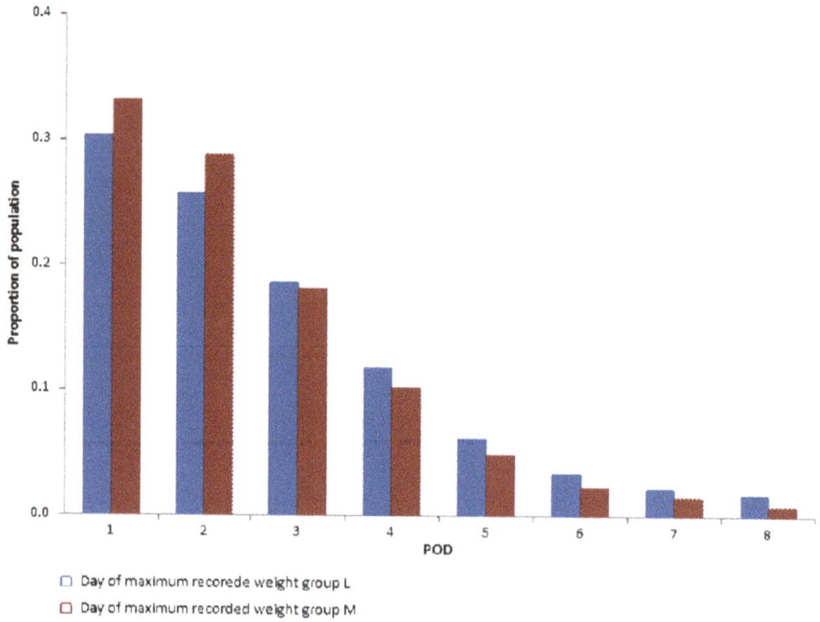

Figure 6. Comparison in day of maximum recorded weight between group L and M.

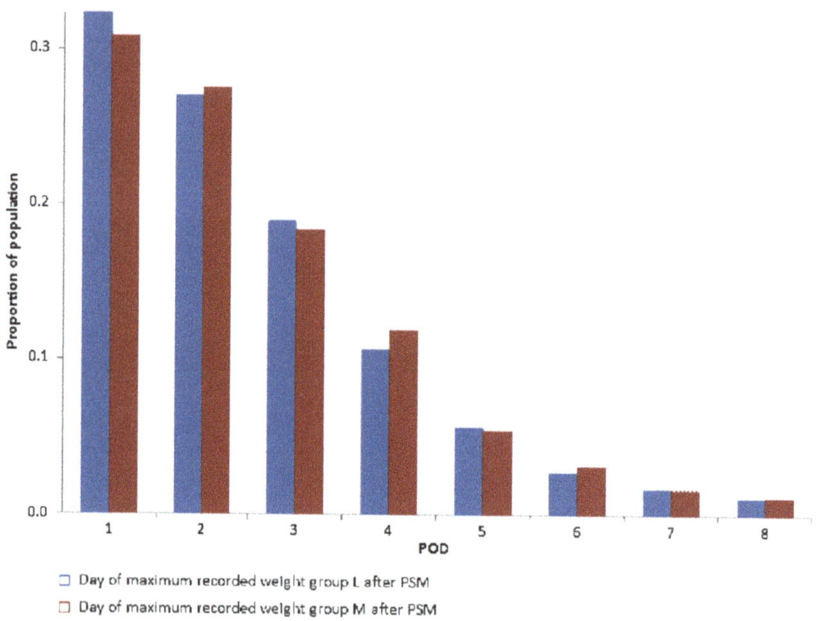

Figure 7. Comparison in day of maximum recorded weight between group L and M after PSM.

Postoperative outcome and mortality are summarized in Table 2. Hospital length of stay was significantly longer in group M (L 8 [3] d vs. M 9 [6] d, $p < 0.0001$). Postoperative acute kidney injury at stages I and II, but not stage III, were significantly higher in group M. AKI was almost twice as high in group M compared to group L.

Table 2. Postoperative outcome and mortality after propensity score matching. Values in mean ± SD or median [IQR] or number (%).

	L n = 857	M n = 857	*p* Value	95% CI	RR
Hospital LOS	8 [3]	9 [6]	<0.0001	0.58 to 0.64	
In-hospital mortality	1 (0.1)	5 (0.5)	0.12		0.19
FTF	81 (9.5)	103 (12)	0.103		0.86
Postoperative acute kidney injury (AKI) total	84 (9.8)	165 (19.2)	<0.0001		0.63
AKI stage I	62 (8.4)	136 (15.8)	<0.0001		0.66
AKI stage II	9 (1)	24 (2.8)	0.013		0.54
AKI stage III	3 (0.3)	5 (0.6)	0.506		0.75
Postop chronic renal impairment	91 (11)	117 (14.5)	0.06		0.86
Any postoperative pulmonary complications	17 (2)	16 (1.8)	0.999		1.0
Number of patients who received 1 or more pRBCs	311 (36)	429 (50)	<0.0001		0.75

RR—relative risk; LOS—length of stay; FTF—fast-track failure; pRBCs—packed red blood cells.

4. Discussion

In our study, 54% of our patients experienced postoperative weight gain ≥7 kg, which was associated with a longer hospital length of stay, increased number of received pRBCs, and higher incidence of postoperative acute kidney injury in enhanced recovery after cardiac surgery. We could find only a moderate correlation between the postoperative change of weight and perioperative fluid balance.

Engelman et al. [2] published the recommendations for ERACS in 2019. Many elements in the recommended bundles are potentially helpful to optimize the postoperative fluid status: perioperative glycemic control, GDT, early detection of kidney stress, early extubation, preoperative correction of nutritional deficiency, continued consumption of clear fluid until 2 h before surgery, and preoperative oral carbohydrates loading.

Unfortunately, there are few studies describing the effects of these elements on perioperative fluid management. GDT in cardiac surgery was described by Osawa et al. [3] and showed positive effects on postoperative major complications and hospital LOS but not on mortality. In comparison to our study, the fluid balance in Osawa et al. [3] was measured only until 8 h postoperatively, and GDT was unexpectedly associated with more fluid intake than the control group. Although a meta-analysis from Aya et al. [5] also showed a positive impact on complications and hospital LOS, it still could not reach a strong conclusion because of the limited data and heterogeneity of the methods used.

Liberal versus restrictive fluid therapy after surgery was also not well studied in cardiac surgery. Parke et al. [4] conducted a randomized controlled trial comparing the two groups after cardiac surgery. The overall fluid balance was lower in the intervention group (319 mL [−284–1274 mL] vs. 673 mL [38–1641 mL], $p < 0.0001$) that received less fluid boluses (1000 mL [250–2000] vs. 1500 mL [500–1500 mL], $p < 0.0001$); however, no impact was found on hospital LOS and postoperative complications. The hospital mortality rate was higher in the intervention group. Again, Parke et al. [4] limited their intervention to 24 h postoperatively, in contrast to our cohort who stayed in the IMC L 25 [46] h vs. M 24 [47] h in addition to a PACU stay L 235 [95] min vs. M 255 [85] min. Myles et al. [7] and Messina et al. [6] studied this issue in major abdominal surgery and found no impact between the two groups on major complications and postoperative mortality.

AKI stage I and II, but not III, were higher in our patients with more volume overload. Although it may be a causal bias (the patients were volume overloaded because of AKI, not vice versa), we do not think so because volume overload would be more obvious in AKI III, which is insignificantly different between both groups. Furthermore, preoperative serum creatinine was comparable between both groups. This is supported by Chen et al. [25] and

Shen et al. [26] who found more AKI in volume overloaded and severely restrictive patients 48 h after cardiac surgery. In contrast, restrictive groups were associated with more renal complications than liberal fluid management in major abdominal surgery [6,7] but not in cardiac surgery [27]. A recent consensus report on adult cardiac surgery associated acute kidney injury (CSA-AKI) [28] mentioned both hypo- and hypervolemia as risk factors for CSA-AKI. They targeted euvolemia using thirteen strategies (pre-, intra- and postoperative) to prevent CSA-AKI. Nevertheless, AKI is an independent factor for prolonged hospital stay after cardiac surgery [29] and may explain the difference in hospital LOS between both groups.

No difference in the postoperative respiratory complications is also consistent with several studies [6,7,27]. The correlation between fluid overload and postoperative major complications was also demonstrated in CABG patients [1], which is in line with our results.

The difference in type of surgery between two groups is striking. There is significantly more aortic valve replacement (AVR) in group M. Patients with AV disease (mostly aortic stenosis) usually presented with LV hypertrophy and a degree of diastolic dysfunction. These patients, with good EF, tend to receive more fluids postoperatively as the sole treatment for any hemodynamic instability. POCUS examination of these patients mostly reveals LV hypertrophy and kissing papillary muscles that mandate fluid therapy. The presence of more on-pump CABG in group L is unexpected because the priming fluid, inflammation, and fluid shift effects of cardiopulmonary bypass may lead to fluid overload. Nevertheless, on-pump CABG is the most common surgical procedure in cardiac surgery, and the physicians may feel more confident in managing these patients, aiming for earlier hospital discharge compared to other types of procedures. Minimally invasive procedures including the thoracotomy approach and partial sternotomy were comparable in both groups. As in most minimally invasive cardiac surgery studies [30,31], these approaches are not inferior to the conventional approach regarding outcome. Olsthoorn et al. [31] showed a longer hospital LOS in a minimally invasive group, but we did not. Our patients were managed with the same ERACS protocol, regardless of type of procedure.

The discrepancy between the calculated and measured fluid balance and the correlation between fluid balance and body weight gain in our study is in concordance with the literature; Eastwood et al. [8] concluded the unreliability of fluid balance to reflect postoperative weight in cardiac surgery. Butti et al. [9] did not find a good correlation between fluid balance and weight gain after major abdominal surgery ($r = 0.214$, $p = 0.19$, vs. $r = 0.4$, $p < 0.001$ in our study). This could be explained by the complex calculation of fluid balance, which is more reliable for human error and is demonstrated in our study by the difference between the calculated and measured fluid balance of 26%. Furthermore, the insensible fluid loss is either ignored or imprecisely calculated. Therefore, we believe that weight gain is more representative of fluid balance after surgery. Köster et al. [20] showed the same results in ICU patients, preferring weight gain over fluid balance measurements.

A higher number of patients receiving transfusion can be noticed in our group M in contrast to group L. As per departmental SOPs, we have a restrictive threshold for transfusion. However, 36% of the group L still received at least one pRBC, which is still in the range of pRBCs transfused in major randomized studies comparing restrictive vs. liberal transfusion after cardiac surgery (52.3% and 25%) [32,33].

Physician compliance and adherence to fluid management protocols could not be assessed because of the nature of retrospective studies. Implementation of fluid management protocols (and all other ERACS elements) are reinforced with regular audits, availability of diagnostic tools (ultrasound machines), and documentation in the local manual for cardiac anesthesiologists. Nevertheless, "lack of compliance" with failure to adhere to the standardized protocol could not be excluded as reason for fluid overload. In the anesthesia setting, implementation of quality indicators was confronted with poor employee compliance [34].

The main limitation of our study is the retrospective design through which we cannot fully exclude the risk of unknown biases. This study did not take into account intraoperative insensible fluid loss and intraoperative bleeding not processed through the cell saver system.

We could not precisely assess adherence to the fluid management protocol. It is difficult to compare hospital LOS in this study with studies from other countries. In Germany, the hospital LOS depends not only on the patients' general condition, but also on the German payment system. Minimum hospital LOS between 4–12 days, according to the cardiac procedure, is required for full payment from health insurance companies. In 2018, the average length of stay for cardiac surgery patients in Germany was 11 days [35,36].

5. Conclusions

Volume overload after cardiac surgery is also quite common within a well-established ERACS program, and it is associated with a prolonged hospital length of stay, higher incidence of postoperative AKI, and blood transfusion. Weight gain is likely to estimate the fluid overload in a better way compared to complex fluid balance calculations. Individual ERACS elements must be prospectively studied to examine its effect on postoperative fluid overload.

Author Contributions: Conceptualization, J.E., W.Z.A.Z. and A.K.; methodology, W.Z.A.Z. and A.K.; software, W.Z.A.Z.; validation, W.Z.A.Z., A.K. and J.E.; formal analysis, W.Z.A.Z. and W.O.; investigation, A.K.; resources, W.Z.A.Z. and J.E.; data curation, W.Z.A.Z., W.O. and A.K.; writing—original draft preparation, W.Z.A.Z. and A.K.; writing—review and editing, A.F.F., J.E., A.J. and M.M.; visualization, W.Z.A.Z., A.J. and A.K.; supervision, W.Z.A.Z. and J.E.; language review, Y.R., A.J. and M.M.; project administration, W.Z.A.Z. and J.E. All authors have read and agreed to the published version of the manuscript.

Funding: This research received no funding.

Institutional Review Board Statement: The study was conducted in accordance with the Declaration of Helsinki and approved by the Local Ethics Committee "Medizinische Fakultät Universität Leipzig" (registration number 552/20-ek).

Informed Consent Statement: Individual patient consent was waived given the retrospective observational nature of the study.

Data Availability Statement: The datasets generated and analyzed during the current study are available from the corresponding author on reasonable request.

Conflicts of Interest: The authors declare no conflict of interest.

Appendix A

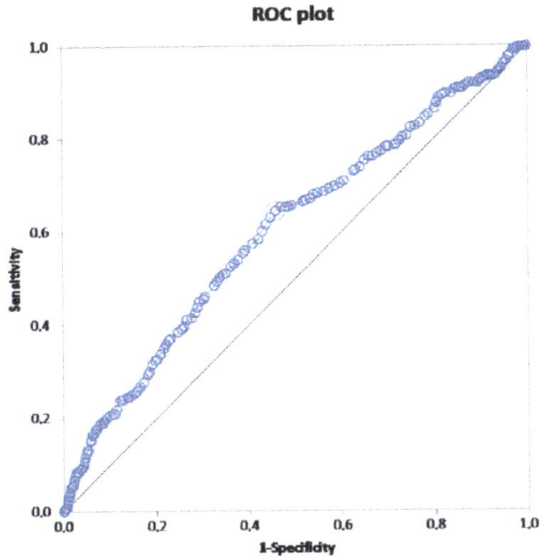

Figure A1. ROC plot for postoperative acute kidney injury.

References

1. Morin, J.-F.; Mistry, B.; Langlois, Y.; Ma, F.; Chamoun, P.; Holcroft, C. Fluid Overload after Coronary Artery Bypass Grafting Surgery Increases the Incidence of Post-Operative Complications. *WJCS* **2011**, *1*, 18–23. [CrossRef]
2. Engelman, D.T.; Ben Ali, W.; Williams, J.B.; Perrault, L.P.; Reddy, V.S.; Arora, R.C.; Roselli, E.E.; Khoynezhad, A.; Gerdisch, M.; Levy, J.H.; et al. Guidelines for Perioperative Care in Cardiac Surgery: Enhanced Recovery After Surgery Society Recommendations. *JAMA Surg.* **2019**, *154*, 755–766. [CrossRef] [PubMed]
3. Osawa, E.A.; Rhodes, A.; Landoni, G.; Galas, F.R.B.G.; Fukushima, J.T.; Park, C.H.L.; Almeida, J.P.; Nakamura, R.E.; Strabelli, T.M.V.; Pileggi, B.; et al. Effect of Perioperative Goal-Directed Hemodynamic Resuscitation Therapy on Outcomes Following Cardiac Surgery: A Randomized Clinical Trial and Systematic Review. *Crit. Care Med.* **2016**, *44*, 724–733. [CrossRef]
4. Parke, R.L.; Gilder, E.; Gillham, M.J.; Walker, L.J.C.; Bailey, M.J.; McGuinness, S.P. A Multicenter, Open-Label, Randomized Controlled Trial of a Conservative Fluid Management Strategy Compared With Usual Care in Participants After Cardiac Surgery: The Fluids After Bypass Study. *Crit. Care Med.* **2021**, *49*, 449–461. [CrossRef]
5. Aya, H.D.; Cecconi, M.; Hamilton, M.; Rhodes, A. Goal-directed therapy in cardiac surgery: A systematic review and meta-analysis. *Br. J. Anaesth.* **2013**, *110*, 510–517. [CrossRef]
6. Messina, A.; Robba, C.; Calabrò, L.; Zambelli, D.; Iannuzzi, F.; Molinari, E.; Scarano, S.; Battaglini, D.; Baggiani, M.; de Mattei, G.; et al. Perioperative liberal versus restrictive fluid strategies and postoperative outcomes: A systematic review and metanalysis on randomised-controlled trials in major abdominal elective surgery. *Crit. Care* **2021**, *25*, 205. [CrossRef]
7. Myles, P.S.; Bellomo, R.; Corcoran, T.; Forbes, A.; Peyton, P.; Story, D.; Christophi, C.; Leslie, K.; McGuinness, S.; Parke, R.; et al. Restrictive versus Liberal Fluid Therapy for Major Abdominal Surgery. *N. Engl. J. Med.* **2018**, *378*, 2263–2274. [CrossRef]
8. Eastwood, G.M. Evaluating the reliability of recorded fluid balance to approximate body weight change in patients undergoing cardiac surgery. *Heart Lung* **2006**, *35*, 27–33. [CrossRef]
9. Butti, F.; Pache, B.; Winiker, M.; Grass, F.; Demartines, N.; Hübner, M. Correlation of postoperative fluid balance and weight and their impact on outcomes. *Langenbecks. Arch. Surg.* **2020**, *405*, 1191–1200. [CrossRef]
10. Grützner, H.; Flo Forner, A.; Meineri, M.; Janai, A.; Ender, J.; Zakhary, W.Z.A. A Comparison of Patients Undergoing On- vs. Off-Pump Coronary Artery Bypass Surgery Managed with a Fast-Track Protocol. *J. Clin. Med.* **2021**, *10*, 4470. [CrossRef]
11. Zakhary, W.Z.A.; Turton, E.W.; Flo Forner, A.; von Aspern, K.; Borger, M.A.; Ender, J.K. A comparison of sufentanil vs. remifentanil in fast-track cardiac surgery patients. *Anaesthesia* **2019**, *74*, 602–608. [CrossRef] [PubMed]
12. Zakhary, W.; Lindner, J.; Sgouropoulou, S.; Eibel, S.; Probst, S.; Scholz, M.; Ender, J. Independent Risk Factors for Fast-Track Failure Using a Predefined Fast-Track Protocol in Preselected Cardiac Surgery Patients. *J. Cardiothorac. Vasc. Anesth.* **2015**, *29*, 1461–1465. [CrossRef] [PubMed]
13. Ender, J.; Borger, M.A.; Scholz, M.; Funkat, A.-K.; Anwar, N.; Sommer, M.; Mohr, F.W.; Fassl, J. Cardiac surgery fast-track treatment in a postanesthetic care unit: Six-month results of the Leipzig fast-track concept. *Anesthesiology* **2008**, *109*, 61–66. [CrossRef] [PubMed]
14. Hasheminejad, E.; Forner, A.F.; Meineri, M.; Ender, J.; Zakhary, W.Z.A. Postoperative Nausea and Vomiting Prophylaxis in Fast-Track Cardiac Anesthesia: A Patient Matched Retrospective before and after Study. *Int. J. Anesthesiol. Pain Med.* **2022**, *8*, 78–85.
15. Korsik, E.; Meineri, M.; Zakhary, W.Z.A.; Balga, I.; Jawad, K.; Ender, J.; Flo Forner, A. Persistent and acute postoperative pain after cardiac surgery with anterolateral thoracotomy or median sternotomy: A prospective observational study. *J. Clin. Anesth.* **2022**, *77*, 110577. [CrossRef] [PubMed]
16. Probst, S.; Cech, C.; Haentschel, D.; Scholz, M.; Ender, J. A specialized post anaesthetic care unit improves fast-track management in cardiac surgery: A prospective randomized trial. *Crit. Care* **2014**, *18*, 468. [CrossRef] [PubMed]
17. GRAß, C.; Stretti, F.; Zakhary, W.; Turton, E.; Sgouoropoulou, S.; Mende, M.; Ender, J. Impact of the post-anesthetic care unit opening hours on fast-track success in cardiac surgery. *Minerva Anestesiol.* **2017**, *83*, 155–164. [CrossRef]
18. Zaouter, C.; Damphousse, R.; Moore, A.; Stevens, L.-M.; Gauthier, A.; Carrier, F.M. Elements not Graded in the Cardiac Enhanced Recovery After Surgery Guidelines Might Improve Postoperative Outcome: A Comprehensive Narrative Review. *J. Cardiothorac. Vasc. Anesth.* **2022**, *36*, 746–765. [CrossRef]
19. Kellum, J.A. KDIGO Clinical Practice Guideline for Acute Kidney Injury. *Kidney Int. Suppl.* **2012**, *2*, 1. [CrossRef]
20. Köster, M.; Dennhardt, S.; Jüttner, F.; Hopf, H.-B. Cumulative changes in weight but not fluid volume balances reflect fluid accumulation in ICU patients. *Acta Anaesthesiol. Scand.* **2017**, *61*, 205–215. [CrossRef]
21. Cagini, L.; Capozzi, R.; Tassi, V.; Savignani, C.; Quintaliani, G.; Reboldi, G.; Puma, F. Fluid and electrolyte balance after major thoracic surgery by bioimpedance and endocrine evaluation. *Eur. J. Cardiothorac. Surg.* **2011**, *40*, e71–e76. [CrossRef]
22. Shiao, C.-C.; Huang, Y.-T.; Lai, T.-S.; Huang, T.-M.; Wang, J.-J.; Huang, C.-T.; Wu, P.-C.; Wu, C.-H.; Tsai, I.-J.; Tseng, L.-J.; et al. Perioperative body weight change is associated with in-hospital mortality in cardiac surgical patients with postoperative acute kidney injury. *PLoS ONE* **2017**, *12*, e0187280. [CrossRef] [PubMed]
23. Hübner, M.; Pache, B.; Solà, J.; Blanc, C.; Hahnloser, D.; Demartines, N.; Grass, F. Thresholds for optimal fluid administration and weight gain after laparoscopic colorectal surgery. *BJS Open* **2019**, *3*, 532–538. [CrossRef] [PubMed]
24. Perko, M.J.; Jarnvig, I.L.; Højgaard-Rasmussen, N.; Eliasen, K.; Arendrup, H. Electric impedance for evaluation of body fluid balance in cardiac surgical patients. *J. Cardiothorac. Vasc. Anesth.* **2001**, *15*, 44–48. [CrossRef]

25. Chen, X.; Xu, J.; Li, Y.; Shen, B.; Jiang, W.; Luo, Z.; Wang, C.; Teng, J.; Ding, X.; Lv, W. The Effect of Postoperative Fluid Balance on the Occurrence and Progression of Acute Kidney Injury After Cardiac Surgery. *J. Cardiothorac. Vasc. Anesth.* **2021**, *35*, 2700–2706. [CrossRef] [PubMed]
26. Shen, Y.; Zhang, W.; Cheng, X.; Ying, M. Association between postoperative fluid balance and acute kidney injury in patients after cardiac surgery: A retrospective cohort study. *J. Crit. Care* **2018**, *44*, 273–277. [CrossRef]
27. Palomba, H.; Treml, R.E.; Caldonazo, T.; Katayama, H.T.; Gomes, B.C.; Malbouisson, L.M.S.; Silva Junior, J.M. Intraoperative fluid balance and cardiac surgery-associated acute kidney injury: A multicenter prospective study. *Braz. J. Anesthesiol.* **2022**, *72*, 688–694. [CrossRef]
28. Brown, J.K.; Shaw, A.D.; Mythen, M.G.; Guzzi, L.; Reddy, V.S.; Crisafi, C.; Engelman, D.T.; Gan, T.J.; Miller, T.; Guinn, N.R.; et al. Adult Cardiac Surgery Associated Acute Kidney Injury: Joint Consensus Report of the PeriOperative Quality Initiative (POQI) and the Enhanced Recovery After Surgery (ERAS®) Cardiac Society. *J. Cardiothorac. Vasc. Anesth.* 2023, *in press*. [CrossRef]
29. Hu, J.; Chen, R.; Liu, S.; Yu, X.; Zou, J.; Ding, X. Global Incidence and Outcomes of Adult Patients With Acute Kidney Injury After Cardiac Surgery: A Systematic Review and Meta-Analysis. *J. Cardiothorac. Vasc. Anesth.* **2016**, *30*, 82–89. [CrossRef]
30. Doenst, T.; Diab, M.; Sponholz, C.; Bauer, M.; Färber, G. The Opportunities and Limitations of Minimally Invasive Cardiac Surgery. *Dtsch. Arztebl. Int.* **2017**, *114*, 777–784. [CrossRef]
31. Olsthoorn, J.R.; Heuts, S.; Houterman, S.; Maessen, J.G.; Sardari Nia, P. Minimally invasive approach compared to resternotomy for mitral valve surgery in patients with prior cardiac surgery: Retrospective multicentre study based on the Netherlands Heart Registration. *Eur. J. Cardiothorac. Surg.* **2022**, *62*, 1–48. [CrossRef] [PubMed]
32. Murphy, G.J.; Pike, K.; Rogers, C.A.; Wordsworth, S.; Stokes, E.A.; Angelini, G.D.; Reeves, B.C. Liberal or restrictive transfusion after cardiac surgery. *N. Engl. J. Med.* **2015**, *372*, 997–1008. [CrossRef] [PubMed]
33. Mazer, C.D.; Whitlock, R.P.; Fergusson, D.A.; Hall, J.; Belley-Cote, E.; Connolly, K.; Khanykin, B.; Gregory, A.J.; de Médicis, É.; McGuinness, S.; et al. Restrictive or Liberal Red-Cell Transfusion for Cardiac Surgery. *N. Engl. J. Med.* **2017**, *377*, 2133–2144. [CrossRef]
34. Ziemann, S.; Coburn, M.; Rossaint, R.; van Waesberghe, J.; Bürkle, H.; Fries, M.; Henrich, M.; Henzler, D.; Iber, T.; Karst, J.; et al. Implementierung anästhesiologischer Qualitätsindikatoren in Deutschland: Eine prospektive, nationale, multizentrische Qualitätssteigerungsstudie. *Anaesthesist* **2021**, *70*, 38–47. [CrossRef]
35. Statistisches Bundesamt. Zahl der Herzoperationen 2018: 23% Mehr Eingriffe Als Zehn Jahre Zuvor. Available online: https://www.destatis.de/DE/Presse/Pressemitteilungen/2019/09/PD19_380_231.html#:~:text=Die%20durchschnittliche%20Verweildauer%20lag%20bei,37b%20f%C3%BCr%202008%20und%202018) (accessed on 30 April 2023).
36. InEK GmbH, Fallpauschalen-Katalog 2021, InEK GmbH. Available online: https://www.g-drg.de/ag-drg-system-2021/fallpauschalen-katalog/fallpauschalen-katalog-2021 (accessed on 29 April 2023).

MDPI AG
Grosspeteranlage 5
4052 Basel
Switzerland
Tel.: +41 61 683 77 34

Journal of Cardiovascular Development and Disease Editorial Office
E-mail: jcdd@mdpi.com
www.mdpi.com/journal/jcdd

www.ingramcontent.com/pod-product-compliance
Lightning Source LLC
Chambersburg PA
CBHW061621210926
51850CB00009B/2393
* 9 7 8 3 7 2 5 8 6 5 2 8 4 *